EDUCATING PHYSICIANS

A Call for Reform of Medical School and Residency

Molly Cooke, David M. Irby,
Bridget C. O'Brien

o

Foreword by

Lee S. Shulman

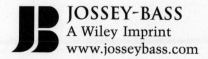
JOSSEY-BASS
A Wiley Imprint
www.josseybass.com

The Jossey-Bass
Higher and Adult Education Series

Published by Jossey-Bass
A Wiley Imprint
989 Market Street, San Francisco, CA 94103-1741—www.josseybass.com

Jossey-Bass books and products are available through most bookstores. To contact
Jossey-Bass directly call our Customer Care Department within the U.S. at 800-956-7739,
outside the U.S. at 317-572-3986, or fax 317-572-4002.

Jossey-Bass also publishes its books in a variety of electronic formats. Some content that
appears in print may not be available in electronic books.

Library of Congress Cataloging-in-Publication Data
Cooke, Molly.
  Educating physicians : a call for reform of medical school and residency / Molly Cooke,
David M. Irby, Bridget C. O'Brien ; foreword by Lee S. Shulman. – 1st ed.
    p. ; cm. – (Preparation for the professions series)
  Includes bibliographical references and index.
  ISBN 978-0-470-45797-9 (hardback)
  1. Medical education–United States. 2. Residents (Medicine)–United States. I. Irby,
David M., 1944- II. O'Brien, Bridget C. III. Carnegie Foundation for the
Advancement of Teaching. IV. Title. V. Series: Preparation for the professions series.
  [DNLM: 1. Education, Medical–United States. W 18 C773e 2010]
  R745.C936 2010
  610.71′173–dc22
                                                                    2010003887

Printed in the United States of America
FIRST EDITION
HB Printing   10 9 8 7 6 5 4 3 2 1

CONTENTS

THE PREPARATION
FOR THE PROFESSIONS SERIES

The Preparation for the Professions Series reports the results of The Carnegie Foundation for the Advancement of Teaching's Preparation for the Professions Program, a comparative study of professional education in medicine, nursing, law, engineering, and preparation of the clergy.

FOREWORD: ON THE
SHOULDERS OF FLEXNER

"The present report on medical education forms the first of a series of papers on professional schools to be issued by the Carnegie Foundation." So wrote Henry S. Pritchett, the first president of The Carnegie Foundation for the Advancement of Teaching, on April 16, 1910, in the opening sentence of his introduction to Abraham Flexner's now-famous Bulletin Number Four, *Medical Education in the United States and Canada*. Having served as Carnegie's eighth president, I now present my own Foreword to this new report on the education of physicians almost precisely one hundred years later. Whereas Flexner's report was among the first issued by the fledgling organization, the current report builds on more than a century of distinguished work, taking its place as the *last* in a series of studies of professional schools conducted by the Carnegie Foundation in recent years.

While Flexner's study of medical education opened a century of work on professional preparation, the present study closes a more recent loop, bringing to completion more than a decade of research on the education of lawyers, engineers, clergy, nurses, and physicians. During the same period, the foundation conducted research on the education of scholars through its studies of Ph.D. programs across a number of fields. In those studies, the doctorate was seen as preparation for a life of "professing" and thus parallel in many ways to other forms of professional preparation. With this body of work on professional education now complete, it seems fitting to look back on a century of research and reflection while also looking ahead to the volume you are about to read and its vision for the future.

On a more personal level, the present volume represents the keeping of a promise I made to Carnegie Foundation board members at my first meeting with them in early 1997. I explained that I admired the accomplishments of the foundation during its then ninety-two years of existence. Nevertheless, I expected that my efforts would be devoted in part to undoing the unintended consequences of some of the foundation's most successful historical contributions to the field of education—including the Flexner Report.

Looking back, it is clear that the foundation's many studies and recommendations created important solutions to major problems at the time. But what is also clear is that the very act of resolving one era's problems often contributed to the dilemmas of the next generation. This dynamic generally entailed transforming what was badly organized or even chaotic by establishing greater standardization and regulation. Thus, the Carnegie Unit addressed the pressing need for a clear distinction between secondary and higher education by setting new and higher standards for both graduation from high school and admission to colleges and universities. It did so by legitimizing a metric that defined the rigor of a secondary school education in terms of the length and intensity of each course that constituted its program. Unfortunately, in doing so it reified the value of "seat time" as a measure of academic rigor instead of looking to students' actual learning as the real gold standard.

A similar dynamic appears in the case of the Flexner Report, which addressed the problem of an utterly unregulated medical education dominated by schools of poor quality. Typically, that poor quality was a function of little or no teaching of modern science, poor prerequisites for admission and promotion, and far too few connections between serious academic work and carefully supervised clinical learning of medical practice in exemplary hospitals. The report was so hard-hitting in its critique and recommendations that within a few years many schools had closed. Flexner reports that, in the thirty years after the publication of his report, the number of American medical schools had been reduced from 155 to about 60 (Flexner, 1943, p. 113). That may be good news for the most part, but the reduction in size brought with it the demise of all but two of the medical schools that prepared black physicians and all but one that devoted its attention to preparing women for medical careers. Ultimately, the "Flexner curriculum" became a problem in itself, one that the authors of the present report address in their work.

Abraham Flexner developed a very special relationship with Henry Pritchett. Although they had never met before that auspicious day in 1908 when Pritchett invited Mr. Flexner to conduct the study of medical education, they subsequently became lifelong friends. So close was their friendship, and so trusting the bond, that upon Pritchett's death in August 1939, his widow asked Flexner to prepare his biography. In that biography, Flexner describes that initial meeting.

> On the basis of a small book, which I had written on the subject
> of the American College and which Pritchett liked, I was fortunate
> enough to be chosen by Pritchett in 1908 to make the study of medical

education in America, subsequently in Europe. At our first interview, he asked me whether I would be willing to study the subject.

I answered, "I am not a physician; aren't you confusing me with my brother Simon at the Rockefeller Institute for Medical Research?"

"No," rejoined Pritchett. "I know your brother well. What I have in mind is not a medical study, but an educational one. Medical schools are schools and must be judged as such. For that, a very sketchy notion of the main functions of the various departments suffices. That you or any other intelligent layman can readily acquire. Such a study as I have in mind takes that for granted. Henceforth, these institutions must be viewed from the standpoint of education. Are they so equipped and conducted as to be able to train students to be efficient physicians, surgeons, and so on?" (Flexner 1943, pp. 108–109)

In his directive to Flexner, Pritchett thus defined the character of Carnegie Foundation studies for the next century. They were not to be studies by insiders for insiders. They were to be conducted by nonspecialists (or, as became more frequently the case, by a combination of specialists and nonspecialists) and addressed to a larger audience than that within the profession alone. Moreover, it would not be sufficient for the study to be conducted by convening a panel of widely admired sages and tapping their acquired wisdom. Instead, Flexner described the process as *ambulando discimus,* "we learn by going about." In this spirit, he engaged in two years of travel, observation, interview, interrogation, espionage, deliberation, and advisement; he learned, in short, by "going about," personally visiting every one of the 155 medical schools in the country. In so doing, he revolutionized our conception of the special report and policy analysis.

I do not, it should be said, use the term "espionage" gratuitously. In one case, Flexner describes the challenge of adequately inspecting the facilities of an osteopathic medical school in Des Moines because, as he toured the facility "in company with its dean, every door was locked and the janitor, who had possession of the keys, could not be found." There were signs on the doors that labeled the locked rooms as "laboratories," "histology," "anatomy," and the like. After getting rid of the dean at the railroad station, Flexner made a stealthy return to the school, finding the missing janitor and using a five-dollar bill to induce him to open every room. The signs on the doors not withstanding, the rooms turned out to be quite empty of any evidence supporting their putative uses. Sometimes, it seems, we learn both by going around and by sneaking

around—though I am confident that the present research team had no
need to employ such methods of investigation.

Among the legacies left by the Flexner Report—beyond its impact on
medical education—is the field-based policy report. Instead of simply
convening a panel of recognized experts to deliberate about an issue of
educational policy, Flexner and Pritchett determined to learn by "going
about," by moving out into the field to visit the places and people in
question. That said, the report was in many ways already shaped before
the first site visit. Flexner had determined that the template for judging
all medical schools would be Johns Hopkins, with its academic rigor, its
teaching hospitals, and the quality of its full-time faculty.

A further legacy of Flexner is the practice of educational evaluation
conducted through the eyes of the legitimate outsider. Once the study
was defined as an educational one, not only was Flexner legitimated as
a judge, but, by the same standard, an exclusively insider's view was
disqualified.

Like Flexner, our research team also accomplished much of its learning
by going about. They visited medical schools across the country that
were selected because we had reason to believe that they were already
employing exemplary practices. We did not use any one of them as a
model of the ideal program, as Flexner had used Johns Hopkins; rather,
the team saw in the schools' varied practices a sort of collective vision
of the possible. Thus, the recommendations in the later chapters are not
pie-in-the-sky dreams but proposals for activities some version of which
are already in place.

In this sense, *ambulando discimus* is not only an apt motto for an
approach to the study of medical education but, ironically, also for the
signature pedagogies employed by the field: the use of clinical rounds and
rotations as the primary basis for physicians to learn medicine by "going
around" with more experienced mentors as well as peers as they move
from patient to patient, from bedside to bedside, from clinic to clinic,
and from hospital to hospital. In this manner, novice physicians study
multiple examples of illness and healing, work with diverse medical role
models and teachers, and engage with a variety of forms of illness and
disability. Like Flexner and his Carnegie successors one hundred years
later, physicians learn by going round and round on rounds and rotations.

The themes that cut through the foundation's other recent studies
of professional education appear vividly in this report as well. Indeed,
we purposely designed the order of our studies to ensure that medicine
came last in the sequence rather than first. Ever since Flexner, medicine has
served as the "model profession," and most other professions and forms

of professional education have been interpreted through the lens of medicine. We began instead with legal education and proceeded through engineering and the clergy before we began our studies of nursing and medical education; the themes that emerged in that sequence pervaded each of the professional fields. In medical education, they included particular attention to the challenge of curricular integration, the essential tension between standardization of curriculum and individualization of instructional opportunities, and the critically central role of professional and personal identity in learning to become a physician.

The challenges of integration are ubiquitous in medical education. As fields mature, they tend to grow through division and multiplication rather than through synthesis and simplification. New domains are added, new topics are identified, and new specializations are added to the canon. For each addition, there must be a new course, a new rotation, and a new set of journals. Yet medical students are expected to learn all these domains and somehow to connect, combine, and integrate them within their own understandings and their own professional identities. Our team repeatedly identified the need for the medical curriculum and its programs to foster more of these integrations rather than leave the work entirely to the students.

Another needed kind of integration, easily as problematic as the intellectual and technical demands of the work, is a synthesis of the cognitive and the moral aspects of professional work. In every field we studied, we concluded that the most overlooked aspect of professional preparation was the formation of a professional identity with a moral and ethical core of service and responsibility around which the habits of mind and of practice could be organized. We first recognized the importance of professional identity in our studies of legal education and developed better language and examples of the process when we studied the education of clergy. Indeed, the very term *formation* is taken from religious education.

Yet, as soon as one recognizes the need for a coordinated curriculum aimed at deep understanding, complex technical competence, and deeply internalized moral responsibility, it becomes apparent that one size will not fit all. The authors of this report address with skill and sensitivity how the standardization of an integrated curriculum must be balanced by the affordances of individual adaptation. An integrated curriculum must provide the basis for the formation of individual professional integrity. This is no small challenge.

○

Quite remarkably, Flexner operated as a solo practitioner. He visited the sites alone and he wrote his report alone, although it was read and critiqued carefully both by leaders of the medical profession and by Pritchett himself. In contrast to Flexner's solo performance, this new Carnegie Foundation study of medical education is an ensemble piece, drawing on multiple disciplines and backgrounds, and involving both insiders and outsiders. Chief among them, as co-leaders of the research program on the education of physicians, are Professor Molly Cooke and Professor David Irby of the University of California, San Francisco (UCSF).

Molly Cooke is a physician who holds the William G. Irwin Endowed Chair as professor of medicine at UCSF as well as serving as director of the Haile T. Debas Academy of Medical Educators at that institution. She has been a pioneer in the treatment of chronically ill HIV/AIDS patients. Her contributions to the teaching of medicine have been recognized through her selection in 2006 as winner of the Robert J. Glaser Award for Excellence in Clinical Teaching by the Association of American Medical Schools, one of the most prestigious national awards in the field of clinical teaching.

David Irby serves as vice dean for medical education at UCSF. He has long been a leader in research in medical education, having been recognized with major awards by both the National Board of Medical Examiners and the American Educational Research Association for his accomplishments in that field. Holding a doctorate in educational research, Irby brings both theoretical and methodological competence to this study that is, like Flexner's, a profoundly educational inquiry.

Bridget O'Brien joined the study team from the beginning as a graduate research assistant while completing her Ph.D. studies in higher education at the University of California, Berkeley. She rapidly became a full partner in the effort, and, when the research was completed, she joined Cooke and Irby on the faculty of UCSF.

As noted above, this study benefitted from being the last in the foundation's series of comparative investigations of education in the professions. Coming on the heels of our studies of legal education, engineering education, and the preparation of Catholic, Protestant, and Jewish clergy, and concurrent with a study on the preparation of nurses, the research drew on insights from other fields. Moreover, the study team regularly invited scholars from other research programs at the foundation to join in their site visits and to become fellow travelers as they learned by going about.

In that spirit, the fingerprints of William Sullivan and Anne Colby can be found on all parts of this work. Sullivan and Colby served as the overall coordinators for each of the foundation's studies of professional preparation. Bill Sullivan is a philosopher whose career has included as much social science as it has philosophical analysis. He was part of the team that authored the landmark studies *Habits of the Heart* and *The Good Society*. The two editions of his book *Work and Integrity* lay out a conception of the moral foundations of professional work. He was senior author of the Carnegie Foundation's report on legal education, *Educating Lawyers*, and its book on undergraduate liberal education as preparation for practice, *A New Agenda for Higher Education*.

Anne Colby is a life-span developmental psychologist whose work on moral development and moral learning in children and adults has had great influence internationally. She is co-author of *The Measurement of Moral Judgment* with Lawrence Kohlberg, and her book with William Damon, *Some Do Care,* is a seminal study of adult moral development. More recently, she is co-author of *Educating Citizens* and *Educating for Democracy,* both books part of Carnegie's program on the role of universities in educating for civic and political engagement.

Thus, in place of Abraham Flexner working alone, a century later we have availed ourselves of the talents of an interdisciplinary team including physicians and medical educators, psychologists and philosophers, and scholars of higher education and of professional education. Nevertheless, the work was possible only because we were able to sit "on the shoulders of Flexner," to build our effort on his, whether viewed appreciatively or critically. And we could pursue the work in the context of a century-old research institution whose credibility rested in large measure on the accomplishments of Flexner and Pritchett.

Henry Pritchett dated his introduction to the Flexner Report on April 16, 1910, which was his fifty-third birthday. Perhaps he viewed the report as a kind of birthday gift from his good friend Mr. Flexner, for no publication before or since contributed more to Pritchett's dream of transforming the Carnegie Foundation from a pension fund into a "great agency" for improving education and teaching in all their dimensions. And what a birthday gift it became! Inspired by the quality of the study and the impact of this kind of field-based policy research aimed at the critical evaluation of educational quality, Mr. Carnegie instructed the leaders of the Carnegie Corporation of New York, his sole philanthropic institution, to add $1,250,000 to the endowment of The Carnegie Foundation for the Advancement of Teaching. In 2010 dollars, this is equivalent to more than $30,000,000 in additional resources for the foundation's work. But even more important, it signaled the formal transformation of the pension program into a world-class research and policy center in education.

Ambulando discimus remains the hallmark of the foundation's work. The gifted scholars who prepared *Educating Physicians* came to the work after "going about" the many fields of study they represent. They sought the advice of many others, both within and outside medicine, and they visited a broad array of institutions, observing and interviewing, surveying and reading. I believe that all those in the field of medical education must take the observations and recommendations of this book seriously and that its insights can be of value to educators outside of the field as well. I commend this fine work to your attention. It has commanded my attention for a number of years. I thank the team and all those who had a part in supporting this superb effort, as I also express my appreciation to Abraham Flexner, on whose shoulders they stand, and to Henry Pritchett, on whose broad shoulders I have been privileged to perch.

Lee S. Shulman, President Emeritus
The Carnegie Foundation for the Advancement of Teaching
Stanford, California

ACKNOWLEDGMENTS

THIS BOOK REPRESENTS more than four years of collaboration. Through fieldwork, generation of ideas, shared writing, and mutual critique, we developed an interdependent process; its product is thus truly a group effort. Accordingly, we list ourselves as authors alphabetically to emphasize that no one of us takes precedence. We hope our audience likewise recognizes and appreciates that in our work and the resulting book we were, and are, an indivisible team.

The team, however, had much by way of assistance, and we gratefully acknowledge the many people who have contributed to the project and book. First among them are the students, residents, faculty members, deans, and hospital CEOs who graciously hosted us; participated in our interviews and focus groups; and allowed us to observe their teaching, medical schools, and teaching hospitals: Atlantic Health; Cambridge Health Alliance; Northwestern University; Henry Ford Health System; Mayo Medical School; Southern Illinois University; University of California, San Francisco; University of Florida; University of Minnesota; University of North Dakota; University of Pennsylvania; University of South Florida; University of Texas Medical Branch, Galveston; and University of Washington.

We also thank our colleagues who offered insightful suggestions midway through the project: Patrick Alguire, Richard Bell, Georges Bordage, Judith Bowen, Paul Friedmann, Robert Galbraith, Kevin Grumbach, Paul Rockey, Gordon Russell, David Shearn, Steve Wartman, and Michael Whitcomb. They also reviewed and commented on our manuscripts, as did Drs. Eva Aagaard, Alan Bleakley, Robert Centor, Carrie Chen, Jordon Cohen, Debra DaRosa, Gurpreet Dhaliwal, Robert Dickler, Karen Fisher, Larry Gruppen, Jeanne Heard, Mike Hindery, Audiey Kao, Darrell Kirch, Richard Knapp, Jack Krakower, Jon Lang, David Leach, Helen Loeser, Kenneth Ludmerer, Bonnie Miller, Gail Morrison, Carol-Anne Moulton, Patricia O'Sullivan, Roy Pea, John Prescott, Glenn Regehr, Arthur Rubenstein, Jed Shivers, Deborah Simpson, Yvonne Steinert, David Stern, George Thibault, Robert Watson, Dan West, Reed Williams, David Wilson, and Paul Worley.

We are especially grateful to The Carnegie Foundation for the Advancement of Teaching for providing a creative and collaborative environment within which to design and complete this project. We thank Lee Shulman, former president of the foundation, for his vision and active engagement. We also thank the foundation's current president, Anthony Bryk, for his continued support for dissemination of this and the other books in the Preparation for the Professions series. We thank William Sullivan and Anne Colby for their continuing guidance; Gay Clyburn, Lydia Baldwin, Ruby Kerawalla, and Molly Breen for their assistance; and Pat O'Sullivan, Arthur Elstein, and Molly Sutphen, external colleagues who participated in our site visits. We also appreciate Ellen Wert's edits of the manuscript.

Finally, we thank The Carnegie Foundation for the Advancement of Teaching and the Atlantic Philanthropies, both of which funded this project; and the University of California, San Francisco, for supporting our participation in this research.

Molly Cooke
David M. Irby
Bridget C. O'Brien

ABOUT THE AUTHORS

Molly Cooke, M.D. Molly Cooke codirected the Study of Medical Education at The Carnegie Foundation for the Advancement of Teaching. She is a professor of medicine and holds the William G. Irwin Endowed Chair at the University of California, San Francisco, School of Medicine. Cooke is a 2006 recipient of the Robert J. Glaser/AOA Distinguished Teacher Award, a national award bestowed by the American Association of Medical Colleges. She is a board member for the National Board of Medical Examiners, which oversees licensing of American physicians. She has been active in the American College of Physicians and currently serves as chair of the Board of Governors and member of the Board of Regents. Cooke is also the director of the Haile T. Debas Academy of Medical Educators, which serves as a community for medical school faculty with significant commitment to medical education, to advocate for teachers in the promotion process and to enhance funding in support of teaching. She earned her medical degree at Stanford University.

David M. Irby, Ph.D. David M. Irby co-directed the Carnegie Foundation's Study of Medical Education. Irby is vice dean for education and a professor of medicine at the University of California, San Francisco, School of Medicine, where he directs undergraduate, graduate, and continuing medical education programs and heads the Office of Medical Education. He is the recipient of the Distinguished Scholar Award by the American Educational Research Association, the John P. Hubbard Award from the National Board of Medical Examiners, the Daniel C. Tosteson Award for Leadership in Medical Education from Harvard Medical School and Beth Israel Deaconess Medical Center, the Distinguished Service Award from Graceland University, and the John E. Chapman Medal Award from Vanderbilt University School of Medicine. He earned a doctorate in education from the University of Washington and a master's of divinity from Union Theological Seminary, and he completed a postdoctoral fellowship in academic administration at Harvard Medical School.

Bridget C. O'Brien, Ph.D. Bridget C. O'Brien was a co-equal participant in the Carnegie Foundation's Study of Medical Education, contributing significantly to all aspects of the project, from framing the conceptual questions through the fieldwork and the writing. She is an assistant professor of medicine at the University of California, San Francisco, School of Medicine and a researcher in the Office of Medical Education. O'Brien conducts research on clinical education and teaches in the Health Professions Education Pathway and the Teaching Scholars Program at UCSF. She has a B.S. from Cornell University, a master's from the Haas School of Business at the University of California at Berkeley, and a doctorate from the Graduate School of Education at UC Berkeley.

INTRODUCTION

IN 1910, ABRAHAM FLEXNER articulated the current blueprint for medical education in North America. His report, *Medical Education in the United States and Canada*, is a comprehensive survey of medical education prepared on behalf of The Carnegie Foundation for the Advancement of Teaching and at the request of the American Medical Association's Council on Medical Education. The basic features outlined by Flexner remain in place today: a university-based education consisting of two years of basic sciences and two years of clinical experience in a teaching hospital. Implementation of that blueprint has brought medical education to a high level of excellence. Yet during the past century, along with enormous societal changes, the practice of medicine and its scientific, pharmacological, and technological foundations have been transformed. Now medical education in the United States is at a crossroads: those who teach medical students and residents must choose whether to continue in the direction established more than a hundred years ago or take a fundamentally different course, guided by contemporary innovation and new understanding about how people learn.

Can medical education's illustrious past serve as an adequate guide to a future of excellence? Flexner asserted that scientific inquiry and discovery, not past traditions and practices, should point the way to the future in both medicine and medical education. Today, this admonition seems even more compelling, given the rapid changes in the practice of medicine and an expanded understanding of human learning. New technologies and drugs are radically altering diagnostic and therapeutic options, and physicians are playing both broader and more specialized roles in an increasingly complex health care system. At the same time, changes in health care delivery, financing, and public policy are leaving millions of Americans without health care, and many health care institutions are gravely underfunded. New discoveries in the learning sciences and

I

changes in the preparation of physicians all argue for the need to reexamine medical education.

Responding to these environmental forces and changes within medicine, virtually every organization within the medical profession is reexamining medical education. The American Medical Association, the Association of American Medical Colleges, the Accreditation Council for Graduate Medical Education, the Accreditation Council for Continuing Medical Education, the Federation of State Medical Boards, the National Board of Medical Examiners, and many specialty boards that license medical specialists are all asking fundamental questions: How can we improve medical education? Can we produce competent and compassionate physicians more efficiently and effectively? How can we reorganize medical education to produce physicians who are able to achieve better health care outcomes for the American people?

It is within this context of self-assessment that, nearly one hundred years after Flexner's landmark study, we undertook an investigation of medical education as part of a larger study of education for the professions, sponsored by The Carnegie Foundation for the Advancement of Teaching. Flexner—his picture hanging prominently in the main room of The Carnegie Foundation for the Advancement of Teaching—became an icon and a companion during our study. As he did, we set out to examine the status of medical education and chart the course for future directions. Following in his large footsteps, we visited medical schools and academic health centers around the country.

Unlike our predecessor, however, we did not find great disparities in the quality of education among the medical schools we visited. Although we were highly selective in choosing which schools to include in our study, and although many of them excel in innovation, we recognize that two important external agents, accrediting and licensing systems.

Without question, medical education today is unlike the enterprise that Flexner investigated in 1909. Today U.S. medical education is characterized by a great deal of educational creativity and innovation. While he would easily understand the current paradigm of physician education as the one he helped to put in place, Flexner would hardly recognize the contemporary practice of medicine,. He would applaud the scientific basis of medicine and the progress that has been made in advancing health. However, he might wonder if the old structures of medical education can continue to support rising challenges, both internal and external, to medical education. As the challenges confronting medical education inevitably increase, a new vision is needed to drive medical education to the next level of excellence. The future demands new approaches to shaping the minds, hands, and hearts of physicians. Fundamental change in medical education will require new curricula, new pedagogies, and new forms of assessment.

Fortunately, this vision is beginning to take shape. Seeds of the future are germinating in innovations in both undergraduate and graduate medical education. As Kenneth Ludmerer points out in *Time to Heal* (1999), the reforms that Flexner advocated were under way well before he issued his critique. Similarly, we observed many innovations in the course of our fieldwork and study of the literature on medical education and the learning sciences. For example, most medical schools have developed integrated coursework for the first two years of study; use web-based learning resources, simulations, and standardized patients for instruction and assessment; have clearly defined competencies and learning objectives; use small groups in a variety of teaching situations; and are guided by effective educational leadership. Likewise, residency programs are using simulation both in teaching and to assess performance; are beginning to take teamwork skills seriously; and are experimenting with using patient outcomes as an element of the assessment of residents.

However, as did Flexner in his time, we find medical education lacking in many important regards. Medical training is inflexible, excessively long, and not learner-centered. We found that clinical education is overly focused on inpatient clinical experience, supervised by clinical faculty who have less and less time to teach and who have ceded much of their teaching responsibilities to residents, and situated in hospitals with marginal capacity to support their teaching mission. We observed poor connections between formal knowledge and experiential learning and inadequate attention to patient populations, health care delivery, and effectiveness. Students lack a holistic view of patients and often poorly understand nonclinical physician roles. At both the undergraduate and graduate levels, there is insufficient attention to the knowledge and skills required to meet the health care needs of the U.S. population. Residents continue to be assigned to clinical settings on the basis of inpatient service imperatives rather than learner educational needs. Across the continuum, we observed that medical education does not adequately make use of the learning sciences. Finally, time and again we saw that the pace and commercial nature of health care impede inculcation of the fundamental values of the profession.

In response to our findings, we offer this book as a way to build on medical education's significant strengths, address its problems, and suggest a vision for the future.

The Study Behind the Book

Our study was part of a larger program of research on preparation for the professions, commissioned by The Carnegie Foundation for the Advancement of Teaching. The work was funded by a grant from the Atlantic Philanthropies, and this resulting book is a companion to reports on educating the clergy, lawyers, engineers, and nurses. (See Benner, Sutphen, Leonard, & Day, 2009; Foster, Dahill, Golemon, & Tolentino, 2005; Sheppard, Macatangay, Colby, & Sullivan, 2008; Sullivan, Colby, Wegner, Bond, & Shulman, 2007; see also Sullivan 2004; Sullivan & Rosin, 2008.) The program was initiated by Carnegie's then president, Lee Shulman, and guided by Carnegie senior scholars Anne Colby and William Sullivan.

Flexner went to all 155 of the medical schools in North America in 1909, and he pioneered the site visit as a research tool. After designing the study protocol and receiving approval from human subject review boards of the Carnegie Foundation and the University of California, San Francisco, we visited 11 of the 130 medical schools and teaching hospitals in the United States currently accredited by the Liaison Committee for Medical Education of the Association of American Medical Colleges and three nonuniversity teaching hospitals. (Osteopathic medical schools, which have somewhat different curricula, cost structures, and accreditation, were not included in the study.) Although each site was selected because of interesting educational innovations, we also wanted to survey medical education across institutional type and geographic location. The institutions thus represent the array of research-intensive and community-based medical schools, academic medical centers, and nonuniversity teaching hospitals where U.S. medical education is located:

o Atlantic Health, Morristown, New Jersey
o Cambridge Hospital, Cambridge, Massachusetts
o Henry Ford Hospital and Medical Center, Detroit, Michigan
o Mayo Medical School, Rochester, Minnesota
o Northwestern University, Chicago, Illinois
o Southern Illinois University, Springfield
o University of California, San Francisco
o University of Florida, Gainesville and Jacksonville
o University of Minnesota, Minneapolis
o University of North Dakota, Grand Forks
o University of Pennsylvania, Philadelphia

- University of South Florida, Tampa
- University of Texas Medical Branch, Galveston
- University of Washington, Seattle

Prior to each site visit, we interviewed approximately ten faculty members, the dean, the education-related associate deans, and the CEO of the teaching hospital. Most site visits lasted three days, included the authors plus other Carnegie scholars, and involved further interviews, focus groups with students, residents, clerkship directors, and residency program directors, and observations of clinical teaching. Over the course of our site visits, we conducted approximately 184 interviews, 104 focus groups, and 100 observations. The interviews and focus groups were transcribed and coded for common themes.

We also reviewed the literature on medical education and the learning sciences as a means of guiding interpretation of our results and our recommendations. Before, during, and after the site visits, we consulted widely with the leadership and staff of the Association of American Medical Colleges, the American Medical Association, the National Board of Medical Examiners, the Society of Directors of Research in Medical Education, and other medical professional organizations; we also convened an expert panel to review our preliminary observations.

In embarking on the study, we envied Flexner because he had a clear template for medical education in mind before he set out on his site visits: medical education should adopt the model recently created at Johns Hopkins. "Without this pattern in the back of my mind," Flexner wrote, "I could have accomplished little. With it I began a swift tour of medical schools in the United States and Canada" (1940, p. 115). We had no such pattern. However, as we conducted our site visits, read widely in the literature of medical education and the learning sciences, and began to share our insights with others, a new vision for the future of medical education emerged, the vision that we offer in this book.

Toward a Vision for the Future of Medical Education

The key findings of our study, which we detail in Chapter One, lead us to recommend four goals for medical education:

1. *Standardization of learning outcomes and individualization of the learning process.* Whereas the Flexner model (two years of basic science instruction followed by two years of clinical experience) has been rigorously maintained through the system of accreditation, medical education should now instead standardize learning outcomes and general competencies and then provide options for individualizing the

learning experience for students and residents, such as offering the possibility of fast tracking within and across levels.

2. *Integration of formal knowledge and clinical experience.* In practice physicians must constantly integrate all aspects of their knowledge and skills. Moreover, physicians educate, advocate, innovate, investigate, and manage teams. Students and residents need to understand and prepare for integration of these diverse roles, responsibilities, knowledge, and skills; their learning in the basic, clinical, and social sciences should be integrated with their clinical experiences. To experience integration of skills and knowledge in a way that prepares for them for practice, medical students should be given early clinical immersion, and residents should have more intense exposure to the sciences and best evidence underlying their practice.

3. *Development of habits of inquiry and innovation.* Commitment to excellence involves developing the habits of mind and heart that continuously advance medicine and health care; this applies to institutions as well as individuals. To help students and residents develop the habits of inquiry and improvement that promote excellence throughout a lifetime of practice, medical schools and teaching hospitals should support engagement of all physicians-in-training in inquiry, discovery, and innovation.

4. *Focus on professional identity formation.* Professional identity formation—development of professional values, actions, and aspirations—should be a major focus of medical education. It should build on an essential foundation of clinical competence, communication and interpersonal skills, and ethical and legal understanding, and extend to aspirational goals in performance excellence, accountability, humanism, and altruism.

These goals, which have their roots in Flexner's model of medical education, reflect many of the strengths of U.S. medical education, address its fault lines, and point to its future. Realizing such a future, however, will entail significant reform within and across programs. Advocacy must change the policies that affect the design and delivery of U.S. medical education.

Consider, for example, undergraduate medical education, the four years of medical school. The progressive and developmental nature of learning calls for greater longitudinal connections to be made among teachers, learners, and patients and across the four years of medical school. The situated and distributed nature of learning suggests the need for a stronger connection between clinical learning in specific contexts and the formal knowledge basic to the practice of medicine. This would suggest the importance of promoting early clinical immersion and continuous connection of formal knowledge to clinical experience, which has consequences for curriculum, pedagogy, and assessment.

However, medical education exists within a web of organizational, financial, and regulatory relationships that both support and challenge educational excellence. The participatory aspect of medical education, for example—long a major strength of medical education at the undergraduate and graduate levels—is now being tested by the financial pressures on the clinical enterprise, which are marginalizing teaching and learning. Not only must new models for teaching and learning be developed but new approaches to financing clinical education will need to be found, entailing policy changes within institutions and in external funding and regulation. Thus, to achieve a new vision for medical education, each of medical education's stakeholder communities will have to work together to examine, strengthen, and align curriculum, pedagogy, assessment, accreditation, licensing, certification, and funding—all toward a common goal of excellence for both the education of aspiring physicians and the care of patients.

The Plan of the Book

The book begins with an overview of medical education and the profession of medicine, the focus of Part One. In Chapter One, we present the historical background and describe the current structure of medical education, including environmental trends and challenges. In Chapter Two we describe the core domains of the physician's work: caring for patients, participating in a professional community, and instigating improvement and inquiry. We review the research on learning that explains how physicians become adept at performing in each of these core domains, and we describe the process of professional formation.

In Part Two, we look at the experience of medical education, of learning to become a physician. In Chapter Three, we examine learning during medical school, and in Chapter Four we describe the experience of learning during residency training. In both chapters we focus on the design and experience of the curriculum, pedagogy, and assessment, looking at strengths and failings as well as promising innovations that build on the former and address the latter.

The complex environment for financing, regulating, and leading medical education is the focus of Part Three. Chapter Five examines the regulation and financing of medical education. Although these external forces have historically inhibited educational innovation, we found that change is afoot in the medical schools and residency programs we visited, sparked by faculty vision, leadership, and creativity and, in some cases, supported by strong institutional leadership and facilitated by innovative uses of regulatory processes to spur change. In Chapter Six, we illustrate the principles of leadership with inspiring examples of transformational leadership we witnessed and learned about during our study.

We close the book with a vision of the possible. Part Four discusses the opportunities for advancing U.S. medical education. Such opportunities abound, and we offer our vision as a set of recommendations that we believe will make medical education the premier professional education in the world. In Chapter Seven, we offer examples of educational programs at the medical student and residency level intended to realize our principles of individualization, integration, inquiry, and improvement and give explicit attention to the formation of professional identity. Because significant reform of medical education will depend on structural changes and creation of a culture of transparency and accountability, we enumerate, in Chapter Eight, a set of recommendations for policy actions that would support medical education in reaching the goals of standardization and individualization, integration, habits of inquiry and improvement, and formation of professional identity. Only through policy changes can this vision for the future of medical education be fully realized.

Using This Book

It is our intention that this book stimulate discussion about the current status and future direction of medical education and advance health globally. We hope that students, residents, and practicing physicians will find that their concerns and hopes are voiced. Deans and associate deans for education, medical educators, and teaching faculty should find direction for curriculum development, pedagogy, and assessment. Educational researchers will find a theoretical base for new areas of scholarship in medical education. Policy bodies charged with accreditation, certification, and licensure will find recommendations for needed changes. Professional organizations will find guidance for future directions of the profession. Hospitals and funding agencies will hear a call for fundamental changes in financing medical education.

Most of all, however, we hope that this book results in much-needed dialogue within and among these groups—dialogue leading to action that strengthens medical education and thus, ultimately, delivers better patient care.

PART ONE

TODAY'S PRACTICE, YESTERDAY'S LEGACY, TOMORROW'S CHALLENGES

I

EDUCATING PHYSICIANS

CONTEXT AND CHALLENGES

CONTEMPORARY MEDICAL EDUCATION would be unrecognizable to physicians in nineteenth-century America. Preparation of doctors then was a relatively informal and unfettered affair: admission standards were lax, and in most instances only a high school education was required. The curriculum consisted of sixteen weeks of lectures, repeated for eight months of instruction. There was no patient contact or laboratory experience, and all matriculants graduated with an M.D. degree regardless of academic performance. Teachers were typically practicing physicians who gave instruction part-time as a means of supplementing their income (Ludmerer, 1985, 1999). Medical schools varied in both organization and quality, ranging from elite university programs to small for-profit enterprises. With no accreditation standards, many of these medical schools were of poor quality indeed. With no certification or licensing requirements, many practicing physicians were marginally competent, if at all. It was virtually impossible for members of the public to know if the medical care they received was quality or quackery.

The document that changed medical education and practice was the Flexner Report of 1910. Challenged by highly variable physician performance and the lack of standards in medical education, the American Medical Association's Council on Medical Education, under the leadership of Dr. N. P. Colwell, conducted a survey of medical schools and found many of them wanting. However, as a membership organization the AMA was in an awkward position if wholesale condemnation of medical education was required. Therefore, in 1908 the AMA sought the help of the newly formed Carnegie Foundation for the Advancement of Teaching to conduct a comprehensive study of medical education in North

America. Henry Pritchett, president of the foundation, commissioned not a physician but an educator, Abraham Flexner, to lead the study. The choice of a non-physician was astute; as Flexner later recalled, "Dr. Colwell and I made many trips together, but, whereas he was under the necessity of proceeding cautiously and tactfully, I was fortunately in position to tell the truth with utmost frankness" (Flexner, 1940, p. 115).

By the time Flexner and Colwell visited all 155 medical schools in the United States and Canada in 1909 and issued his report in 1910, the basic framework of contemporary medical education was already taking shape. The transformation that shifted medical education to its current rigorous, science-based form began in the mid-nineteenth century with the rise of experimental medicine in German universities, where research laboratories empirically confirmed or disproved hypotheses about mechanisms of disease. This experimentalist approach challenged the established medical culture, in which both learning and practicing medicine were based on tradition and the works of ancient physicians. American physicians, attracted to Germany and laboratory research, returned from visits abroad imbued with this spirit of scientific medicine and determined to adopt the model for preparing physicians at their universities, which included Chicago, Cornell, Harvard, Michigan, Pennsylvania, and later Johns Hopkins, where the empirical approach to medicine achieved its zenith. Through the efforts of these reformers, medical education was brought into the university and medical laboratories were established along with teaching hospitals (Ludmerer, 1985).

In preparation for his site visits, Flexner visited Johns Hopkins, where his brother Simon had studied medicine before becoming the first director of the Rockefeller Institute for Medical Research. There he spoke to leading physicians who had strong opinions about what a medical school should be, having created one only twenty years earlier. Flexner adopted the Johns Hopkins model as his standard, comparing the schools that he visited to it.

During his site visits, Flexner encountered a number of excellent university-based programs of medical education that met his criteria. Flexner believed that medical practice must be firmly rooted in the foundation of science, not in superstition, speculation, and uncritical empiricism. He saw inculcation of scientific curiosity and methods of investigation as essential to medical education, drawing a parallel between research and practice: "No distinction can be made between research and practice. The investigator, obviously, observes, experiments, and judges; so do the physician and surgeon who practice their art in the modern spirit. At bottom the intellectual attitude and processes of the two are—or should be—identical.... If this position is sound, the ward and the laboratory are logically, from the standpoints of investigation, treatment, and education, inextricably intertwined" (Flexner, 1925, pp. 4, 6).

The Flexner Report

Because medicine is a science-based practice, Flexner argued, medical schools should be housed in universities, which should also have teaching hospitals, and scientific inquiry should be the modus operandi from the laboratory to the hospital. To ensure that all North American medical education achieved the desired standards, Flexner proposed a number of features of a four-year M.D. degree, which have become common requisites:

- High admissions standards, including requiring a bachelor's degree with a strong science focus, rather than merely a high school degree, as was typical at the time
- A university-based medical school to train students to think like scientists, furnishing two years of basic science instruction instead of a mere eight months of lectures
- Two years of supervised clinical experience by university-based physicians in a teaching hospital
- Experience in investigation through supervised immersion in laboratories and clinical settings
- Instruction by physician-scientists who could move effortlessly from the research laboratory to the bedside and back

In his report, Flexner identified a number of medical schools that did not fit the Johns Hopkins University template, generally small proprietary schools that appalled him, as the acerbic characterizations in his report make clear. He decried their poor quality of instruction, facilities, faculty members, students, administrators, and clinical training. The impact of Flexner's report was amplified by the muckraking journalists of the era, and within a decade approximately one-third of the 155 medical schools closed or merged with other schools. Unfortunately, several of the schools that closed had offered the only access to medical education available to women and African Americans, a situation that was not rectified until the 1970s.

The Medical Profession's Response

Within a decade of publication of the Flexner report, accreditation, certification, and licensing procedures were put into place to protect the public and monitor (and, when necessary, sanction) schools of medicine.

Accreditation processes for schools of medicine were fortified, and the National Board of Medical Examiners (NBME) established the NBME Part Examination program. State medical boards, which had begun to license practicing physicians in the mid-1880s, reorganized their coordinating entity, formerly the National Confederation of State Examining and Licensing Medical Boards into the Federation of State Medical Boards (FSMB), founded in 1912. The current licensing sequence, the United States Medical Licensing Examination (USMLE), was introduced in the early 1990s and replaced the NBME Part Examination and the FSMB's Federation Licensing Examination (FLEX) program. Founded in 1915 in response to the call of the Flexner report to assure the public that all graduates of U.S. medical schools were competent, NBME saw its scope of authority as covering five years: four years of medical school plus one of internship. Likewise, the AMA's Council on Medical Education regarded its role as extending through this fifth year, and in 1919 it published "Essentials for Approved Internships" and a list of "approved" internships. By 1923, there were enough intern positions to accommodate all graduates of U.S. medical schools.

Specialization and Graduate Medical Education

For the first half of the twentieth century, most physicians worked as general practitioners, caring for adults and children, performing surgeries, and delivering babies. Consequently, for most physicians the general internship year was appropriate preparation, and there was no need for a period of training devoted to specialization. However, some graduates of the internship sought more advanced clinical education. At that time, specialty training was seen as preparation for those graduates who planned careers as faculty members and clinical investigators. This advanced training was accomplished mainly through completion of a program in a degree-granting school of graduate medical education or by pursuing further intensive university-based clinical training, called residency. Both routes had a strongly academic character. In 1925, only twenty-nine hospitals in the United States offered residencies, and even up to World War II a small minority of medical school and internship graduates sought residency training (Ludmerer, 1985).

Reminiscent of the variability of undergraduate medical education prior to Flexner, rigorous advanced residency programs coexisted through the 1920s along with inadequate "short courses," as brief as two weeks, after which a physician would declare himself a specialist. Beginning in 1917, but predominantly during the 1930s, specialty boards were founded, with their major goal to define and standardize the duration and content of advanced training and to administer a specialty examination after which a physician could call himself a specialist. By the end of the 1930s, hospital-based residency programs supplanted the freestanding schools of graduate medical education, but still 75 percent of medical school graduates pursued an internship only and practiced as general practitioners.

After World War II, residency positions increased dramatically, and residency programs, which had been a pyramid shedding trainees who were perceived to be less academically promising along the way, were restructured so that essentially everyone who began a residency could complete the course of training. The advanced clinical training and preparation for a career in clinical investigation that before the war had been the purpose of residency training was shifted to a postresidency phase called *fellowship*. Then, in the early 1950s, graduate medical education underwent systematic expansion. A number of factors underlay this growth. The advent of private, employer-based insurance during World War II increased the demand for care at teaching hospitals and generated enthusiasm on the part of teaching hospitals for resident manpower; the higher prestige of specialty, and ultimately subspecialty, medicine decreased interest among medical school graduates for classical general practice; and even in those relatively early days of modern medicine, the complexity of the field made competent practice over the broad array of primary specialties difficult.

Since 1938, the number of first-year residency positions has consistently exceeded the number of graduates of U.S. medical schools; the difference is made up by graduates of U.S. schools of osteopathy (which were not part of this study) and the graduates of allopathic medical schools outside the United States. Residency positions and the dependence of teaching hospitals on resident participation in patient care have continued to the present.

Postwar Expansion

The period after World War II saw expansion in medical schools, more biomedical research, and growth in residency education. Medical schools expanded in size and number in response to increasing federal support for research, primarily through the National Institutes of Health (NIH). This funding went primarily to research-intensive medical schools and their associated university teaching hospitals. Consequently, smaller community-based medical schools that had no teaching hospitals and community hospitals did not undergo this expansion (Association of American Medical Colleges, 2008).

In the 1960s and 1970s, federal and state governments funded major expansion of medical schools in response to a perceived physician shortage. This was also a time of curricular innovation, with creation of the organ-system curriculum at Case Western Reserve University and the problem-based curriculum at Michigan State University, McMaster University in Ontario, and the University of New Mexico (Papa & Harasym, 1999), approaches that we describe in Chapter Three. Another significant trend emerged in this period: creation of offices of medical education to bring faculty members from schools of education into medical education to help with evaluation, faculty and curriculum development, and, later, educational technology. Offices of medical education are a unique phenomenon in education for the professions; as we describe in Chapter Six, they have helped to guide many curricular reforms.

Medical schools were also reshaped by the rising demand for medical care and expanded federal funding of Medicare and Medicaid, a trend that continues, as we describe in Chapter Five. Prior to 1965, the year in which Medicare was created, medical schools were small organizations with few faculty members; clinical practice revenues accounted for less than 3 percent of total school revenues (Watson, 2003). In contrast, by 2007 clinical revenue had increased to 40 percent of total revenue, and the number of faculty members in clinical departments expanded comparably (Association of American Medical Colleges, 2008). Medicare and Medicaid funding has not only moved the country toward a one-class system of care but has also transformed teaching hospitals from providers of charity care to providers of care to the poor, covered by Medicare or Medicaid. This change in the financing of clinical service set in motion a gradual shift in medical schools toward more direct patient-care, a larger number of clinical faculty, and dependence on clinically generated revenue. This growth in the clinical enterprise offered expanded learning opportunities for students and residents because of the greater number of patients seen and the emerging medicines and technologies available (Ludmerer, 1999).

This expansionary era led to soaring health care expenditures in the 1970s, which in turn ushered in an era of cost containment and a variety of regulations designed to limit expenditures by Medicare and Medicaid. This placed great pressures on teaching hospitals in the 1980s to reduce costs, increase efficiency, and become more price-competitive, thus challenging their ability to offer a quality learning environment for medical students and residents. As a result, university teaching hospitals became an increasingly difficult place within which to learn because of shortened lengths of stay, growing acuity of patient problems seen in inpatient settings, and expanding use of complex technological and therapeutic modalities in patient care.

Quality Improvement in Patient Care

By the 1990s and the first decade of the twenty-first century, it became evident that these external pressures on medical schools and teaching hospitals had led to deterioration of the conditions under which clinical education takes place, sparking concern about patient safety, resident duty hours, and minimum competencies of medical graduates. Several Institute of Medicine studies called for greater attention to the quality of patient care and reduction of errors, stimulating improvement efforts across the continuum of medical education and in hospitals nationally (Committee on Quality of Health Care in America, 2000, 2001; Committee on the Health Professions Education Summit, 2003; Association of American Medical Colleges, 2004). Simultaneously, the long duty hours of residents and the lack of sleep associated with working up to 120 hours a week were connected to patient safety concerns and resident well-being. Under threat of congressional legislation, the Accreditation Council for Graduate Medical Education (ACGME) imposed rules on resident duty hours, resulting in a cap of eighty hours a week. Many residency program directors and clinical faculty resisted this constraint because they were concerned that residents would not have enough experience to competently perform difficult procedures, care for a variety of patients, and assume professional responsibility for their patients. Many hospitals resisted because they were dependent on cheap labor from residents and changes would raise their fixed costs. However, all have accommodated this new rule and are working to mitigate its potential adverse effects on education.

Quality improvement in patient care has now become a major move-ment in American medicine. It is incorporated into the ACGME com-petencies for all residents. Two of the six competencies relate to quality improvement: practice-based learning and improvement (learning from one's own patients and improving their care), and systems-based practice (working within and improving health care systems of practice). The other competencies are medical knowledge, clinical reasoning, patient communication, and professionalism. Medical schools have elected to use similar competencies for undergraduate medical education as well. Competencies identify general, nondomain-specific areas of performance expected of all trainees at every level of development and have stimulated curricular innovations in graduate medical education and undergraduate medical education (Irby & Wilkerson, 2003).

Increased Specialization

During the 1990s and early twenty-first century, funding for biomedical research from NIH doubled. The result of this expansion was a more intense focus on molecular medicine and breakthroughs in diagnostic and therapeutic modalities. As more knowledge and technology developed, physicians began to narrow their areas of focus, resulting in subspecialization and sub-subspecialization. Prior to 1970, there were nineteen specialties and ten subspecialties approved by the American Board of Medical Specialties (ABMS). Today, ABMS recognizes 24 specialties and 121 subspecialty members (http://www.abms.org/About_ABMS/ABMS_History/).

With ever-increasing specialization, new clinical roles and relationships unimagined by Flexner have arisen. Physicians care for patients in partnership with a variety of other health professionals, such as nurse anesthetists, physician assistants, and clinical pharmacists. As specialization proliferates, companion phenomena have emerged: interdisciplinary patient care teams and research. Although frequently identified with outpatient primary care, generalist physicians who can identify key clinical priorities and integrate input from specialists play a greater role in the hospital as well. Known as hospitalists, these physicians work exclusively in the hospital, caring for patients and coordinating care between a variety of hospital specialists.

The Business of Medical Education

Regardless of specialty or subspecialty, physicians are educated and practice within systems of health care. At the macro level, health care in the United States is a $2.1 trillion business annually and consumes about 16 percent of the gross domestic product. This industry is uncoordinated, and in spite of spending approximately twice as much on health care as do other developed nations, the United States achieves health outcomes unsatisfactory by many standards (Ginsburg et al., 2008). Even among those patients with private or public health insurance, outcomes are substandard due to defects in the delivery system. Moreover, 47 million Americans remain uninsured. In this environment, university teaching hospitals carry a disproportionate share of care for the uninsured while also constituting a learning environment for the next generation of physicians and conducting clinical research. The multiple missions of patient care, care for the poor, teaching, and research—all vying for limited resources—have placed many teaching hospitals at a competitive disadvantage in the health care marketplace. In this context, medical students and residents learn within systems that are often suboptimal for delivering quality care.

On the broader cultural level, the rise of consumerism and expectations for accountability and transparency are powerfully influencing how medicine is practiced and taught. Information on the performance of hospitals, clinics, and individual physicians is now being collected and made available to the public. Benchmarks of performance are being formulated and results published even though such measures are not always valid indicators.

Finally, a wave of expansion is currently taking place in response to a projected physician shortage for the United States. New medical schools are being established, and existing medical schools are increasing enrollment. However, this is unlikely to meet future demand because of inadequate numbers and quite uneven distribution, in terms of geography and specialties, of physicians. Rural and inner-city communities are unable to attract physicians to practice there, and too many students are choosing procedural specialties rather than primary care. These problems will inhibit appropriate deployment of physicians to areas of need.

The Current Model of Medical Education

Today, there are 130 accredited M.D.-granting medical schools in the United States. The purpose of the four years of undergraduate medical education is to accomplish the general professional education of the physician and to ready physicians-in-training for supervised practice during residency training.

Premedical Education and Admission

Preparation for medical education begins with a bachelor's degree and a common set of science courses. These standard courses are a Flexnerian legacy and include one year of biology, two years of general and organic chemistry, one year of physics, and in some schools one year of mathematics. This grounding in the sciences has long been viewed as important to success in medical school because of the intensity of science instruction in the first two years of the curriculum. However, there is much debate about what coursework should be required for entry into medical school (Dienstag, 2008). Recent work by the AAMC and the Howard Hughes Medical Institute recommends changes in the scientific competencies for premedical and medical school students, an expanded set of prerequisites that more accurately reflect the integrated nature of the basic, clinical, and social sciences and more broadly represents the core competencies expected of a physician (Association of American Medical Colleges & Howard Hughes Medical Institute, 2009).

In 2007, the total number of applicants to U.S. medical schools offering an M.D. degree rose to some forty-two thousand for eighteen thousand total positions (Association of American Medical Colleges, 2008). Admission decisions are made in large part on the basis of the student's grade point average in science courses and performance on the Medical College Admission Test (MCAT). This exam is oriented toward scientific knowledge and reasoning, expected outcomes of a premedical course of study. Although these criteria predict performance on examinations in the first two years, they do not correlate highly with performance in clerkships or later licensing examinations (Kreiter, Yin, Solow, & Brennan, 2004). In an effort to assess the personal qualities of applicants essential to the practice of medicine, such as compassion, trustworthiness, and dependability, medical school admissions committee and residency selection committee members interview applicants. These interviews are time-intensive and notoriously unreliable (Kreiter et al., 2004). Alternative interviewing practices are beginning to emerge that more accurately assess noncognitive factors in the selection process (Eva, Reiter, Rosenfeld, & Norman, 2004a, 2004b; Eva, Rosenfeld, Reiter, & Norman, 2004).

Those who are selected for the study of medicine discover that their classmates are accomplished and diverse. This diversity was not a feature of medical education in Flexner's day, especially after several schools that educated women and African Americans closed in the wake of his report. Even until the early 1960s, virtually all physicians in training were white men. Diversity in medical education is now enhancing the quality of education for all learners and translating into more effective and culturally competent physicians who are better prepared to serve an increasingly heterogeneous patient population. In addition, minority physicians are more likely to practice in underserved areas and be proficient in languages other than English, thus helping address linguistic and cultural barriers that may hinder provision of quality care (Coleman, Palmer, & Winnick, 2008).

Undergraduate Medical Education

Once admitted to the study of medicine, students begin the two years of classroom-based coursework that is designed to constitute the foundation of formal knowledge on which clinical practice is based. The majority of medical schools offer this in integrated courses organized in discrete time blocks around organ systems or topics (cardiovascular, renal, respiratory, genetics, cancer). This foundational coursework is followed by two years of clinical practica, organized into specialty blocks called clerkships. During the third year, students rotate through a series of clerkships, typically for four to eight weeks, in the core specialties of family medicine, internal medicine, neurology, obstetrics and gynecology, pediatrics, psychiatry, and surgery. Following these required clerkships and subinternships (advanced clerkships), the fourth year is primarily elective.

Within this broad framework of undergraduate medical education (often referred to as UME, which we describe in depth in Chapter Three), some schools have created unique learning experiences to align with their school's mission; some schools focus on primary care in rural communities, others address public health issues, and others prepare future researchers and academics. Some medical schools offer specialized tracks within their curricula, allowing students to pursue areas of interest such as biotechnology, clinical and translational research, molecular medicine, and global health; such focused programs affording opportunities for students to tailor learning experiences to their interests are responsive to the need for individualization.

Graduate Medical Education

In their fourth year of medical school, students interview at multiple residency programs around the country in their chosen specialty. Residency, or graduate medical education (usually referred to as GME, the subject of Chapter Four), programs largely consist of extensive and intensive clinical experience organized to promote progressive development of knowledge and skills within the resident's chosen specialty; each specialty also requires some didactic education. Residency training spans three to seven years, depending on the specialty. For example, residency programs in internal medicine, family medicine, and pediatrics are three years. Surgical specialties and radiology are at least five years.

Like medical schools, residency programs may have specific goals, such as training individuals to meet the health care needs of a particular region, preparing academic leaders, or setting a clinical foundation for a research career. At completion of residency education, graduates are ready for unsupervised practice within their specialty or may elect to take a fellowship within a subspecialty. Virtually all of the larger clinical specialties have subspecialties; preparation for certification in subspecialties requires another one to three years of training. The great majority of internal medicine residents go on to subspecialize in areas such as cardiology, gastroenterology, geriatrics, and hematology/oncology. Fellowships follow the structure developed after World War II: typically a year of clinical experience and a year or two of research.

Currently, residency training programs in primary care specialties—particularly family medicine and internal medicine—are having great difficulty in filling the available positions they offer because students are choosing procedural specialties. This is driven by many factors, including inequities in pay among medical specialties, increasing student debt (in 2008 average student debt was $140,000 from medical school alone), and a desire on the part of students to achieve work-life balance and controllable work hours while still earning enough to retire their debt. As a result, fewer and fewer students are choosing primary care specialties, and residency programs in these areas are having difficulty filling their positions with U.S. medical graduates.

In 2008, there were 107,851 residents in 8,490 ACGME-accredited programs training in the United States (Accreditation Council for Graduate Medical Education, 2009). The majority of residency programs are in community-based teaching hospitals, although, because they are larger, university-based residencies train the majority of residents in the U.S. (This is in contrast to Canada, where university medical schools oversee all GME.) The demographics of residents differ from those of medical students because there are 1.3 times as many first-year residency positions as graduates from U.S. medical schools. As an illustration, in 2003, there were some twenty-four thousand first-year residency positions available, yet only fifteen thousand U.S. medical school graduates. The difference is made up by graduates of U.S. schools of osteopathy (6 percent of residents) and international medical graduates (27 percent of residents). International medical graduates practicing in the United States typically attended medical school in India (20.3 percent), the Philippines (10.7 percent), Mexico (6.2 percent), Pakistan (4.5 percent), China (3.3 percent), and the Republic of Korea (2.7 percent) (Hart et al., 2007). A growing percentage of international medical graduates are U.S. citizens trained abroad, predominantly in for-profit schools in the Caribbean. Many residency programs in rural and less desirable inner-city communities have less success in attracting U.S. medical graduates and are therefore especially dependent on international medical graduates.

Given rapid changes in the practice of medicine, physicians must find ways to continuously update their knowledge and learn new skills and procedures. Continuing medical education (CME) programs supply those ongoing educational opportunities, and participation in such programs is a condition for maintaining licensure in many states and continued certification in many specialties. CME is beyond the scope of this book but has a considerable research literature (Davis, 2005; Davis et al., 1999).

Medical Education's Key Challenges

There is no question that the reforms of undergraduate medical education promoted by Flexner, the development of a phased program of graduate medical education from internship through fellowship, the investments made in biomedical science through the NIH, and the public funding of care for the elderly, disabled, and indigent have in the aggregate produced a remarkable system of health care and, along with it, an exceptional educational program for preparation of physicians. However, the shortcomings of the health care system in the United States in the first decade of the twenty-first century are pervasive and severe (McGlynn et al., 2003). Embedded as it is in the health care system, medical education also has severe shortcomings that require immediate and vigorous corrective action.

In the course of our fieldwork, we saw many instances of foundational knowledge poorly linked to experience; well-thought-out, integrated teaching subverted by inappropriate assessments; and missed opportunities for allowing learners to participate in the important nonclinical roles physicians play within health care and more broadly in society. We also saw exciting innovations through which students and residents were given authority to improve the settings in which they learn and to improve outcomes for patients; and we observed inspiring examples of institutional culture supporting and advancing the humanism and professional values of learners.

In our review and observation of medical education, we were as well influenced by research in the learning sciences and medical education. Much of this research has been distilled in *How People Learn: Brain, Mind, Experience, and School* (Bransford, Brown, & Cocking, 1999) for the National Academy of Sciences. In medical education, research on physician knowledge, reasoning and action, and investigations into workplace learning have contributed to our arguments for change. We review this research in our discussion of practice in Chapter Two, and throughout the book we use it as a lens for our critique of current practices in medical education and make recommendations for future directions.

As we explain in the Introduction, our fieldwork and review of the learning sciences led us to identify four goals for medical education: (1) standardization and individualization, (2) integration, (3) insistence on excellence, and (4) formation of professional identity. Although these

Table 1.1. Flexner's Recommendations for Educating Physicians in 1910

Goals	Challenges	Recommendations
Standardization	Lack of standard, rigorous educational program Poorly prepared students Heterogeneity in student achievement	Insist on a four-year college degree as a prerequisite to medical studies. Standardize a four-year curriculum in 2+2 design. Establish accreditation process for medical schools.
Integration	Limited science in the curriculum No connection between practice and science	Integrate advances in the laboratory with practice at the bedside. Provide clinical training in university teaching hospitals.
Habits of inquiry and improvement	Excessive emphasis on rote memorization rather than on learning by doing in the laboratory and hospital Faculty tradition-bound rather than scientifically oriented	Train physicians to "think like scientists." Require medical education to be taught by scientifically trained faculty members within university settings.
Professional formation	Teaching by unqualified faculty members Role modeling by physicians with varying competency, in many proprietary and for-profit schools	Immerse medical education in university culture. Facilitate close and sustained contact between learners and scientifically based faculty role models.

four goals are consistent with and can be understood as an extension of Flexner's work, they are also the basis for a new agenda for change. Accordingly, we base our descriptive analyses of the various facets of medical education on them.

Table 1.1 describes the goals in terms of the major challenges Flexner found in 1910 and his recommendations for addressing them. Table 1.2 presents them in the context of our findings, along with a summary of our recommendations for the future of medical education, which we present in detail in Chapters Seven and Eight.

Table 1.2. Recommendations for Educating Physicians, 2010

Goals	Challenges	Recommendations
Standardization and individualization	Medical education is: ○ Not outcomes-based ○ Inflexible ○ Excessively long ○ Not learner-centered	Standardize learning outcomes through assessment of competencies. Individualize learning process within and across levels. Offer elective programs to support development of skills for inquiry and improvement.
Integration	Poor connections between formal knowledge and experiential learning Fragmented understanding of patient experience Poor understanding of nonclinical and civic roles of physicians Inadequate attention to the skills required for effective team-delivered care in a complex health care system	Connect formal knowledge to clinical experience, including early clinical immersion and adequate opportunities for more advanced learners to reflect and study. Integrate basic, clinical, and social sciences. Engage learners at all levels with a more comprehensive perspective on patients' experience of illness and care, including more longitudinal connections with patients. Provide opportunities for learners to experience the broader professional roles of physicians, including educator, advocate, investigator. Incorporate interprofessional education and teamwork into the curriculum.
Habits of inquiry and improvement	Focused on mastering today's skills and knowledge without also promoting knowledge building and an enduring commitment to excellence	Prepare learners to attain both routine and adaptive forms of expertise. Engage learners in challenging problems, and allow them to participate authentically in inquiry, innovation, and improvement of care.

(Continued)

Table 1.2. (*Continued*)

Goals	Challenges	Recommendations
Habits of inquiry and improvement (cont'd.)	Limited and often pro forma engagement in scientific inquiry and improvement exercises Inadequate attention to patient populations, health promotion, and practice-based learning and improvement Insufficient opportunity to participate in management and improvement of the health care systems within which they learn and work	Engage learners in initiatives focused on population health, quality improvement, and patient safety. Locate clinical education in settings where quality patient care is delivered, not just in university teaching hospitals.
Professional formation	Lack of clarity and focus on professional values Failure to assess, acknowledge, and advance professional behaviors Inadequate expectations for progressively higher levels of professional commitment Erosion of professional values because of pace and commercial nature of health care	Promote formal ethics instruction, storytelling, and symbols (honor codes, pledges, and white-coat ceremonies). Address the underlying messages expressed in the hidden curriculum, and strive to align the espoused and enacted values of the clinical environment. Offer feedback, opportunities for reflection, and assessment of professionalism in the context of longitudinal mentoring and advising. Promote relationships with faculty who simultaneously support learners and hold them to high standards. Create collaborative learning environments committed to excellence and continuous improvement.

Standardization and Individualization

To promote high academic standards, Flexner argued for standardization based on structural requirements: a bachelor's degree with a rigorous science background for admissions, two years of university-based basic science courses, and two years of clinical experience in a university teaching hospital. Another approach to standardization has been to focus on learning outcomes and the general competencies of the graduates. Two major issues have arisen around the competency movement: how to define and assess complex competencies, and how to promote excellence when competencies are targeted at "good enough" or minimal standards of performance.

Although Flexner's uniformity of structure raised academic standards, a companion problem has emerged: lack of sufficient flexibility in the length of training. In Flexner's day and through the 1940s, most physicians were prepared for practice within five years of graduation from college. Thus physicians began their career at age twenty-six or twenty-seven. Currently, the minimum preparation for independent practice requires seven years after college, and physicians in a long residency and those preparing for an academic career may be in their midthirties before they complete their formal education. Clearly the field of medicine is enormously more complex than it was in Flexner's time, but other factors have contributed to the ever-lengthening process of medical education. Undergraduate medical education has been managed using time-and-process metrics: four years and sometimes longer if a student chooses to extend the period of study to do research, pursues cocurricular or personal interest, or requires remediation. In general, students are not able to "test out" of a significant amount of introductory work, regardless of their undergraduate major and premedical experience. There has been little sustained exploration of approaches that might increase the efficiency of medical education. With the exception of short tracking in internal medicine, where residents in good standing may skip the third year of medicine residency program and go directly into fellowship training, there has been minimal experimentation in allowing medical learners to more rapidly proceed through various levels of education.

Likewise, residency programs have been designed to maximize the likelihood that all, or close to all, residents who proceed through the specified number of months, and across the specified clinical activities and settings, will emerge competent to practice without supervision. By adopting this approach, it is inevitable that some residents will have achieved this level of global competence before the end of the stipulated period and could be advanced more rapidly. According to one study, residents undergoing a rigorous competency-based training program could become competent in about one-third less time than is currently required in a time-based rotation system (Long, 2000). When we talk about individualization in this regard, we mean the ability of educational programs to adjust to meet students' and residents' learning needs and offer educational experiences that acknowledge differences in background, preparation, and rate of mastering concepts and skills, in contrast to the current one-size-fits-all approach.

Another argument for increasing the efficiency and decreasing the duration of medical training is that the vast majority of students preparing to become physicians acquire extraordinary indebtedness; this debt burden is creating a serious barrier to entry into the profession and is skewing the specialty choice of those who do elect to become physicians. The average medical student debt at graduation has risen, increasing from $80,000 in 1998 to $140,000 in 2007; this does not include premedical school debt (Association of American Medical Colleges, 2008). A well-educated physician workforce is a clear societal need and an important social good (Starfield, 1992). Thus society must take a compelling interest in ensuring that the composition of the physician workforce is appropriate to meet the needs of the public. Career choice is complicated and multifaceted; however, addressing medical student debt is critical to ensuring a socioeconomically diverse group of graduates who choose broadly among medical specialties and subspecialties.

Integration

The formal knowledge foundational to medical practice is not well integrated with acquisition of experiential knowledge over the continuum of medical education. The premedical requirements overemphasize some scientific fields, such as physics, to the detriment of the social sciences and nonscience domains. Early in medical school, even in schools that have fairly extensive clinical exposure, students rarely have clearly defined and authentic clinical roles, and their classroom formal learning is poorly linked, if at all, to what they have experienced in clinical settings. This lack of integration results in early-stage medical students typically failing to appreciate the relevance and clinical context for the information they encounter in their classroom work. The other side of this issue is that, once in a clinical environment, students struggle to recognize the relationships between what they have been taught in the classroom and the problems patients present, and so they feel they have to learn everything all over again. Learning facts disassociated from patients results in a 30–50 percent loss in knowledge by the time students reach the clinical setting and requires students to reorganize their knowledge in memory from a basic science disciplinary perspective to a patient-centered clinical perspective (Custers, 2008). In addition, students must learn to connect and integrate multiple forms of reasoning (critical and creative thinking, and pattern recognition) and types of knowledge (formal knowledge and case knowledge) in order to care for patients.

The balance between and integration of formal knowledge and experiential learning continues to be challenging in the residency phase of education, although the tables turn. In GME, clinical experience is ascendant; residents often suffer from inadequate time and encouragement to reflect on what they have seen in the course of patient care, to read, to discuss, and to wonder. The shortened length of patients' hospital stays, increased clinical acuity of hospitalized patients, and discontinuity in relationships among faculty, residents, students, hospital staff, and patients have conspired to increase the pace and complexity of the resident's day to the point that it often becomes inimical to learning. The lack of longitudinal relationships creates an inefficient and haphazard system for learners and clinical teachers and less-than-optimal care for patients. Thoughtful attention must be given to both the tempo of the clinical learning environment and the appropriate balance between formal and experiential learning over the entire continuum of medical education.

A second distinct aspect of integration entails an understanding and appreciation of the multiple roles physicians play beyond provision of one-on-one clinical care. Medical school matriculants have often had experience in international health, advocacy, and research. Others are deeply engaged in the humanities and want to explore the connection between their work as a clinician and their experience as a poet or musician. Furthermore, physicians play a key role in the leadership of health care systems, from small practices to hospitals, to managed care organizations, and to insurance companies. We believe medical students and residents should be exposed to these broader roles that physicians play in health care and in society, and they should have the opportunity to explore in a sustained way the integration of the clinical role with these other roles. Currently, these other roles are underemphasized in most schools and residency programs, compromising learners' appreciation and experience of the full dimension of being a physician.

Inquiry and Improvement

Medical education overemphasizes factual medical knowledge and underemphasizes the importance of both clinically driven curiosity and the complex system in which physicians must function. We see curiosity as the engine of lifelong learning; all physicians, no matter how well educated at completion of residency, must relentlessly question the validity of what they think they know, accept received truths with skepticism, and wonder with every patient what improved understanding or novel therapy is just around the corner. An educational program that continuously prepares its graduates to think in these ways will foster not rote learning, mnemonics, and a tyranny of facts and associations but curiosity, exploration, skepticism, and wonder. Instead of simply presenting scientific concepts as facts, medical education should entail some exploration of the frontiers of science and should examine the controversies within the field. By mastering the tools of scholarship in one area of investigation (for example, molecular medicine, clinical and translational research, medical education, global health sciences, health disparities), physicians-in-training can develop the skills and the habits of mind that will allow them to advance their practice over a lifetime of engagement with the problems and challenges of clinical work.

Medicine is practiced within a complex health care system with many imperfections. Medical education should prepare physicians to address, analyze, and improve the systems within which they work. In some cases, these advances will flow out of large research projects or state- or national-level policy work, but physicians also need to see the daily adaptations they make in practice to better meet the needs of their patients as important ways to advance the field of medicine (Mylopoulos & Scardamalia, 2008).These frequently small practice-based improvements require originality, commitment, effort, and skill and are important steps in improving patient care.

Professional Formation

Curriculum, and often teaching and assessment practices, tends to neglect the fundamentally moral nature of medical practice and consequently of medical education. Even though considerable progress has been made over the past thirty years in including ethics courses in medical school and residency curricula, and in detecting and attempting to remediate lapses in ethical comportment, medical education is still squeamish about addressing the aspirational dimension of medicine, specifically the critical importance of inculcating a desire to be more compassionate, more altruistic, and more humane. This commitment to excellence is a dimension of the moral identity of the physician as well.

Students typically enter medical school with only a superficial understanding of the values underpinning the medical profession and how these values inform every step of the educational process. Whereas students are expected to learn these values through direct instruction, modeling, and socialization, their practical application is not obvious. For example, how do professional values apply to conflict among team members about patient issues or disruptive behavior of faculty members in the operating room? Or what should a male student do if he is asked by his resident to practice a pelvic exam on an anesthetized woman who has declined male examiners? Typically, the clinical setting is where students observe positive and often negative interactions of physicians with patients and with other health professionals.

Unfortunately, moral development of physicians-to-be is often described as arrested or regressing during medical school and residency training (Branch, 2000; Branch, Pels, Lawrence, & Arky, 1993). Students report having great difficulty accommodating to and being assimilated into the hospital culture (Branch, Hafler, & Pels, 1998). Students often feel trapped between their moral ideals and the desire to conform to the norms, values, and actions of their team. Without a forum to share and reflect on their moral choices, students feel isolated and unable to resolve their identity and ethical conflict. This can lead to depression, loss of empathy, and moral regression (Branch, 2000).

By the time medical learners reach residency, they have been immersed in clinical environments for two or more years and much acculturation has already occurred. However, residency remains the forge that molds and tempers the physician-to-be. Three elements of resident work account for the importance of this phase of medical education: teaching, team leadership and teamwork, and the nature of the resident's role in patient care.

The fact that residents are expected to teach signals the shift in their position in the learning community; although not yet ready for independent patient care, the resident has enough formal knowledge and experience that she is expected to monitor and support the learning of more junior trainees. As we discuss in Chapter Four, residency is also the time when every medical learner is called on to deploy the leadership and management skills demanded by the team leader role. Although the attending physician is responsible for the clinical decisions made by the team under her supervision, the quality of the team interactions and the nature of the work and learning environment are largely determined by the resident. The interactions that a resident has in the team leader role, with subordinates, peers, and superiors, can be positive or equally negative; in either case, they are powerfully formative. Finally, the resident's role in patient care is different from that of the students, and in most programs from interns as well; residents frequently make clinical decisions that are not double-checked in real time. When a fourth-year student detects an unexpected physical finding, his exam will be repeated and the finding confirmed or refuted within minutes or a few hours. Likewise, when an intern admits a patient, develops a management plan, and writes admission orders, her admit note and orders will be reviewed, and amended and corrected if needed, by the resident who is in the hospital and working in parallel with the intern. In contrast, although the attending physician will see each patient every day, there may be an interval of hours between the resident's assessment of and response to a clinical development and the attending physician's verification. Supervision is always a phone call away, but the resident must recognize when she needs assistance. The sense that the patient's well-being hangs in the balance and that the resident's judgment counts powerfully molds the character of the young physician.

Of course, there are negative influences that threaten to countervail the positive effects of teaching responsibilities, assuming leadership for a team, and being responsible for knowing when help is needed in the absence of real-time supervision. Failure in any of these key domains can shake the resident's confidence. Moreover, residents, like students, receive mixed messages about the core values of the medical profession and see many examples of behavior that should not be emulated. The importance of making formation of an appropriate professional identity a major curricular goal is underscored by recent research showing that lapses in professionalism demonstrated by students during medical school and as residents in training are associated with professional sanctions later in practice (Papadakis, Arnold, Blank, Holmboe, & Lipner, 2008; Papadakis, Loeser, & Healy, 2001; Papadakis, Hodgson, Teherani, & Kohatsu, 2004; Papadakis, Osborn, Cooke, & Healy, 1999; Papadakis et al., 2005). A major, and too-often-neglected, challenge of medical educators is finding the best ways to promote professionalism in medical school and residency training (Stern & Papadakis, 2006).

One of the major ways of promoting professional formation is to immerse trainees in a setting that embodies the highest values of the profession: excellence, collaboration, respect, and compassion. The clinician teachers who work in such communities shape the practices there. Faculty development programs and academies of medical educators seek to create a space where a community of teachers can share their ideas about teaching and learning. This involves building a culture that values continuous learning and the scholarship of teaching and learning, a communal space also known as a "teaching commons" (Huber & Hutchings, 2005; Irby, Cooke, Lowenstein, & Richards, 2004): "As *Scholarship Reconsidered* (Boyer, 1990) made clear, the professional responsibility of educators was to engage continuously in their own efforts to study the quality of their work, its fidelity to their missions, and its impact on students intellectually, practically, and morally" (Shulman, 2005a, p. vi). Therefore, teachers and learners are powerfully shaped by the values and practices of their professional communities.

Yesterday's Legacy, Tomorrow's Practice

Medical education and the practice of medicine have come a long way in the past hundred years. Although he would easily understand the current paradigm of physician education, Flexner would hardly recognize the contemporary practice of medicine. He would applaud the scientific basis of medicine and the progress that has been made in advancing health. However, he might wonder if the old structures of medical education can continue to support the rising challenges to the curriculum, pedagogies, and assessment of medical education. Accordingly, in the next chapter we examine the practice of medicine and the nature of learning, an essential discussion that must preface any description of how medical education is—and should be—structured.

2

BEING A DOCTOR

FOUNDATIONS OF PROFESSIONAL
EDUCATION

DISCUSSION OF MEDICAL EDUCATION has long emphasized the vast knowledge base of medicine, from cutting-edge science to the tricks of the trade, and the high level of technical proficiency that students and residents must attain for practice. However, clinical education involves far more than outfitting individual physicians with scientific knowledge and technical skills. The clinical work and the other professional activities of physicians are social practices, and physicians must be prepared to work in relationships with their patients and with other professionals and nonprofessionals in clinics, medical centers, and communities. Care of patients is an interpersonal endeavor, involving transactions between clinicians and patients, which even in a simple clinical situation involves many people, let alone in more complex settings where an array of specialists from a variety of fields are engaged.

We focus this chapter on practice and learning for practice. We begin by considering a brief moment from the daily work of two practicing physicians—a trauma surgeon who is five years into licensed practice, and a family medicine physician who is more than twenty years into practice—using these exemplars to describe the activities and competencies associated with the domains of the physician's work. We then consider the relevant learning theories, conceptual frameworks, and research that have informed our understanding of the process by which medical students become physicians adept in these domains and the professional formation that is deeply entwined with this process. We close by highlighting some of the implications for curriculum, pedagogy, and assessment—topics we address in detail in Chapters Three and

Four and to which we return in Chapter Seven, as we explore future possibilities in medical education.

Domains of Physicians' Work

○

Dr. Sam Caldwell, a thirty-eight-year-old trauma surgeon, is called to the emergency department in anticipation of the arrival of a woman gravely injured in an automobile accident. He has learned that, initially trapped in her car, the woman was extricated using the Jaws of Life. At the scene, the paramedics described a moaning woman who appeared to be in her midtwenties with crush injuries to her torso, and particularly her pelvis. By the time she was ready for the ten-minute transport to the hospital, she had developed signs of shock.

One of the things Dr. Caldwell enjoys about trauma surgery is that each patient's injuries are unique. Providing expert care requires the on-the-spot integration of what he knows of the field, the formal knowledge and the experience he has acquired over his residency and the five years he has been in practice, with the particulars of each patient's situation. As he hurries to the emergency department, he anticipates what this woman's care is likely to require of him immediately: the ability to lead the emergency department team, nurses, respiratory therapists, X-ray technicians, and others in the patient's initial assessment and stabilization; surgical skills to address traumatic injuries within his expertise and recruitment of other specialists to manage her possible orthopedic and urologic injuries; and the capacity to establish a connection and communicate effectively with her distraught family.

Assuming that she survives the night, he will need to work with the hospital's intensivist and the highly skilled nurses in the intensive care unit (ICU) to participate in the hospital's campaign to reduce ventilator-associated pneumonias. Later, when his patient is ready, he will bring in a physical therapist, and possibly a physiatrist.

Dr. Caldwell's hospital is near a major highway, and he briefly reflects on the number of alcohol-related accidents they see. He has been active in his community's schools, talking about injury prevention in general and underage drinking and driving in particular. As he is wondering if he might be more effective at the community level, the paramedics race in with his patient. He asks for two large-bore IVs and begins the trauma assessment.

○

Dr. Susana Alvarado is a fifty-one-year-old family physician with a largely Latino population. Arriving at her modest office at 7:15 a.m., she glances at her schedule for the morning: twelve patients, including a well-baby check for a six-month-old, an octogenarian who had a bad fall recently and is doing poorly at home, and a college student who wants contraceptive and sexual health counseling. Dr. Alvarado notes that there are five diabetics to be seen, including two patients for medication adjustment referred from the self-management group her nurse runs with a medical assistant, and a sixty-three-year-old man three weeks post-op from a below-the-knee amputation. She shakes her head sadly: Why hadn't she been able to get Ramón Gutierrez more engaged in controlling his blood sugar or attentive to his foot care? This amputation was preventable.

Some years ago, Dr. Alvarado became concerned about the effectiveness of the diabetes care she and her partners were providing. An "early adopter," she worked with like-minded colleagues in her community to identify an electronic health record (EHR) with the functionalities that best met their needs. Collaborating across practices, they were able to persuade their community hospital to adopt the same platform so that information could be shared across care settings.

This EHR has multiple functions that allow her to generate registries of patients with asthma, to automatically create prompts to telephone patients two weeks after initiation of antidepressant therapy and to remind patients who are overdue for being seen to call for appointments. Monthly, she and her partners review their practice's performance on standard measures as well as some they have chosen themselves as pertinent to their patient population; the practice nurse and front-desk staff are included in the performance review and actively contribute to the discussion about how the practice might be more effective in meeting its goals for patients. It was noted that many patients have persistently elevated HA1c measurements, a test that had not been developed at the time Dr. Alvarado completed her residency. The nurse and the office manager agreed to add some group visits focused on increasing patients' self-management skills and efficacy. Meanwhile Dr. Alvarado considers whether an option such as sitagliptin would be appropriate for these poorly controlled patients. This therapy was submitted to the FDA for new drug approval in 2006, more than twenty years after she completed her training. Despite all these advances, some patients, like Sr. Gutierrez, do not do as well as she would like. As she sits down to review the morning's charts, she asks herself what additional changes she and her practice colleagues might make to increase their effectiveness.

Why begin a discussion of medical education with these snapshots of physicians at work? These scenarios describe the three key domains of physicians' work: caring for patients, engaging in inquiry and innovation, and participating in professional communities. The performance of exemplary doctors such as Caldwell and Alvarado has much to tell us about how education should be structured to support development of physicians whose work is outstanding in these key dimensions. The fundamental goal of medical education is professional formation, the hallmark of which is commitment to making things better for patients and, more broadly, the public—an aspiration to excellence across the domains of practice. This is, in our view, the essence of professionalism.

To become practitioners like Dr. Caldwell and Dr. Alvarado, medical students and residents must integrate themselves into unfamiliar social structures, accustom themselves to the range of physician roles, deduce the expertise and scope of practice of a host of nonphysician protagonists, make sense of various representations of medical work, and become proficient in use of an array of medical tools and artifacts. The complexity of this undertaking, of becoming a full participant in the work of medicine, may be underestimated by teachers of medicine and by learners, in part because of a dramatic increase in the complexity of medical science and medical care over the past forty years, but also because older conceptualizations of learning medicine overemphasize the individual learner's acquisition of the knowledge and skills of medicine as the principal form of learning.

Caring for Patients

As the snapshots of Drs. Caldwell and Alvarado at work suggest, *caring for patients* includes both caring for individual patients and caring for patient populations. Many physicians like Dr. Alvarado must also manage a practice and monitor group-level outcomes over time. Traditionally, medical education has focused almost exclusively on care of individual patients, with emphasis on data gathering (history and physical exam skills, communication and interpersonal skills), diagnosis (reasoning and pattern recognition), formulation of a plan of care (treatment, patient education and counseling), and skillful performance of procedures. However, effective performance of physicians' professional activities also depends on solid preparation in knowledge, skills, and values related to care of populations and improvement of the delivery system. These areas are as legitimate, important, and intellectually challenging as diagnosis of an obscure condition or a technically demanding operative procedure.

Engaging in Inquiry and Improvement

Inquiry and improvement are daily aspects of the physician's practice. On a personal level, physicians keep their knowledge and skills current by scanning specialty journals; attending local, regional, and national conferences and meetings; consulting with colleagues; reading in depth about new treatments and technologies; preparing for lectures and teaching sessions; and listening to and observing their patients. Their fund of knowledge changes regularly with every new insight and understanding. Physicians who exclusively care for patients manage their fund of knowledge on such multiple fronts as pharmacology, genetics, and policy changes that affect their patients. To the extent they are also involved in nonclinical activities, physicians manage their knowledge and skills in scientific, policy, and pedagogical as well as clinical domains. Keeping up with and integrating new knowledge and advances in the field is a professional obligation and a necessary routine. The greater goal is for the individual practitioner to use this new knowledge to tackle more complex or persistent problems in practice.

On an interpersonal level, physicians also contribute to a shared, or distributed, knowledge and skills base. Although they engage in some activities for the sake of their own learning, they also participate in many activities that make what they know visible and accessible to others, often resulting in changes in practices, team or group functioning, and a new level of understanding among all members. For example, when Dr. Alvarado discovers a coverage gap for a medication she regularly prescribes to patients, she emails all the other physicians, nurses, residents, and students working in the clinic to alert them to the gap; lists the alternatives (as well as any significant warning associated with the alternatives); and asks her administrative assistant to send a request to software support staff to add a pop-up reminder to the system whenever a physician selects this medication from the menu. Ultimately, the knowledge she acquires is made public in a way that has the potential to change a suboptimal patient care practice occurring in the clinic. Of note is the number of individuals contributing to the development and flow of the knowledge and information that is ultimately distributed to all members of the clinic.

On a systems, or societal, level, physicians contribute in many ways to improvements in the operations of a practice or clinic, of an educational program, of health center policies or public policy. In some cases, they do so through such scholarly activities as clinical, educational, policy, and health services research. In other cases, it occurs through creative and thoughtful systems redesign or through participation in professional organizations, committee work, or visionary leadership. The point is an active commitment to achieving a higher level of performance or better outcomes, rather than a passive acceptance of the status quo.

Innovation can occur at any of these levels—personal, interpersonal, or systems—and in many domains. For example, a physician who creates a handout that can be used to guide discussion about weight loss and can be given to patients as a resource is engaging in systematic improvements in daily practice. Other examples of innovation are design and implementation of new educational practices such as biweekly interprofessional quality-improvement rounds, development of a clinical research proposal, reading about new developments in treatment for congestive heart failure, and participation on a local or national health care policy advisory committee. In all these examples, a physician or group of health care professionals is attuned to or is regularly monitoring important outcomes and processes, with an eye toward new possibilities or opportunities for improvement.

Participating in a Professional Community

As the snapshots of Dr. Caldwell and Dr. Alvarado illustrate, whereas physicians work and live in professional communities, they are also professionals in a larger social world, and they work to help their patients in medical environments where there are other professionals and nonprofessionals. We regard both the social nature of physicians' work and the character of medicine as a profession as critical dimensions of medical practice and education. Physicians function in complex social networks, collaborating in the care of patients with onsite and distant colleagues and interacting with other stakeholders in health care whom they have never met. They use a variety of tools of the trade and other material resources, and if they do not find a ready-made resource to their liking they are apt to fashion one of their own. They participate in their communities and societies as physicians, identifying and responding to health care needs and challenges and being sought out for their expertise and leadership. Finally, collectively they participate in ceaseless refinement of the social contract that underlies medicine's standing as a profession, in response to changes in the conditions under which medicine is practiced.

Some advocacy and service roles are entirely familiar to physicians; they tend to be so closely linked to patient care that they may be perceived more as a practice hassle than as political work. A perhaps too-familiar example is the frequent need to call an insurer or pharmacy benefits manager to contest denial of coverage or to request provision of a nonformulary medication. Physicians also play roles outside the exam room when they participate in governance and administration of their clinical settings; hospitals and medical centers depend on the willingness of physicians and other members of the organization to serve on committees, such as the ethics committee, and ad hoc groups to address issues as they emerge. These roles are important because they afford physicians the opportunity to improve services for individual patients and groups of patients efficiently through systems-level interventions.

Beyond this, physicians have traditionally been expected to be leaders in their local community and at the state or national level. Although this tradition is perhaps fading out in highly urbanized environments, it continues in more rural settings. Leadership is an important part of the physician's work, and its atrophy reflects a limited, reductionist, and overly technical conception of what physicians do—or should do.

Implications for Education

As Dr. Alvarado and Dr. Caldwell illustrate, the role of the physician is broader than simply the activities he or she undertakes with patients one at a time, in the exam room, in the operating room, or in the emergency department. It is not just the medical researcher, clinic medical director, or leader in organized medicine who has this broader role; full-time practitioners like our exemplar physicians must be prepared to play a role in their community and work to improve health and the health care system. The goal of educating physicians who are competent practitioners at completion of their formal training is an ambitious one, but the U.S. system of medical education system faces far more daunting challenges. Society requires caring, compassionate physicians with a high level of expertise and commitment to constantly growing and refining that expertise, and who are engaged citizens of their profession and their community, working to improve health and health care. In addition to the breadth of these goals, physicians must be prepared to train and retrain others, and train themselves again many times over the course of a professional lifetime in medicine as their field is transformed and expanded. If that is the end goal, how should the education of physicians be designed and conducted to produce it?

Professional Formation

The experiences of medical school and residency transform laypersons into physicians. Though still considered learners, students and residents participate in the complex interactions of health care in the role of and with the responsibilities of physicians and are present with patients and families at moments of crisis and death, as professionals endowed not only with their own learning and experience but with the knowledge, experience, credibility, and professional standing of their forebears. They engage with society more broadly, directly as individuals or through professional and civic organizations, but always as physicians. This forging of a professional identity, or formation, is both a process of personal development and a social enterprise, a process of becoming and contributing.

Earlier in this chapter we set the stage for our discussion of learning in the three domains of physicians' work by highlighting professional formation as the fundamental goal of the learning process. By professional formation we mean "an ongoing, self-reflective *process* involving habits of thinking, feeling, and acting" (Wear & Castellani, 2000, p. 603). These habits of thought, feeling, and action ideally develop in ways that allow learners to demonstrate *"compassionate, communicative, and socially responsible physicianhood"* (Wear & Castellani, 2000, p. 603, italics in original). The physician we envision has, first and foremost, a deep sense of commitment and responsibility to patients, colleagues, institutions, society, and self and an unfailing aspiration to perform better and achieve more. Such commitment and responsibility involves habitual searching for improvements in all domains—however small they may seem—and willingness to invest the effort to strategize and enact such improvements. If Dr. Caldwell and Dr. Alvarado functioned only as providers of medical services without a deeper sense of purpose and social responsibility, it is unlikely that they would conceptualize "patient care" as something more than providing medical services to individual patients, or invest the effort to examine communities and health care systems as possible sources for improving the health of patients as a individuals or as groups.

However, defining professional formation only by looking at individual processes suggests a more limited understanding of the concept than we intend. Instead, professional formation, much like other learning processes, must be understood in the context of interpersonal relationships and cultural values. This point is well articulated by Lave and Wenger:

> As an aspect of social practice, learning involves the whole person: it implies not only a relation to specific activities, but a relation to social communities—it implies becoming a full participant, a member, a kind of person. In this view, learning only partly and often incidentally implies becoming able to be involved in new activities, to perform new tasks and functions, to master new understandings. Activities,

task, functions and understandings do not exist in isolation; they are part of broader systems of relations in which they have meaning.... Learning thus implies becoming a different person with respect to the possibilities enabled by these systems of relations. To ignore this aspect of learning is to overlook the fact that learning involves the construction of identities [1991, p. 53].

Learning Patient Care

Learning to care for patients has long been recognized as fundamentally an experiential process; likewise, advancing skills of caring for populations of patients and tuning the performance of a practice to achieve desired outcomes for patients is driven by the experience of doing it. However, learners' experiences as they engage in patient care activities are far more complex than is implied by conventional notions of "experience." For students who have received most of their education in the classroom, learning in a clinical setting demands new ways of preparing for, engaging in, and reflecting on activities that are both educational and practical. Moreover, if it is challenging for students and residents to convert skills for classroom learning to patient care settings, it is even more difficult for them to imagine patients in the aggregate, in locations distinct from more familiar clinical settings, to muster the skills for population-level analysis and intervention, and to borrow from fields such as management, health care law, and systems design to improve clinical outcomes.

Just as Dr. Caldwell learned basic surgical skills before tackling complex procedures, dealing effectively with the complexity of levels of "caring for patients" as an educational domain requires the ability to coordinate educational experiences with learner readiness. The learning and development that occur through practical experience at these levels require consideration of the kinds of activities in which learners engage, the social and cultural context in which these activities occur, and the individual cognitive and affective processes involved. To frame our understanding of the experience of caring for patients, from the perspective of both practitioners and medical students and residents, we draw on four complementary perspectives: expertise as a progressive process, the dynamic and situated nature of knowledge and expertise, multiple forms of knowing and reasoning, and distributed intelligence.

EXPERTISE AS A PROGRESSIVE PROCESS.   Expertise in medicine has been studied in a variety of ways, including comparison of experts and novices with respect to content knowledge (Boshuizen & Schmidt, 1992; Schmidt

& Boshuizen, 1993), knowledge structures (Bordage, 1994; Bordage & Lemieux, 1991), approaches to clinical reasoning tasks (Norman, 2005; Norman, Eva, Brooks, & Hamstra, 2006), and performance of procedural skills (Hatala, Brooks, & Norman, 2003; Grantcharov, Bardram, Funch-Jensen, & Rosenberg, 2003; Megali, Sinigaglia, Tonet, & Dario, 2006). The goal of this work is typically to understand what constitutes expertise in various domains, thus supplying valuable information about the goals and desired outcomes of medical education.

However, this view of expertise is limited in its implications for the design of education because it fails to address questions about the means by which expertise is achieved, and it treats expertise as a static, relatively universal end state. This second set of issues has been explored through studies of the processes by which one becomes an expert (Dreyfus & Dreyfus, 1986; Nelson et al., 2002; Benner, 1984) and by comparison of those who do and do not achieve expertise, even after years of experience (Bereiter & Scardamalia, 1993; Ericsson, 2002, 2004).

We are particularly interested in these latter explorations of expertise. They frame learning as a progressive trajectory and are useful in helping us understand the processes involved in becoming more advanced or expert in the routine aspects of patient care as well as the complex, nonroutine aspects. This necessarily involves competent performance in multiple domains of activity, such as gathering and processing information, treating patients in ways that are respectful and empathic, negotiating possible courses of action with patients and families, and observing outcomes and developing plans for improving them.

By way of example, we can imagine some of the processes that led Dr. Caldwell to his current level of expertise in responding to each trauma patient who comes through the emergency department. In medical school, he learned the roles and responsibilities of the members of the trauma team, he trained his mind to focus on the ABCs of trauma resuscitation, and he observed various ways of comforting families during a time of crisis. In his internship, he became increasingly able to manage patients recovering from trauma surgery, which afforded some opportunity to notice different outcomes among trauma patients and begin thinking through possible reasons for the varied outcomes. As he progressed through residency, he became more adept at responding to each trauma patient, and eventually he knew what to do, seemingly without thinking.

Now, five years into licensed practice, he regularly finds new challenges in his work as a trauma surgeon, including ways of improving coordination among members of the trauma team, keeping up with new technologies and protocols that expand the range of options for treating trauma injuries and help reduce ventilator-associated pneumonias and other complications. The key point is that his experiences are cumulative; as phenomena associated with most or all trauma care become more familiar, he is afforded more opportunity to notice and grapple with complexities and challenging aspects of situations. His learning spans many domains, and even though these domains may seem distinct early on, they become more deeply entwined as he begins taking more responsibility for the care of patients.

DYNAMIC AND SITUATED NATURE OF KNOWLEDGE AND EXPERTISE. As is evident in the examples of Drs. Caldwell and Alvarado, expertise is not an end state that, once attained, requires no upkeep. Expertise in patient care is a dynamic phenomenon, shaped by new developments in biomedical knowledge, societal values and expectations, health care policy, organization of health care services, and technology. When Dr. Alvarado began practice twenty years ago, the incidence of diabetes among her clinic patients was much lower than it is now, and there were few tools available to measure and monitor the health of her patients with diabetes. Furthermore, there were far fewer medications, support groups, and other resources available to assist patients in their efforts to control their blood sugar levels. Similarly, despite the fact that Dr. Caldwell is only five years out of residency, he has already seen his practice changed by the advent of new devices, surgical approaches, and critical care processes and procedures.

This dynamic view of expertise, derived from recognition that the nature of physicians' knowledge and ways of knowing is continuously evolving and changing, warrants a shift in thinking about curricular content and learning objectives. What aspects of Dr. Alvarado's education and experience enable her to provide ongoing expert care to her patients? From a cognitive perspective, we might point to her flexibility (Feltovich, Spiro, & Coulson, 1997), her motivation and ability to notice opportunities for improvement, her willingness to frame a problem from another perspective, or draw on other domains of knowledge to improve her understanding of an ambiguous or uncertain situation. With relatively little difficulty, she is also able to integrate new knowledge and skills with her existing capabilities. From a sociocultural perspective, we can point to the values and commitment to the service of patients and society that she has internalized through many years of training and practice as well as to values and commitments embedded in the context of her work. Dr. Alvarado works with other individuals, physicians as well as nurses and front-desk staff, who are willing to devote time, effort, and resources to reviewing performance, identifying opportunities for improvement, and taking action to do things differently even if the outcome is not guaranteed to be a success. In a broader context, she also works in a practice that has sufficient resources to allow her to make important (although sometimes expensive) changes in her practice that draw on advances in technology, biomedical knowledge, public health, and other arenas.

MULTIPLE FORMS OF KNOWLEDGE AND REASONING. Physicians exploit many forms of knowledge and use a variety of reasoning strategies in the course of caring for patients (Eva, 2005). Over the continuum of medical education, emphasis on certain types of knowledge and ways of knowing and reasoning shifts from an intensely scientific, biomedical orientation to a more pragmatic orientation. The biomedical orientation emphasizes facts, conceptual understanding, and causal reasoning; the pragmatic orientation uses practical intelligence and other forms of tacit and explicit knowledge that are available and relevant to a particular situation to guide action (Montgomery, 2006). In addition, as students and residents advance through training they use a combination of analytical and nonanalytical reasoning strategies according to the knowledge and experience they bring to a case or clinical encounter (Eva, 2005).

Taking Drs. Caldwell and Alvarado as examples, we can identify—and infer—many kinds of knowledge in use. Most obvious is their general know-how. Dr. Caldwell knows exactly what he will do when the patient arrives. His initial observations will guide his subsequent actions. Most likely, what he observes will be similar to conditions he has seen in previous patients; hence his ability to predict his first steps even before he sees the patient. Many of the cues he will observe are subtle and difficult to articulate. They are part of his tacit or implicit knowledge. If, however, he notices something out of the ordinary that does not seem to fit any of the patterns he recognizes, he will revert to more formal, explicit knowledge resources, perhaps running through a list of possible diagnoses and ruling them in or out (analytical reasoning) or focusing on a particular finding that concerns him and thinking through possible causes (causal reasoning). Likewise, as Dr. Alvarado reflects on Sr. Gutierrez's case, she shows clear examples of formal knowledge acquired since her residency but also of practical intelligence and reasoning.

A central question for medical education is how best to facilitate development of these forms of knowledge and reasoning as well as the ability to move fluidly among them at the appropriate moment. Experienced physicians tend to revert to causal or analytical reasoning when they encounter unfamiliar, difficult problems that elude routine processes and customary approaches. However, many of the errors and oversights that occur in patient care result from failure to notice when things are deviating from the usual course and when more analytical reasoning may be needed (Croskerry, 2005). Although universities and other academic settings have become quite good at transmitting bodies of knowledge and advancing learners' causal reasoning skills, many questions remain about the relationship between this type of knowledge, reasoning, and the learning processes it requires and development of learners' clinical reasoning during actual patient care.

Some argue that learners must first build a foundation of factual knowledge and then progress toward conceptual knowledge in which facts are organized in a way that allows deeper understanding. Only after this knowledge becomes sufficiently well structured will it be accessible in practice for clinical reasoning (Anderson, 1980). This view is most consistent with the traditional, discipline-structured, classroom-based curriculum. Others argue that learners construct conceptual understanding through opportunities to use factual knowledge in multiple ways and through exposure to a variety of cases that present factual knowledge in a number of ways (Feltovich et al., 1997). This view is most consistent with integrated disciplines and case-based curricula. Yet another perspective emphasizes experiential learning, suggesting that through guided observation and supported participation in day-to-day clinical scenarios, learners develop sophisticated conceptual understanding, pattern recognition, and clinical reasoning or problem-solving processes (Billett, 2002, 2006). Over time, as increasingly complex and unfamiliar circumstances are encountered, conceptual understanding necessarily must be expanded and elaborated through facts, theoretical knowledge, and further conceptual understanding. Medical education has traditionally favored mastery of factual knowledge over experiential learning, though there is a notable shift toward a more balanced approach that recognizes both as providing important and complementary cognitive resources.

DISTRIBUTED INTELLIGENCE. We view medical knowledge as distributed throughout the clinical environment in which patient care occurs (Greeno, 2006; Hutchins, 1995; Salomon, 1993). In contrast to physicians of a hundred, or even fifty, years ago, Drs. Caldwell and Alvarado live in a world that is characterized by not only a massive increase in the amount of medical knowledge and skill but also far broader distribution of those assets. Many more people know things, have skills, and contribute to the care of individual patients and populations of patients than formerly. Some of the relationships among these individuals are formal and structured (for example, with the consulting cardiologist or the physical therapist), others are professional but less structured (the nursing home supervisor or the pharmacy technician in the community drugstore), and still others are informal or involve a layperson (a daughter-in-law whose mother has a similar condition, a spouse who has been on the Internet, or a concerned neighbor). All of these individuals have information, perspectives, and experience that may be applied to the care of the patient. In addition, there is expertise embodied in artifacts and material resources such as the self-sheathing venipuncture needle, the consult referral form, and of course the medical information system. Thus successful care of individual patients and patient populations regularly depends on collective knowledge and understanding, not solely on knowledge housed in the mind of the individual physician. When Dr. Caldwell leads a team in the emergency department, he depends on the members to know their roles, engage their expertise, and communicate information effectively so the initial assessment is completed in a thorough and time-efficient manner. The knowledge and practices of others shape the quality of his decisions at least as much as his personal knowledge and practices do.

The concept of distributed intelligence is important for several reasons. To begin, it explains why a clinical setting can be a particularly rich learning environment for learners of all levels. There is more knowledge available in a clinical setting than any single individual can possess. Correspondingly, there are endless opportunities for learners to push the boundaries of their knowledge and understanding in a range of domains, so long as learners have sufficient guidance and motivation to direct their learning meaningfully and significantly and opportunities to interact with the repositories of intelligence, both human and otherwise, in their surroundings. In the knowledge-rich environments in which patient care typically occurs, learning necessarily involves knowing where and how to access useful knowledge as well as how to use and build on this knowledge for future improvements in practice. Developing expertise in the practice of medicine is, or should be, characterized by increasingly sophisticated recognition and use of capabilities distributed throughout the patient care environment in the form of nonphysician staff, consultants, patients and their circles of friends and families, forms, instruments, and even the layout of the clinical environment.

Recognizing knowledge as distributed also acknowledges that the knowledge, practices, and artifacts of patient care activities are socially, culturally, and historically constituted or defined. For example, the protocol that Dr. Caldwell and his team follow when assessing each newly arrived trauma patient and the performance benchmarks selected by Dr. Alvarado and her colleagues reflect standards of care that have evolved over time through experience, careful observation of processes and outcomes, and fine tuning. In the future, these tools will undergo further changes reflecting new knowledge and understanding. Current medical students, residents, and practitioners benefit from the years of knowledge and understanding embedded in these tools, and they must take seriously their responsibility to carry on the legacy.

Finally, the concept of distributed intelligence is a framework for consideration of health systems, safety, and quality improvement. The physician proficient in caring for patients appreciates that responsibility for patient safety and quality improvement is collective and requires a collaborative effort. Many situational and experiential factors are recognized as influencing decision making and judgment. To the extent that certain susceptibilities are recognized, such as cognitive biases and limitations of working memory, there are opportunities to develop ways of reducing reliance on memory, training for awareness of common biases and lapses in judgment, and designing ways of improving the availability of real-time information and performance feedback (Croskerry, 2003). Fortifying the capacity of the settings and systems of care by skillful use of the distributed nature of intelligence in it has the potential to protect against inevitable blind spots in individual cognition.

IMPLICATIONS FOR EDUCATION IN PATIENT CARE.   Successful performance of patient care activities requires solid preparation in medical school and residency as well as lifelong growth and advancement beyond competence. For nearly a hundred years, the importance of scientific knowledge and understanding of biomedical concepts has been acknowledged as a central pillar of the practice of medicine. Clinical wisdom and practical know-how, humanism and integrity, innovation in care delivery, and civic engagement are often represented as less significant or inferior contributors to medical practice and thus as areas of development that require less explicit and dedicated attention in medical education. This may be due, in part, to the fact that most of these areas draw on tacit knowledge and are commonly thought to be learned best through experience rather than through formal curriculum and instruction. Consequently, efforts to think systematically about ways of facilitating learning and development in these areas lag far behind efforts to teach scientific knowledge. At the same time that we argue that the medical curriculum at undergraduate and residency levels needs to accommodate new content, we recognize it is already overstuffed, having attempted to include many of the exciting discoveries of the past fifty years. Furnishing a learning experience that appropriately represents the dynamic and situated nature of physicians' work will require a perspective that recognizes the importance of physicians' capability beyond formal scientific knowledge as well as vigorous management of curricular content and appropriate sequencing of learning challenges.

Both formal knowledge and working experience in the care of individual patients and patient populations are necessary. Learners require thoughtfully staged educational experiences that allow them to develop skills in, and to see the connections between, for example, caring for a patient with diabetes, assessing their effectiveness in improving the health of a group of patients under their care with diabetes, and working at the community level to identify affected individuals who do not know that they have diabetes and to prevent diabetes in the first place. Learning experiences must be organized in ways that are developmentally appropriate and occur in the company of effective teachers and role models. Furthermore, the literature on expertise suggests that opportunities for regular practice using knowledge and skills in similar, but not identical, scenarios coupled with focused feedback on performance is most effective for improving learners' efficiency and accuracy in many activities (Ericsson, 2007).

Inquiry and Improvement

When people think of expertise, they tend to think of individuals who perform exceptionally well at a particular kind of activity. Expertise is not typically associated with innovation or continuous improvement of personal and collective performance unless the expertise is in research-oriented, competitive, or creative activities. We propose, instead, a broader conception of expertise that recognizes *improving* care for patients as part of physicians' professional responsibility and, correspondingly, as an essential part of their expertise. To understand how physicians develop this aspect of expertise, we turn to theories and concepts that explain differences in approaches to difficult situations or problems and ways of recognizing opportunities for improvement.

The focus of our earlier discussion on learning to deliver patient care was on development of skillful performance characterized by the ability both to perform common or routine activities easily and to respond effectively to unfamiliar and nonroutine situations, in caring for individuals and groups of patients and populations. However, becoming an expert physician requires development of efficiency in a core set of competencies, characterized by the ability to respond effectively in complex situations, and the capacity to expand the depth and breadth of one's competencies, characterized by the ability to innovate (Hatano & Oura, 2003; Schwartz, Bransford, & Sears, 2005). Thus we focus on the adaptive dimension of expertise, particularly on development of strategies for continuous learning and improvement among individual physicians and communities of clinicians.

ADAPTIVE EXPERTISE.   One of the primary goals of medical education is to ensure that students and residents are "prepared for future learning" (Schwartz et al., 2005, p. 32) so that they can deploy their prior knowledge and skills to approach and develop solutions to difficult, complex, or novel problems—the kind of problems that may not have a single (or even a known) solution. This goal is contrasted with another goal of medical education, involving development of more routine problem solving that allows learners to *apply* what they already know to solve new instances of common problems efficiently (Schwartz et al., 2005). In essence the difference is between the kinds of creative processes that generate new approaches or alternate ways of thinking about problems, as, for example, when Dr. Alvarado ponders the reasons for Sr. Gutierrez's unfortunate outcome, despite many advances in practice, and thinks of what to try next or what to invent for use with similar patients, and the more routine expertise that is typically used to handle a familiar set or type of problem, as with Dr. Caldwell's ability to respond to the unique needs of each trauma patient.

As we see it, an educational program has failed to achieve a key part of its mission if it produces physicians who perform routine work skillfully but rarely see new possibilities or greater complexity in their daily practice. When such "experienced, nonexpert" physicians (possibly routine experts, but not adaptive or dynamic experts; they are experienced nonexperts by Bereiter and Scardamalia's definition because they do not engage in knowledge building or, in our terms, inquiry and improvement) encounter unfamiliar problems or situational constraints, they tend to draw on preexisting knowledge and work within existing systems and frameworks to find a best-fit or "satisficing" solution—one that will usually get the job done under the circumstances. By contrast, when an adaptive expert physician faces situational constraints or unfamiliar problems, he or she reframes the problem or systematically investigates the situation in greater depth in an effort to develop a way of achieving better outcomes—an optimizing strategy (Bereiter & Scardamalia, 1993; Mylopoulos & Regehr, 2007).

EXPERTLIKE LEARNERS AND PROGRESSIVE PROBLEM SOLVING.   What kinds of learning processes and educational activities are likely to enhance learners' development of adaptive expertise? In other words, how can we help medical students and residents develop the ability to respond flexibly to situational variations, modify established practices or develop new ones to improve performance, and cross conventional domain boundaries to explore new perspectives and develop novel solutions to persistent problems in a given domain (Hatano & Oura, 2003; Alexander, 2003)?

Several perspectives are relevant to these questions. There are a set of metacognitive processes, or approaches to learning, that are more consistent with development and maintenance of adaptive expertise than other approaches are. Studies have explored these processes by comparing how individuals approach very difficult or complex problems. For experienced physicians, this might be the kind of persistent, perplexing, and unresolved problem or challenge that interferes with delivery of patient care or limits patient outcomes in their own practice or community or more broadly within their specialty. These are the "constitutive problems of the domain" (Bereiter & Scardamalia, 1993, p. 97), the kinds of problems that are endlessly complex and never definitively soluble, but against which progress can always be made. In medicine, the overarching constitutive problem is elimination of disease; physicians work on this problem in many ways but without an expectation that all disease will actually be eliminated. Research into disease pathogenesis and development of novel therapies exemplify rejection of received understandings and progressive problem solving to build knowledge. But Dr. Alvarado and Dr. Caldwell are grappling with other constitutive problems as well: Dr. Alvarado when she attempts to attract the attention of state legislators to the struggles of her underinsured, perhaps undocumented patients, in the face of competing political priorities; and Dr. Caldwell when he tries to make the case against risk taking to his community's high school students.

Bereiter and Scardamalia suggest that there are a few identifiable expertlike approaches to problem solving and learning that can appear even early on among learners. One is a knowledge-building orientation when a situation or problem is novel or unfamiliar. In these situations, expertlike learners are highly cognizant of the limitations of their knowledge and of their uncertainty. Consequently, they recognize their interpretation as provisional rather than conclusive, their questions are open rather than closed, and they actively pursue more complete understanding rather than assuming they already know the most important things, and as a consequence becoming indifferent to what more remains to be learned (Bereiter & Scardamalia, 1993; Scardamalia & Bereiter, 2006). In addition, there may be personal, social, and cultural factors that influence students' tendency toward this knowledge-building approach. Learners vary with respect to their self-concept and beliefs about their ability to tackle new and difficult problems (Dweck, 2000; Grant & Dweck, 2003), their source of motivation to invest the requisite effort—that is, sense of responsibility or pleasure; perceived benefits or fear of consequences—and the rules and norms modeled and reinforced by peers, role models, or even task structures and assessment systems.

Another important expertlike approach involves reinvestment of effort, as some activities and types of problems become more familiar and routine and can be performed with less and less effort. As more cognitive space becomes available through pattern recognition and automation, the progressive problem solver or knowledge builder identifies new challenges or reframes a recurrent problem in a more complex way to take advantage of the available space (Guest, Regehr, & Tiberius, 2001; Regehr & Mylopoulos, 2008). For example, rather than viewing her octogenarian patient as yet another elderly woman who fell at home, broke her hip, and waited many hours before someone found her, Dr. Alvarado contemplates more effective ways to identify patients in her community at risk of falling and to deploy what is known about fall prevention in a population of patients, many of whom suffer from social isolation and economic limitations.

The practice of medicine is dynamic and carries far more unknowns and uncertainties than confirmed facts and evidence-based best practices. Correspondingly, there are always opportunities to reinvest the effort conserved through facile performance in one domain to a new domain of practice or to more complex or challenging aspects within the same domain. For example, a first-year resident might initially focus narrowly on all the details involved in knowing how to work up anemia. After several cases, multiple discussions with colleagues, and focused reading on anemia, the resident is quite comfortable working up anemic patients. The nature of the resident's questions about anemia now shift toward strategies for identifying asymptomatic anemic patients in the population (for pediatricians especially), decreasing risk factors for anemia in the population, exploration of the literature to better understand current efforts to address the problem among populations, and cost-effective solutions for the health care system. This example suggests two additional areas in need of investigation and elaboration as we develop a framework for understanding physicians' innovation and improvement. First, how does the resident, or any practitioner, notice opportunities for learning and improvement, select appropriate ones to pursue, and develop a reasonable approach? To explore this question, we turn to insights from the literature on reflective practice and self-assessment or self-regulated learning. Second, what explains the resident's willingness to think about anemia from a different perspective, in other words, to invest the effort necessary for an optimizing strategy as opposed to a satisficing one? We explore this question later in this chapter as we discuss a broader concept of professionalism.

REFLECTIVE PRACTICE. Embedded in Bereiter and Scardamalia's model of "progressive problem-solving" is an implicit expectation that practitioners are able to identify and engage in opportunities for improvement or problem solving (as when Dr. Alvarado pondered Sr. Gutierrez's outcome, or when Dr. Caldwell thinks about strategies to reduce the number of alcohol-related accidents) and can frame "messy," nonroutine, or complex aspects of practice so as to make them more manageable or approachable. Schön's work, *Educating the Reflective Practitioner*, is concerned with precisely the aspects of professional practice that call for solutions outside the ordinary realm (Schön, 1987). Following Schön's model, we understand that when medical students start out in clinical settings most of their effort is devoted to development of "knowing in action," the kind of experiential knowledge or skilled know-how needed to perform routine, day-to-day practice. Schön emphasizes that knowing in action is something different from the knowledge taught in professional schools. The relationship between the two is still not well understood: "Ordinary knowing-in-action may be an application of research-based professional knowledge taught in schools, may be overlapping with it, or may have nothing to do with it" (Schön, 1987, p. 40).

In medical education, this knowing in action often exists along with a substantial body of conceptual knowledge. With guided practice and coaching, students are able to perform more tasks and activities with less investment of cognitive effort as they recognize patterns, form scripts and schemas, and make procedures routine. At this stage, learners can begin training for "reflection in action"—the true art of professional practice and the mark of expertise. It is through reflection in action that a physician like Dr. Caldwell responds to a subtle cue in his patient's course and deviates from his standard method of examining and treating the patient. As Schön describes, it is "the cases of problematic diagnosis in which practitioners not only follow rules of inquiry, but also sometimes respond to surprising findings by inventing new rules, on the spot. This kind of reflection-in-action is central to the artistry with which practitioners sometimes make new sense of uncertain, unique, or conflicted situations"(Schön, 1987, p. 35). However, there is some evidence to suggest that with increasing experience many presumed experts become less reflective and willing or open to exploration of alternative explanations (Eva & Cunnington, 2006). These findings highlight the importance of not only instilling a reflective, knowledge-building approach early on in learners but also reinforcing this approach throughout a physician's career.

Schön identifies three important components of efforts to train learners for reflection in action. The first is learning by doing. Depending on the level of the learner, this involves practicing common tasks (such as history taking, physical exam, diagnostic reasoning, and creating a management plan) in simulated, controlled, or closely supervised environments. The second is coaching by teachers and peers, which primarily involves demonstrating, advising, critiquing, and questioning. The teacher engages the learner in challenging tasks that require framing or reframing problems, developing and testing new strategies of action, and generating new understanding. If the learner gets stuck, the teacher or peers turn to the third component, reflective dialogue, to help the learner see another approach or consider an alternate strategy. The point is to foster opportunities for learners to practice making sense of unfamiliar, uncertain, or conflicting situations of practice.

SELF-REGULATED LEARNING AND FEEDBACK FOR IMPROVEMENT. How do individuals and teams know when performance could be improved and better outcomes could be achieved? How do they develop strategies for improvement? Engaging in inquiry and improvement necessarily requires the ability to notice things such as incomplete understanding of a concept or phenomena (asking such questions as "Why should we wait until a patient's CD4 count falls below 350 cells/μL to initiate antiretroviral therapy?"), suboptimal performance (reflections such as "Patients often seem uncomfortable with me, and I often have to ask a question several ways before I get the information I need"), or improvable outcomes (for example, wondering "Why do so few patients in our clinic schedule follow-up appointments within the desired timeframe?").

Despite enthusiasm for teaching learners to be better self-assessors and more self-directed in their learning, the literature on self-assessment and self-regulated learning in the health professions suggests that these may be unreliable motivators for continuous learning and improvement. If we cannot depend on self-assessment, we must increase our focus on assisting learners in becoming open to, and adept at seeking, reliable external assessments of their performance and skilled at responding to it constructively. If the goal of the training process is to cultivate habits of mind such as curiosity, self- and situation awareness, and flexible but persistent pursuit of better outcomes for patients and populations, we must be more thoughtful and effective in teaching medical learners how to use external sources of information, benchmarks, and feedback to improve performance and in reliably offering a diverse array of credible and clear sources of information regarding learner performance (Eva, Cunnington, Reiter, Keane, & Norman, 2004; Eva & Regehr, 2005).

Early on, students necessarily rely heavily on guidance and feedback from others to notice opportunities for improvement in their own understanding or performance and to identify fruitful strategies for subsequent learning and improvement. As they progress through residency, learners are expected to take greater responsibility for monitoring their own performance and managing their own learning. As they become more familiar and comfortable with various aspects of clinical performance, learners must develop habits of mind that enable them to notice when routine practices are no longer sufficient to handle the situation at hand (reflective practice) and compel them to act on the shortcomings or complexities they notice (progressive problem solving).

IMPLICATIONS FOR EDUCATION IN INQUIRY AND IMPROVEMENT. Encouraging learners to seek improvement in their own performance as well as in the performance of the groups, teams, and systems in which they work must begin early in medical school and must be reinforced in residency and beyond. Although part of learning necessarily involves performing routine practices reliably and efficiently, another part involves recognition of situations that call for nonroutine practice and novel approaches or solutions. Medical students need coaching and guidance to distinguish between these types of situations, but practice in both is recommended so that inquiry and innovation become well-established habits of mind as they move on to residency. By the time of residency, the challenge is to move beyond service demands and established routines, actively identifying how care for patients can be improved and collecting the information needed to evaluate whether the goals and desired outcomes have been achieved.

Participating in a Professional Community

Classical cognitive perspectives on medical learning, though powerful in analyzing how individual physicians solve diagnostic puzzles and manage the vast landscape of changing facts and concepts on which medical understanding is based, give short shrift to the process of becoming a functional member of the community of physicians and a colleague among health care professionals. Equally, or perhaps more so, the social and public dimension of being a physician is not captured by analyses that focus exclusively on the interactions between individual physicians and their patients' problems. Correspondingly, medical education attends poorly to the experience of this process from the standpoint of medical learners and may trivialize outcomes having to do with the effectiveness of medical students and residents as collaborative agents in workplace communities and their engagement in the larger world as "physician-citizens."

The social world of medical practice and the critical social dimensions of medical learning come into high relief when viewed through the lens of sociocultural theories of learning. These theories emphasize the inextricability of learning from doing, the immediacy and authenticity afforded to learning when in the context of real-world activities, the essentially social nature of learning even when individuals appear to be acting on their own, and the role in learning of peers and others not classically regarded as teachers. Sociocultural theories also recognize the environment and its resources as playing an important role in learning by mediating (or structuring and supplying cues for) activities, and by distributing assets necessary or helpful for accomplishing a task across a number of people and material artifacts. These theories are informative in analyzing how physicians work together to care for patients; how physicians and nonphysicians, including both health care professionals and nonprofessionals, collaborate; and, of course, how new practitioners are brought into the complex systems and practices of health care.

In addition, physicians' work has an important social and participatory dimension beyond the workplace and local professional community, as is exemplified by Dr. Caldwell and Dr. Alvarado. The former speaks in his neighborhood high school; the latter has testified before her state senate's health committee at the request of her professional organization on the challenges her monolingual Spanish-speaking patients experience in receiving adequate services for their diabetes and the need to support culturally appropriate community-based services for them. Although our two doctors may or may not be participants in communities of practice as they engage in these activities, these roles raise issues of community engagement and the scope of responsibilities for physicians, and the role of professional organizations and physicians in them. To the extent that we expect that all or most physicians will be active in their communities and participating in the collective activities of their specialty, those expectations must be conveyed during training and students and residents must be given the opportunity to experience these roles.

COMMUNITIES OF PRACTICE. The term *community of practice* describes a set of people with complex interrelationships working together to accomplish a shared objective. Who participates in the practice defines the community; the participants, their history, social relationships, and the artifacts they use define the practice (Wenger, 1998). As all people do, physicians participate in many communities of practice, some related to their work and others linked to personal concerns such as play groups, hobbies, and civic organizations. Every community of practice is characterized by mutual engagement, meaning a network of interrelationships and variably strong connections; joint enterprise, or shared work with collaboratively constructed goals and a sense of mutual accountability;

and a common or shared repertoire of resources, artifacts, beliefs, and approaches (Wenger, 1998). A community clinic; a residency training program; a ward team; and the office of a solo practitioner, his or her office manager, and the office nurse might all constitute communities of practice. For an individual, proficiency in the work of a community means the ability to fully engage in its central activities or practices (Lave & Wenger, 1991). However, not all contributions at the center of the community of practice are identical. Therefore, Dr. Caldwell recognizes the respiratory therapist, the critical care nurse, and the unit secretary as central contributors to patient care in the intensive care unit, although he does not aspire to their roles, nor do they to his.

Learning in a community of practice involves moving from a peripheral position with respect to the activities of the community toward the center. Still, even for the established members, life in their community of practice is not static. Everyone in a community of practice is always learning because the nature of the joint enterprise, how participants engage with one another to advance the joint enterprise, and how they appropriate, modify, and discard tools, approaches, language, and stances is always changing; thus, communities of practice are always emergent. Consider Dr. Alvarado's practice: she, her partners, and their staff continuously negotiate and renegotiate their goals for their diabetic patients. As they find themselves frustrated by disappointing outcomes, they deploy a new format for patient care—the group visit—changing both the participation of the front desk staff and the practice nurse, and consequently their engagement with the physicians.

Because healthy communities of practice are emergent structures, it can be a simple matter for a newcomer to arrive at the periphery and be drawn in to the center of the joint enterprise. However, communities of practice are just as good at excluding participation as they are at inviting it. To be afforded access, newcomers must be regarded as legitimate, that is, having the potential to become full participants. Peripheral participation, even in a capacity that may seem insignificant or passive, such as listening in and observing, can be educationally powerful for newcomers and intermediate practitioners (Billett, 2001; Rogoff, Paradise, Arauz, Correa-Chavez, & Angelillo, 2003). From the edge of the practice, beginners are engaged, invited in, and centripetally drawn to full participation; "the transformation of newcomers to old-timers [is] unremarkably integral to the practice" (Lave & Wenger, 1991, p. 122). The ability to move toward full participation in medical practice may be less a matter of command of the high knowledge of medicine and more a matter of knowing who is who and how things are done. This is not to say that the high knowledge is unimportant, but it is difficult to deploy fluently or effectively without experiential familiarity with the practice. To some extent, elements of practice can be simulated and separated from the actual work environment, but practice is inherently complex, underdetermined, and emergent. By reducing or eliminating these hallmarks, simulations may limit their own effectiveness. From the perspective of communities of practice, invitation of the old timers and intentional structuring and sequencing of the work is the pedagogy, and progression of learners through the practice to central participation is the curriculum of learning a practice.

THE PHYSICIAN AS ADVOCATE AND COMMUNITY LEADER. Doctors must engage as physician-citizens in their communities and their profession. The first level of this engagement is not qualitatively different from that expected of other members of society, although perhaps it is greater in degree by virtue of the assets physicians possess: access, financial resources, leadership skills, and education. At this level, many physicians are, say, members of their neighborhood association, serve on the board of a community organization, and are active in their temple or congregation.

Physicians have particular perspectives and expertise, which militate for special roles in the community in addition to the general ones just enumerated. Social problems often underlie health problems for individuals and populations; doctors are uniquely positioned to point out to the larger public the social hazards and inequities that result in health problems in the community. Often by virtue of the standing of physicians compared to those afflicted, they are far better positioned both to witness and to advocate than are those directly affected. Dr. Caldwell's reflections on alcohol-related motor vehicle accidents in his community and his response are straightforward examples of this level of community engagement and social responsibility.

The strategies to properly address health problems arising in the community are, like the problems themselves, complex and require special expertise, some of which physicians can and should contribute. The challenge vexing Dr. Alvarado, the rising incidence of diabetes in her Latino patient population, requires sophisticated understanding of the genetic and acquired factors leading to development of diabetes, the efficacy of primary prevention efforts, the science underlying human behavior change, dietary and other cultural practices of the affected community, the socioeconomic conditions of the individuals affected, and organization of the health care delivery system both locally and nationally. Neither community-based programs nor local, state, and national policy response will be effective without the expertise physicians can bring to the table to help tackle these problems. These contributions may take the form of educating the public about particular health issues, serving as a board member or advisor to a community-based advocacy or service organization, or, as Dr. Alvarado's testimony before her state legislators illustrates, more direct political action.

Finally, like any other concerned citizen, a physician is likely to be more effective, particularly in the political process, when working collectively. It has been said that "although individual action is laudable, collective action is a hallmark of professionalism" (Gruen, Pearson, & Brennan, 2004, p. 97). Participation in the broader professional community, either through membership and activity in specialty organizations such as the American College of Surgeons or in cause-related organizations such as Physicians for Human Rights, creates a forum for discussion of matters of professional identity and purpose, amplifies and unifies the voices of individual physicians, and makes clear to the public what the profession stands for. Through policy development in these organizations, physicians clarify and articulate the values of the profession; this is a critical process for promoting cohesion and coherence in the profession as times and conditions change and (to borrow from the language of communities of practice) the nature of the joint enterprise necessarily shifts. This process of renegotiation and re-articulation of collective professional values must precede, or at least occur simultaneously with, public negotiation of the priorities of medicine and health care in the context of other societal needs and values.

IMPLICATIONS FOR EDUCATION: PARTICIPATING IN PROFESSIONAL COMMUNITIES.   The interactions within a community of practice are rich and complex. Not only are proficient members of the community examples of desirable attributes and actions that junior members of the community can, and should, emulate; they are an important source of information for learners on how close or far the learner's approximation of professional performance is from the performance expected at her level. When we think about physicians' work as a collaborative and social practice oriented toward optimal patient outcomes, the role of feedback becomes central for the community of practice as a whole as well as the individuals contributing to the community. Feedback becomes a personal responsibility of the members on two levels: first, so they can ensure they are contributing to the community's effort to the best of their ability and scope of their role; and second, so they can monitor and facilitate the performance of other members.

At its heart, medical practice is about what can be accomplished on behalf of patients. Focusing on the outcome for the patient or for populations of patients, rather than on the attributes or qualifications of the physician, highlights the fact that capable medical practice requires skillful participation in a complex system and effective interaction with other actors and resources in the system, including technology, health care workers, community assets, and the patients' friends and family. Just as learners become skilled in patient care through opportunities to participate, initially on the periphery and then progressively at the center but always authentically, in patient care activities and in the company of skilled teachers and role models who expect learners to use their clinical experiences to fuel acquisition of further formal knowledge and to prompt reflection, students and residents can learn how physicians contribute as members of their health care systems, as engaged physician-citizens in their community, and as advocates by having opportunities to do so that are developmentally appropriate. Conceptions of learning that emphasize its social and cultural dimensions create a broad frame that is helpful as we consider how to organize the education of physicians.

A Broader Conception of Professionalism

We began this discussion by identifying professional formation as the purpose that should guide medical education and drive the learning process. Now we revisit the question we posed earlier: What are the hallmarks of the physician that society wants a student or resident to become? What processes support and promote this transformation of identity?

The public needs more from medicine than competent performance; the toll of illness and the burden of human suffering demand it. A broad conception of the physician's work extends beyond the care of individual patients to engaged participation in professional organizations and in medical and nonmedical communities, and experimenting and innovating to understand health problems better and improve outcomes. Across all domains of professional work, physicians must strive to achieve a level of performance that is, in the end, unattainable. True professional excellence is grounded in a deep sense of commitment to healing and improving the health of individual patients and populations of patients and personal responsibility. The commitment to doing more and better for the health of people links the three domains of physician work, and this devotion to excellence across the three domains is the hallmark of professionalism.

Professional formation can occur both intentionally and unintentionally, but efforts to make the process and the ideals more explicit allow a carefully monitored and thoughtfully guided process. We suggest self-awareness (Epstein, 1999), interpersonal relationships (Haidet et al., 2008), and acculturation (Hafferty & Franks, 1994) as three aspects of professional formation warranting explicit attention. Although we acknowledge that external guides such as moral and ethical codes of conduct and skills such as communication and moral reasoning play a part in professional formation, our focus is more on the heart and soul of professional development than on demonstration of knowledge, skills, and behaviors. We identify a deep sense of commitment to healing and improving the health of individual patients and populations of patients as the foundation and the guiding and motivating force for the physician's work. Medical educators must ask: What is the source of this commitment? How is it cultivated and sustained?

SELF-AWARENESS AND REFLECTIVE PRACTICE. When students enter medical school, they bring along a set of interests, commitments, and conceptions of what it means to be a physician. These are the "internal goods" with which each novice professional begins the formative process (Benner, Tanner, & Chesla, 1996). As medical students encounter new knowledge, skills, and perspectives, their capacity to function in the world of medicine expands. As they listen to the stories of patients—the joys, the concerns, the fears, the motivations—as they experience the feeling of being viewed by a patient or family as a doctor, and as they observe physicians in practice, students develop a deeper, more sophisticated understanding of what being a physician truly involves. They begin to appreciate the kinds of information physicians use, the power as well as the limitations of what physicians can offer patients and the public, and the responsibilities physicians hold. They must also confront and reconcile differences between their initial assumptions and beliefs about being a physician and the realities and new understandings that surface through exposure to the field and experience in practice.

Self-awareness occurs as learners develop the capacity to recognize and engage with perspectives different from their own and use these alternate perspectives as a window for examining their own beliefs, assumptions, and emotions. This self-awareness enables professionals to be present with others, make difficult decisions with clarity, acknowledge strong feelings, and act rather than react. Self-awareness has been described as essential to the physician's ability to express core values of medicine such as empathy, compassion, and altruism (Epstein, 1999). The idea is that physicians must be able to separate their own emotions and perspectives from those of the patient in order to communicate with compassion, acknowledge the patient's needs, and respond in a way that prioritizes the patient's needs over their own beliefs, values, and emotional reactions.

Self-awareness also involves conscious attention to personal strengths and limitations, which can then be used to seek feedback, guide learning, and engage in improvement-oriented activities or practices. Such self-awareness develops through reflective processes and through access to external sources of feedback that can be used to gauge performance. These are, by and large, metacognitive skills that allow learners to critically examine their own processes of thinking and approaches to learning. Coming to terms with the realities of medicine and with an honest appreciation of personal limitations in the context of a formative process that exhorts the young professional to perform better and achieve more is a demanding experience. The self-awareness encouraged in medical education must be partnered with support for development of a capacity for resilience and forgiveness. These are both individual attributes and features of organizational and educational culture.

RELATIONSHIPS. Relationships play a major part in students' professional development. Although the patient-physician relationship has received much attention in medical education—as evidenced by curricular content for patient-centered communication, interviewing and physical exam skills, and diagnostic reasoning—new attention has been given to other types of relationships that play a significant role in professional formation. Relationship-centered care, a term coined by the Pew-Fetzer taskforce on advancing psychosocial health education, acknowledges the formative role of relationships among health professionals and between physicians and the communities, systems, and institutions in which they practice (Tresolini, 1994).

Professional formation occurs through relationships with patients. From the early stages of medical education through practice, relationships with patients involve experiences with attachment, strong emotions, and resolution of conflicting points of view or dilemmas. These experiences shape personal values and commitments so as to cultivate a sense of agency and a desire to advocate for the patient's best interest (Ratanawongsa, Teherani, & Hauer, 2005). Bleakley and Bligh (2008) have gone so far as to say that "deep, collaborative relationships between students and patients" ought to be treated as "the primary locus for knowledge production" (p. 91) because such relationships are the motivation to understand the patient's condition from both the patient's own perspective as well as from a biomedical and psychosocial perspective. Moreover, they can reinforce the curiosity and desire for more knowledge or improved care that is an essential part of a physician's work.

Professional formation also occurs through relationships with other physicians and health professionals. Dr. Caldwell still remembers the day on his surgery clerkship when the attending surgeon turned to him and asked what he thought should be done for a post-op patient who had unexpectedly taken a turn for the worse. He recalled a long conversation with a very skilled and knowledgeable nurse the night before. She had generously helped him understand just how much was at stake for this patient and how important it was to make wise decisions over the next twelve hours. As a result, he had pushed past his fatigue to learn as much as possible about the clinical situation and come up with a plan for his participation as a third-year medical student. He wanted to contribute in some way, despite being a novice.

Medical care today rarely involves just a patient-physician relationship. Instead, teams of health professionals, including multiple levels of learners, must coordinate efforts and communicate effectively to deliver appropriate care. These interprofessional relationships have a strong influence on learners' understanding of the roles and responsibilities of different types of health professionals, the extent to which they value the contributions of various professionals, and their own identity as a physician on a team.

Through the process of working with others to achieve shared patient care goals, students and residents develop and expand their professional identity (Forsythe, 2005), confidence, and motivation to learn and improve their practical competence (Dornan, Boshuizen, King, & Scherpbier, 2007). As participants in communities of practice, students and residents are both taking in and contributing to the shared values, commitments, social and intellectual resources, and responsibilities of the community. Within these communities some colleagues serve as guides, mentors, and role models, calling for higher performance and achievement from themselves and others, helping co-participants believe they are capable of better outcomes, and exemplifying resilience in the face of disappointment and failure. These relationships can inform learners' developing professional judgment, career choices, and decisions about personal life and are powerfully formative.

Lastly, professional formation occurs through relationships with communities and systems. Why does Dr. Alvarado work in private practice and accept Medicare while many of her peers from medical school and residency work in larger systems in which they have a guaranteed salary and have institutional policies that determine which patients they can and cannot see? Early on in medical school, she found herself drawn to opportunities to work with underserved populations. Some of her most memorable role models were physicians, social workers, and clinic nurses who relentlessly sought ways to improve care and quality of life in these communities.

Physicians' work and training carries physicians into many communities and systems of care, from home visits in a neighborhood that looks nothing like the one in which they live to private hospitals and offices that serve patients who pay for customized care, and to rural villages in developing countries. Learning to function effectively as a professional in these settings requires willingness to listen, observe, and adapt to the needs of the community, which can at times require setting aside one's own beliefs and judgments. Physicians' experiences traversing diverse communities give them unique appreciation for the changes needed to improve the health and well-being of communities that may lack the resources and capacity to advocate for change. There are many ways in which physicians can fulfill these advocacy roles and earn the trust of communities to which they do not directly belong. Cultivating such relationships and supporting students' and residents' exposure to these roles is essential to inculcate a sense of responsibility to become a citizen of the community and serve its values.

ACCULTURATION. Beyond the self and interpersonal relationships, there are norms and values of the community and the larger institutional context (including the profession at large) that contribute to professional formation. The espoused values of most practice settings and institutions suggest appropriate commitments to quality of care, safety, and ongoing training. However, just below the surface learners find discrepancies and disappointments. Health professionals regularly encounter tensions between compliance with policy or administrative processes and efforts to satisfy the needs and best interests of particular patients. Pressure to see as many patients as possible comes at the expense of time for exploring patients' beliefs and perspectives, which may in turn influence patients' perceived quality of care. Inefficiency and breakdowns in systems of care can breed frustration and cynicism among health professionals.

Novice professionals tend to adapt to and internalize the dominant values of the clinical environment in which they are immersed. A setting in which health professionals are committed to quality of care, patient-centered approaches, safety, and continuous learning and improvement is clearly desirable but not always available for all learners. The deleterious consequences of placing learners in a clinical environment in which the espoused values, or the values taught in the formal curriculum, are discordant with the enacted values must not be underestimated. Hafferty (1998) describes the enacted values, especially when discordant with the stated values, as the "hidden curriculum," and the inimical effect on professional formation is well documented. Yet Dr. Alvarado and Dr. Caldwell undoubtedly encountered some learning environments with suboptimal cultures and still managed to emerge as esteemed professionals. How is this possible?

One answer is that these two physicians developed and maintained, as many do, a strong sense of purpose and commitment that guided them through particularly challenging environments and situations. Where this commitment and purpose comes from is unclear, but it likely involves some combination of the individual processes and interpersonal relationships described just above. Another answer is that there were times during their training when they succumbed to the pressures of the dominant culture or power structure, but they did not internalize these values and make them habitual practice. They learned from them, examined the consequences, and moved on.

We believe that transformation of identity should be the highest purpose of medical education. If the naïve enthusiasm of entering medical students can reliably be tempered and forged into a commitment to do better for patients and populations, partnered with the recognition that this work is never done, and fortified with the resilience to carry on through disappointment and failure, the more familiar goals of medical training will largely take care of themselves. The aspiration to do better, coupled with commitment and a sense of personal responsibility, will drive knowledge seeking and enhanced procedural proficiency, not only in training but over a lifetime. Moreover, because relief of suffering, not merely prevention or mitigation of illness, is a key goal of medicine, our physicians' concern for their patients' experience as human beings and their ability to empathize will grow in parallel. The insistence on doing better for patients, exemplified by Drs. Alvarado and Caldwell, promotes resourceful and flexible engagement in the various social relationships through which patients are cared for, and the health of communities is improved and underlies a restless resistance to "good enough" care. This is the essence of professionalism.

Learning for Practice

To this point, our discussion of practice and learning for practice has focused on the three key domains of a physician's work and professional formation. Now we return to the question posed earlier in this chapter: If the end goal of medical education is making things better for patients, and professionalism is commitment to excellence across the domains of caring for patients, engaging in innovation and improvement, and participating in communities, then how should this education be designed and conducted? Our consideration of the achievement of high-performing physicians and our study of the contributions of the learning sciences suggests three premises about learning, and with those premises, implications for curriculum, pedagogy, and assessment.

Premise One: Learning Is Progressive and Developmental

Implicit in our descriptions of development of expertise with respect to formal knowledge, experiential knowledge, clinical performance, and innovation is an understanding that knowledge is dynamic—constantly reshaped, recombined, expanded, and elaborated in ways that create new understanding or improve performance in the care of individual patients and patient populations. For example, a beginning student can execute each step of a pulmonary exam with a high level of precision but completely miss what might be, to a senior student, an obvious constellation of findings. The senior medical student might become interested in the relationship between pesticide spraying and migrant worker respiratory problems, which might lead to a project in public health policy research and advocacy. Students arrive in medical school as twenty-one-year-old college graduates or as thirty-year-old career changers, many with little exposure to illness, care of patients, or the work of the physician. Four years later they graduate, having done about five hundred complete physical examinations, made three hundred clinical notes on patients with health problems requiring hospitalization, assisted at the delivery of ten to thirty babies, and sat, perhaps three times, at a bedside as someone they had cared for died. The transformative power of these experiences must not be underestimated.

The transformation that takes place across the residency years is, if anything, greater. Despite their experiences, medical school graduates begin residency as neophytes, having spent as little as eight to ten weeks caring for patients within their chosen specialty. Much as the third year of medical school gives students a general overview of the care of patients in a variety of settings and across the range of clinical specialties, so the early years of residency afford an overview of a specialty and its care settings and activities, and they offer an opportunity for beginning residents to tackle the fundamental tasks and master the basic activities of the specialty. Residents late in training are looking ahead to independent practice in six to twelve months; their concerns are with advanced procedural skills, subtle diagnostic distinctions, and acquiring the judgment that comes from experience. A graduating resident must be able to provide competent care for most conditions—from straightforward to complex—within her specialty area, accurately and readily detect those situations where she needs the assistance of a more seasoned colleague to deliver optimal care, and consistently marry a solid knowledge base and technical competence with compassion, dedication, and altruism. This about-to-be-independent clinician has come a long way.

Ultimately, what an individual knows and can do depends on prior knowledge and understanding in the domain as well as features of specific situations that afford access to additional knowledge and deeper understanding. Continuously building new knowledge and developing deeper understandings of practice are essential for improvement of individual and collective performance; it is this intentional and relentless building upon that we mean when we say that learning is progressive. Medical education that is aligned with this premise will include:

A curricular structure that connects formal knowledge and experiential knowledge and integrates content longitudinally. A variety of curricular features support this progression from neophyte in the specialty to independent clinician, but a common theme is a match between what the learner needs to tackle next and the opportunities available in the clinical workplace. Accomplishing this productive match involves a combination of selecting suitable activities and responsibilities and appropriate sequencing of these activities and responsibilities. Educators achieve an effective learning trajectory by balancing the students' and residents' need to learn to make increasingly high-stakes decisions and perform more demanding procedures with the requirement for close supervision and safe patient care, and perhaps, most challenging, by exercising the flexibility to allow individual learners to remain at a given level for a longer or shorter period of time according to the inevitable differences in how each individual needs to master a particular set of facts, concepts, and skills.

Pedagogies that accommodate individual learning needs by using longitudinal mentoring and oversight and promoting opportunities for learners to participate in the direction of their own learning. Pedagogies that acknowledge the progressive and developmental nature of medical education allow every learner to participate in the direction of his learning. However, because the goal is an independent clinician who recognizes both what he can tackle on his own and when he is at the limit of his capabilities, pedagogies that create a learning space in which the learner can consider how much help he needs and how to recruit the additional expertise needed to deal with a clinical problem, within the bounds of excellent patient care, are paramount. Similarly, teaching strategies that model and promote capitalizing on patient care as a stimulus for curiosity can help establish habits of learning that build toward expertise.

An integrated system of assessment that tracks learners' progress in multiple domains over time. Assessment approaches that support progressive learning emphasize that learners' responses to what they do not know are at least as important as their factual knowledge. All domains in which medical learners must progress and develop must be explicitly addressed with credible methods. Learners should be actively engaged in the feedback process, identifying areas in which they are trying to improve their own performance, and thus increasing the odds that they will value and respond to the insights they receive about their performance.

Premise Two: Learning Is Participatory

Values, identity, and skillful performance are formed through participation in professional communities. The members of these communities are engaged in meaningful, goal-oriented, collective activities such as identifying important learning objectives for a case, setting priorities for a home visit to a patient, coordinating trauma care for a severely injured patient arriving at the emergency department, or addressing a patient's concerns and needs during a clinic visit. By working alongside others who have skills and abilities different from or more advanced than their own, by taking responsibility for specific tasks that challenge their level of performance, and by receiving guidance and feedback, students make progress in their ability to perform patient care activities, communicate effectively with colleagues, and engage in ethically sound and culturally valued practice.

A distinctive feature of learning at the graduate level of medical education is the complete transformation, from the beginning to the end of residency, of the medical learner's ability to participate in the activities of patient care and a corresponding transformation in her relationship with co-participants. Neophyte residents spend much time observing more proficient physicians engage in high-stakes aspects of patient care and undertake only the most routine components on their own; by the end of graduate medical education, residents are capable of independent patient care within their specialty, applying knowledge, judgment, technical skills, and compassion. Although continuing to observe and emulate those more seasoned, they now do this as peers and colleagues as they teach more junior residents. Because of the distance learners travel over the course of residency training, from novice with respect to their specialty to competent practitioner, their relationships with other actors in clinical settings and the nature of their co-participation in caring for patients evolve markedly. On the other hand, because residents spend the vast majority of their time in the care of hospitalized patients, the opportunity to experience other dimensions of the work of physicians, even clinical work in nonhospital settings, is severely constrained. The implications of this premise for medical education will include:

A curricular structure that sequences tasks and activities to allow meaningful and valued contributions to patient care, and explicit attention to collaborative practices and communication processes. It would furnish learners with sufficient formal instruction and opportunities for skill development such that they can participate effectively and to good effect in nonclinical activities of physicians.

Pedagogies that involve inviting learners into the community, guiding and coaching, communicating clear roles and responsibilities, and giving feedback on performance. In addition, proximity to physician role models offers important examples of how to interact and co-participate with physician and nonphysician colleagues.

Assessment that is performance-based in a variety of domains (for example, knowledge, reasoning, communication, system improvement) and that captures individual and collective performance. Assessment approaches supporting participation in the full range of physician activities would attend to which activities learners choose to participate in, the depth and commitment of their participation, their interactions and collaborations with physician and nonphysician colleagues, and the outcome of the collaborative effort.

Premise Three: Learning Is Situated and Distributed

The clinical settings is a potentially rich learning environment, offering opportunities for calling on existing knowledge, achieving deeper understanding, improving performance, and developing personal and professional values. Students and residents learn a great deal by observing day-to-day patient care activities in a clinical setting, using technologies that facilitate patient care, and participating in complex systems that support physicians' work. Yet, with so much information and so many resources available in clinic settings, learners (especially early learners) can easily be overwhelmed, overstimulated, and left unfocused. Therefore, supplying sources of guidance such as more experienced colleagues or specific learning cues and benchmarks is important to help students focus their attention and identify and access appropriate resources. Improving the effectiveness and efficiency of clinical education depends significantly on recognizing and capitalizing on the hidden clinical knowledge that rests in particular settings and people, particularly in light of the rapid pace of change in the technology that supports patient care.

A dimension of effective functioning in health care settings depends on appreciation of the capacity of nonphysicians—respect for what others know and can do. On this foundation rests the ability to participate skillfully with nonphysicians in the care of patients. As physicians in training become more skilled and knowledgeable, and as they assume ever more central roles, they require an increasingly sophisticated understanding of how to marshal or coordinate resources for patient care in areas beyond their immediate experience and capabilities. Although the importance of this ability to collaborate productively with a physical therapist or a social worker without a deep command of what those clinicians do may seem obvious, this skill is not well represented in the ethos of medical education. Rather, the predominant ethos in medical education tends to celebrate individual mastery and achievement. This hierarchical representation of clinical care is problematic; it can lead to discounting of the contributions of nonphysicians to patient care and underdevelopment of residents' skills in bringing resources to their work. It may also lead medical students to avoid specialties in which the ability to collaborate with a complex cast of nonphysicians over time is especially important. Some have suggested that it is related to burnout.

Thinking about knowledge as something that is shared or distributed among colleagues or team members and that is embedded in routine actions and technology, and recognizing performance as a collaborative outcome, raises important questions about licensing and certification processes. These processes will continue to be important ways of verifying individual competence, but this premise highlights the need for ways of monitoring and verifying an adequate level of group, team, and system performance. Medical education that is aligned with this premise will include:

A curricular structure that offers opportunities for learners to encounter problems, content, and experiences multiple times in differing contexts or situations; curriculum that focuses more on ways of approaching problems and using information than on memorizing facts; and strategies for giving learners access to or making visible the hidden knowledge in clinical settings. Education aligned with this principle will have a curriculum that involves learners in patient care in a variety of settings, supporting development of a sophisticated understanding of the resources available in disparate clinical locales. Though not intended to undermine learners' sense of their own developing capabilities, work across a variety of settings can help learners appreciate the importance—sometimes the predominant importance—of the expertise of nonphysicians.

Pedagogies that involve guided observation and reflection, encourage inquiry and discovery, and engage learners in discussion that makes their assumptions and understanding more transparent and congruent with experts in the field. Pedagogies that deemphasize, where appropriate, the information that the teacher holds in his head and model mining the environment for the intelligence distributed across other people and artifacts will support this aspect of learning.

Assessment that takes note of efficient and effective use of physical and social resources and networks, collective performance, and individual contributions to collective performance. Assessment attending to the situated and distributed nature of clinical intelligence or information will assess the learner's ability to function collaboratively and efficiently in complex environments: can the learner make fluent, timely use of resources that come from nonphysician collaborators and nonhuman resources, such as information available at the point of services?

The Work Ahead: Preparing for Practice

Our consideration of the three core domains of physicians' work— patient care, inquiry and innovation, and participation in professional communities—suggests that medical education should build on the learning theories and research that explain both how physicians become adept in each of these core domains and the professional formation that is deeply entwined with this process. To understand why and how these ideas could be used to improve preparation of tomorrow's physicians, we now turn to a description of current U.S. medical education. As we look, in Chapters Three and Four, at undergraduate and graduate medical education, we keep in mind that learning is progressive and developmental, participatory, and situated and distributed. As we consider current models of education in relation to these premises, we suggest new models that address the nature of learning and the nature of practice.

PART TWO

LEARNING THE PHYSICIAN'S WORK

3

THE STUDENT'S EXPERIENCE

UNDERGRADUATE MEDICAL EDUCATION

A STRIKING TRANSFORMATION OCCURS during medical school. Students arrive excited, anxious, and full of many untested assumptions about what it means to be a physician; by the time they leave medical school they have become relatively knowledgeable, confident, and able to perform selected roles of a physician under supervision. How does this considerable change in understanding, performance, and character occur? To answer the question, in this chapter we describe current curricular models, pedagogical practices, and assessment methods in U.S. medical schools.

In Flexner's day, because students went immediately into practice upon graduation, the purpose of the undergraduate period (referred to as UME) was to prepare physicians for practice. Today, UME prepares students for entry into the extended period of specialty training known as graduate medical education (GME). However, because medical specialties vary so widely, determining what general knowledge and which skills are needed for entry into every specialty is challenging. Moreover, as we explain in Chapter Two, regardless of specialty the physician's work demands skills in and commitment to caring for patients and patient populations, inquiry and improvement, and participation in a professional community. Therefore, UME should equip physicians in training with the foundational knowledge, skills, and professional values to relentlessly pursue excellence in the practice of medicine within their chosen specialty.

As we describe the curricular models, pedagogies, and assessment prevalent in UME, we keep in mind the demands of today's practices, that is, practices and trends that point to tomorrow's, and we also keep in mind that (detailed in Chapter Two) learning is progressive and developmental, participatory, and situated and distributed. Accordingly, along the way we offer examples of innovative approaches that address both contemporary medical practice and the nature of learning.

UME Curricular Structures

With the goal of producing graduates capable of entering specialty-specific GME, most medical schools organize their instruction along one of three curricular models for preclerkship education: discipline-based, organ-system or integrated medical sciences, and problem- or case-based. Clerkship, or clinical, education generally employs sequential specialty block clerkships, longitudinal integrated clerkships, and mixed models. These models have gone through several phases of reform (Papa & Harasym, 1999), each of which has tended to add new instructional design, pedagogy, and assessment while preserving some prior elements. We focus on these structures because they are generally representative of UME in the United States (we observed all of these curricular structures in our site visits, but we do not intend them to portray the curriculum of any particular school).

Preclerkship Curriculum Structures

Flexner's model of medical education was designed to ensure that all practicing physicians had a solid foundation in biomedical sciences. Flexner recognized the need to connect advances in biomedical knowledge with medical practice and the need to train students for problem solving, critical thinking, and self-education rather than for mastery of facts that would quickly become outdated or irrelevant (Ludmerer, 1999). However, as the knowledge available to inform clinical medicine expands, medical education struggles with questions about the extent to which students need to learn scientific principles and clinical information before discovering the practical relevance of the same principles and information in the care of patients. Moreover, problem solving and critical thinking are now better understood through the lens of situated learning, meaning they are context-specific cognitive processes that rely on a combination of knowledge and experience, rather than as general knowledge and skills that can be learned independently of content and transferred to any situation. This understanding of problem solving and critical thinking raises questions about the optimal sequence for learning scientific principles and clinical information. The premise that learning is progressive and developmental implies the need for careful planning and design of curriculum to coordinate and sequence content and experience in order to build new and more sophisticated understanding as well as better performance. Correspondingly, the various curricular structures used in preclerkship education take differing approaches to organizing and presenting scientific principles and to balancing these concepts with clinical practice.

THE MEDICAL DISCIPLINES MODEL. In the discipline-based curriculum structure recommended by Flexner, which prevailed until the 1960s, students typically learn normal structures, functions, and processes of the body organized by disciplines such as anatomy, physiology, microbiology, histology, and biochemistry, followed by pathophysiology and disease management. Discipline-specific courses are taught in parallel with other disciplinary courses; too often, we found, there is little coordination or reference to clinical relevance. Over time, new content areas such as evidence-based medicine, genetics, and medical ethics have been added as independent, concurrent courses.

The purpose of being immersed in science is not just to understand the human body, according to Flexner, but also to ensure that physicians in training would learn to use scientific reasoning, or the hypothetico-deductive reasoning process. Although this approach is plausibly related to learning to think through certain kinds of difficult problems, major challenges have arisen with expansion of knowledge and proliferation of disciplines. Learning in the medical curriculum today is difficult because of the overwhelming amount of potential information to be mastered and uncertainty about which information will be most relevant for the future. Students struggling with factual overload may adopt learning strategies such as rote memorization that are inimical to scientific reasoning and inquiry.

Accordingly, today very few schools structure the curriculum entirely around separate discipline courses. One feature of this curricular approach that we found to be of particular concern is that it requires students to be the integrators of knowledge and find appropriate application to clinical medicine. The curricular format does not integrate content sequentially, leaving students to determine how the content in one domain relates to another, and how both relate to patient care. Curricula organized this way do not honor the premise that learning is progressive and developmental. Students voice frustration with the lack of coordination among lecturers who are unaware of the content covered in preceding lectures or who fail to acknowledge and build on students' existing knowledge. Students are also critical of lecturers who fail to discuss the relevance of scientific concepts to the practice of medicine.

A second problem with this curricular structure is its inefficiency. Students are required to learn the content two entirely different ways, first organized around basic science content and later organized around patient signs and symptoms. As a consequence, students arrive in the clinical setting with abstract knowledge that is difficult for them to access and apply to patient care. This curricular structure is inconsistent with the premise that learning is situated and distributed; it fails to capitalize on the richness of the clinical context early on and to engage learners authentically in using their knowledge and skills in the care of patients.

Third, the pedagogies employed in the discipline-based model often rely heavily on lectures that do not actively engage learners in constructing conceptual understanding. Because the practical and experiential aspects of the curriculum are segregated from the biomedical content, many students fail to understand and appreciate the interconnectedness of these forms of knowledge. Students have little sense of the context of the knowledge they are acquiring and the various means by which it can be used in practice. Finally, the assessment system typically focuses narrowly on scientific content knowledge and ignores such other important domains of performance as synthesis, integration, and evaluation of information and domains beyond bioscience, such as professionalism, clinical skills, and systems improvement.

ORGAN SYSTEMS AND INTEGRATED MEDICAL SCIENCES MODEL.   In the 1950s, Case Western Reserve University designed a new curriculum intended to be more closely aligned with the knowledge base used by physicians in practice. The goal was to integrate knowledge of basic and clinical sciences by organizing the preclerkship curriculum around organs or body systems. The expectation was that such early integration would make formal knowledge more accessible to students when they entered the clinical setting. In this model, students spend a block of time studying a system, for example the cardiovascular or musculoskeletal system, through the lenses of anatomy, physiology, biochemistry, pathophysiology, pharmacology, and epidemiology.

Designed to encourage conceptual integration, the organ-systems curriculum forces faculty members to work together with their counterparts across departments to determine what content is relevant and important, the appropriate level of depth, and how the content can be connected. However, because of the amount of faculty time required for planning and coordination, many medical schools that adopted an organ systems curriculum in the 1960s and 1970s returned to a disciplinary approach for the first year of courses and used the organ-systems approach for the second year. This design covered the normal structure and functions of the human body in year one and abnormal or pathophysiology in year two. This mixed model was the norm until the 1990s, when the disadvantages of disconnected content in parallel courses reemerged and curricula oriented toward conceptual integration once again became the norm. Today discipline-specific, departmentally controlled, parallel courses are found in a small minority of schools; the reigning curriculum model is the integrated curriculum organized around organ systems and content themes such as genetics or cancer.

The more recent version of integrated curricula seeks to advance student learning by helping students connect diverse content areas with patient care. Students are immersed in one topic or organ system at a time and examine normal and abnormal functions of that system from the molecular level to the societal. This allows students to use a compare-and-contrast learning strategy, which has been shown to facilitate learning in certain domains and is helpful in developing strong conceptual frameworks (Bordage & Lemieux, 1991; Nendaz & Bordage, 2002).

This curricular structure is an advance over the discipline-based structure because it guides students' integration of knowledge and situates learning in a clinically oriented conceptual framework. However, with this approach there is still an imbalance between the large volume of formal scientific information to be learned and knowledge gleaned from clinical experience. Although students often enjoy the clinical skills courses and clinical preceptorship experiences of the preclerkship years, they tend to perceive them as "soft," leading to marginalization and underappreciation of the content. Students in clinical settings early in medical school often do not have authentic roles or responsibilities and may be passive observers. This underpowered clinical engagement is exacerbated by an assessment system that tends to focus on knowledge acquisition and, correspondingly, influences students' priorities and commands the majority of their attention. In addition, lack of clinical experience poses a challenge to understanding because of the perceived lack of clinical relevance—knowing why and how the knowledge being acquired in the classroom can be used in caring for particular patients. The net result is lack of experiential knowledge to accompany and guide learning of formal knowledge. There are clear indications that, from the learner's perspective, such efforts are coming up short with respect to the intended effect of a true clinical context. Furthermore, the model tends to be rigid in structure, affording limited opportunity to take learners' own developmental needs and abilities into account.

PROBLEM-BASED AND CASE-BASED LEARNING MODEL.   Introduction of problem-based learning (PBL) occurred in the late 1960s and early 1970s as a few medical schools, in particular McMaster University and later the University of New Mexico, introduced new curricula based on learning principles from education and cognitive science (Neufeld & Barrows, 1974; Johnson & Finucane, 2000). A number of medical schools adopted this integrative curricular structure in the 1980s and 1990s, and many others include PBL tutorials as one of many pedagogical methods used in the curriculum.

PBL is the essence of discovery learning (Sweeney, 1999) and is aligned with the premises that learning is participatory and distributed. In PBL, the case serves as a stimulus for small-group and self-directed learning. The "problems" are patient cases that are studied over the course of a week or several weeks by small groups of six to eight students, a faculty facilitator, and sometimes a near-peer tutor. The cases are carefully designed to give students an opportunity to learn basic and clinical science content in the domains covered in more traditional curricula. The core feature of this model is a "progressive framework of problems unconstrained by subject divisions" (Maudsley, 1999, p. 180). An advantage of this model is that students encounter each problem without knowing what the primary focus of the problem is. There is no cuing from the topic of the course itself (as in, "Since this is a cardiovascular unit, the case must be about a heart problem"). Although faculty members write PBL cases to address specific learning objectives and students typically pursue those objectives, students are not given the objectives at the outset because this would impair the discovery learning process.

In the PBL model, students start with the presenting complaint or situation and are progressively given small portions of the case. For example: "Mr. Smith is a twenty-two-year-old man who arrived in the emergency room unconscious following a motorcycle accident." Starting with this limited amount of information, the group begins sharing hypotheses about the patient's problem, defining learning objectives, determining what further clinical information is needed and why it might be important (history, physical exam, laboratory or radiology results), and where the group needs to improve its collective understanding of underlying basic science, clinical processes, or health care systems. This successive disclosure of the case with the attendant iterative hypothesis generation drives collaborative discussion and problem solving.

PBL tutorials typically last one and a half to two hours and occur two or three times a week. Individual study occurs in between group meetings, and each student shares his or her results with other group members, usually before the next meeting so that group time can be spent discussing the case rather than presenting what every person learned about the case. The process continues until the basic learning objectives are completed and the case is finished, typically two or three sessions on a single case. Some schools present a progression of PBL cases beginning with written cases, moving to DVDs of cases with videotaped actors, and finally to working with standardized patients. This last variation offers the opportunity to practice interviewing, communication, and physical exam skills while also learning the biomedical content. Some schools, such as McMaster University and the University of California, Los Angeles, provide additional short cases at the last session of every case to help students generalize knowledge gleaned from the more extreme individual case.

The intent of PBL is to empower students to engage in self-directed, clinically prompted learning and to collaboratively share their developing understandings with one another. As students move through the case sequence, they necessarily draw on knowledge and concepts from prior cases to make sense of new cases and build new understanding. The model may also facilitate students' development of multiple reasoning strategies that more closely approximate the reasoning strategies used by physicians in practice (Albanese, 2000; Koh, Khoo, Wong, & Koh, 2008; Sweeney, 1999; Vernon & Blake, 1993).

Like the curricular structures based on disciplinary categories as well as those based on organ systems or integrated medical sciences, the PBL model focuses more on formal knowledge acquisition and clinical reasoning than on patient care skills and professional formation. Without a focused effort to connect formal knowledge and problem-based reasoning skills to relevant clinical experiences and skills, the challenges associated with integrating and situating knowledge authentically remain. However, even when it is not an explicit focus, professionalism is often part of the informal curriculum in PBL's small groups; consequently, these groups can be an excellent forum for dealing with issues associated with professional behavior, communication, and identity. In most schools using PBL, assessment of learning focuses primarily on the individual student, thus missing an opportunity to evaluate collective performance and reinforce the participatory and distributed nature of learning. An additional curriculum model pioneered at the University of Calgary in 1991 and adopted by others later is called the clinical presentation model (Mandin, Harasym, Eagle, & Watanabe, 1995; Mandin, Jones, Woloschuk, & Harasym, 1997; Papa & Harasym, 1999; Woloschuk, Harasym, Mandin, & Jones, 2000). This curriculum takes a somewhat different approach to use of problems by pushing learning down to the level of presenting signs and symptoms (for example, chest pain) for 125 clinical presentations. Faculty members developed conceptual schemas for each clinical presentation that outlined the key information and concepts needed to understand, diagnose, and treat the condition. Students are expected to learn to solve clinical cases by examining and using these schemas. The advantage of this approach is the efficiency of the structure and learning process; students see the relationships between basic and clinical science, work on using both in more authentic ways, and subsequently need to invest less effort restructuring their knowledge when they enter clerkships.

Research using a variety of outcome measures on all of these curriculum models has found relatively few differences among them, perhaps attributable to the high quality of students and the need to pass high-stakes licensure exams (Colliver, 2000; Norman & Schmidt, 2000). However, there is some evidence about the positive impact that problem-based learning formats compared to nonproblem-based learning have on later self-perceptions and behaviors of practitioners, demonstrating positive effects on such things as teamwork, personal well-being, and communication skills (Koh et al., 2008).

Clerkship Curriculum Structures

The third year, dedicated to patient care and investigation of clinical problems presented by hospitalized patients, is a legacy of the Flexnerian reforms, although the lengths of rotations have shifted and many new rotations have been added to the original three of medicine, surgery, and obstetrics. Flexner proposed clerkships as an opportunity to apply the scientific model of thinking and reasoning to the care of patients. Physicians who brought the most advanced laboratory-based scientific knowledge to bear on patient care staffed teaching hospitals. Patients stayed in the hospital for an extended period of time, which created excellent learning opportunities for students in a relatively relaxed and longitudinally guided atmosphere.

Today, the third year of medical school is devoted to full-time clinical learning, typically organized into a series of specialty-specific block rotations ranging from four to twelve weeks. The core clerkships are internal medicine, surgery, pediatrics, obstetrics and gynecology, and psychiatry, and they often include family medicine, neurology, and other specialties. These are required rotations, their duration established by state licensing boards.

Regardless of which preclerkship curriculum structure their school uses, students enter their clerkship year with little practical experience in patient care. Consequently, many medical schools end the formal curriculum with a "transition to clerkship" course. Such courses furnish more practical instruction related to the clinical tasks students will per-form once they enter the clinical environment. This includes working with an electronic medical record, writing notes in patient charts, understand-ing how ward teams function, figuring out when to show up and when to go home, whom to report to, and whom to call in an emergency. This practical information is often lacking in the heavily content-focused preclerkship curriculum. Thus, transition courses attempt to bridge the divide between the learner-centered classroom environment and the patient-centered clinical work environment (Poncelet & O'Brien, 2008).

The purpose of the core clinical clerkship experience is to allow students to progressively take on more responsibility for patient care with appropriate guidance, support, and practice. Over the course of their clerkship, students are expected to come to understand and take on the role and identity of a physician, develop basic proficiency in assessing and treating patients with common problems, and expand their clinical skills and abilities to work in teams.

Most clerkships are offered in the inpatient setting, which is a more challenging setting within which to learn than ever. Today's hospitals are filled with extremely sick patients who stay for a short period and who are cared for by an army of specialists. Students struggle to learn in highly complex and technologically advanced hospital environments with acutely sick patients. When a patient is hospitalized, typically the diagnosis has been established in the outpatient clinic or emergency room. As a result, students rarely see undiagnosed patients or follow the natural course of disease; nor do they see the impact their treatments have on patients. In such a short-stay and intensive clinical environment, authentic participation in patient care is difficult to achieve.

Students' tenuous grasp on their patients' illnesses and the events of brief hospital stays is exacerbated by the lack of faculty time to orient, teach, observe, and evaluate medical students. Faculty members struggle with how to meet rising clinical productivity standards while maintaining research and teaching responsibilities. Given these competing responsibilities, their engagement in clinical practice has been reduced to shorter and more intense periods (down from one month to one or two weeks at a time); there is much less opportunity to get to know students. As a result, mentoring relationships may be fragile or nonexistent, and progressive advancement of student competencies is not well guided across the curriculum. Despite all of the problems with the clerkship learning environment, students do emerge from the third year with expanded knowledge and skills. However, the toll on students is high, raising the question of how the core clinical clerkship experience can be improved.

The predominant curricular structures in clinical clerkships are sequential, disciplinary block rotation; longitudinal integrated clerkship; and a mixed model with some longitudinal integration and some block rotation. In our site visits, we observed all three models.

DISCIPLINARY BLOCK ROTATIONS. Discipline-specific clerkship rotations, the norm in U.S. medical schools, present opportunities for students to experience the practice of one specialty at a time by joining an inpatient care team and participating in outpatient clinics within a teaching hospital or community clinic. Students are assigned full-time to a specific clinical site and specialty service for one to three months. Once the rotation ends, the students move on to the next specialty service and clinical site. The content of the curriculum is derived from the patients seen and the instruction associated with them. These disciplinary block rotations do a good job of exposing students to the hospital environment, immersing them in the inpatient practice of the specialty, giving students a chance to work directly with resident teams, and offering powerful and dramatic clinical experiences.

However, in disciplinary block rotation students are repeatedly overwhelmed by the rapid transition from one discipline to another, from one patient population to another, from one setting to another, from one team and teacher to another, from one set of tasks to another, from one set of shorthand language to another, and from one culture to another. As a student in a focus group described the experience, "At the very beginning I found myself [thinking], 'What planet have I landed on today?' Because every four weeks or every six weeks or every two weeks you're changing and you have different people who have different expectations, you have a different role, you have a different set of diagnoses to be considered, a different physical, a different history, different forms, different nurses."

The burden of anxiety and stress that this constant churning of people, tasks, and sites imposes is substantial and is rarely appreciated by the faculty (O'Brien, Cooke, & Irby, 2007). Student learning accrues through immersion in practice communities (Lave & Wenger, 1991), in ways that can be more or less participatory, and it is strongly influenced by patient census, time sensitivity in the environment, and the multiple and conflicting commitments of resident, faculty, and staff participants in the practice (Dornan, Hadfield, Brown, Boshuizen, & Scherpbier, 2005; Hoffman & Donaldson, 2004). Moving from specialty to specialty and hospital to hospital repetitively disrupts nascent workgroups, impeding establishment of longitudinal relationships between teachers and students.

It challenges the ability of teachers to appropriately guide students' developmental progression and give feedback on their performance.

To strengthen the connections between students and faculty members over time and decrease the imbalance between inpatient and outpatient experience, some schools have created longitudinal clinical experiences that span block rotations. A typical format is half-day sessions once per week with a longitudinal clinical preceptor throughout the clerkship year (Schneider, Coyle, Ryan, Bell, & DaRosa, 2007). These experiences afford closer, more personal working relationships between faculty members and students, offer opportunities for career guidance and mentoring, and help connect students with patients over time. Although these approaches improve longitudinal relationships, they operate in conflict with the inpatient clerkships that, as the students recognize, have much more import for their grades.

To increase curricular continuity, a number of schools offer "intersessions" in the third year to periodically bring students back to campus, typically three or four times a year for a week at a time, to advance their core knowledge and skills and reflect on their clinical experiences. The curriculum of the intersession is designed to ensure that all students have access to essential knowledge in such areas as health care systems and health policy; quality improvement and error reduction; evidence-based practice; advances in medical sciences, ethics, and professionalism; and communication and procedural skills. Intersessions can reinforce progressive learning and sequencing of content over time and can be a powerful way to integrate ideas across clinical experiences.

LONGITUDINAL INTEGRATED CLERKSHIPS.   A small number of schools have broken out of the discipline-based block rotation model to create longitudinal integrated clerkships. This curricular design is intended to reduce the amount of discontinuity students experience in their clerkships, present an integrated curriculum across the third year, and offer developmentally appropriate educational experiences and longitudinal assessment of core competencies (Hirsh et al., 2006; Hirsh, Ogur, Thibault, & Cox, 2007; Irby, 2007; Ogur, Hirsh, Krupat, & Bor, 2007). In this model, students are assigned to a group of faculty in various specialties for six months to a year, and the students accrue a panel of patients whom they follow longitudinally.

The Consortium of Longitudinal Integrated Clerkships (CLIC) identifies these core elements of the longitudinal model:

o Participation in the comprehensive care of patients over time

o Continuing learning relationships with these patients' clinicians o Meeting, through these experiences, the majority of the year's core clinical competencies across multiple disciplines simultaneously

Every week, students might have patient care experiences organized around half-day clinics in a variety of specialties with the same set of preceptors, taking calls one evening a week in the emergency department or urgent care center, participating in weekly tutorials, and interacting with an assigned mentor who oversees the student's development and reviews student self-reflections and case diaries. At some schools, students participate in a yearlong clinical procedures course as well.

Students are assigned longitudinally to outpatient practices in internal medicine, neurology, psychiatry, pediatrics, obstetrics and gynecology, and surgery. The patients a student sees are carefully selected, when possible, by the preceptor to give each student appropriate exposure to the major illnesses and conditions seen in the specialty. Locating the primary experience in outpatient clinics rather than inpatient services allows students to see patients over time and participate in diagnosis, treatment, and management of important clinical problems in each specialty. A typical panel of fifty to one hundred patients might include about fifteen patients from internal medicine, ten from pediatrics, and five to ten from surgery, psychiatry, neurology, and other areas.

In such an integrated model, students gain a broad perspective on what the various medical specialties actually do for patients; students often accompany their patients to appointments in specialty clinics and inpatient services, and they work closely with their assigned preceptors over an extended period. Students can appreciate what practicing physicians in the various specialties do, as opposed to what residents in those specialties do, and this may help them imagine themselves in a number of medical and surgical specialties.

Integrated clerkship models are consistent with the understanding of learning that we describe in Chapter Two. In these models, learning is guided by faculty progressively and developmentally, students experience sustained immersion in a community of practice such that their participation is increasingly significant, and students learn that knowledge is situated and distributed in settings of practice. However, as the major responsibility for teaching and supervision is shifted from residents to faculty preceptors, these clerkships require added resources, particularly faculty time as well as skillful teaching and mentoring.

MIXED MODEL CLERKSHIPS. In our observations and study, we also noted a hybrid of the longitudinal integrated and block rotation models. Some programs merge multiple clerkships into single, larger blocks, often combining neurology and psychiatry or surgery and surgical specialties, or a variety of specialty ambulatory rotations such as internal medicine, family medicine, pediatrics, and women's health.

Hybrid models are often used to give interested students sustained experience in a particular setting (most commonly rural environments). This can be done by compressing inpatient core block rotations into a shorter timeframe of three to six months, and offering the remainder of the year as an integrated, ambulatory, longitudinal clinical experience (Hansen et al., 1992; Ramsey, Coombs, Hunt, Marshall, & Wenrich, 2001; Schauer & Schieve, 2006). These programs are built on an apprenticeship model in which students are assigned to a primary preceptor, typically a family physician, and then work closely with other specialists as well.

Clerkship structures, whether sequential specialty-block, integrated, or mixed model, influence both the nature of the experience and the support for learning. Of the three models, the integrated clerkship offers the greatest longitudinal relationships among faculty members, patients and students; it also seems to afford the best opportunity for progressive, guided learning over time.

Fourth-Year Advanced Clerkship Curriculum Structures

During the fourth year of medical school, students have an opportunity to advance their knowledge and skills in caring for patients on hospital services, explore professional interests, examine career options, conduct research, and prepare to become an intern. Much of the fourth year is elective, and requirements vary with the school. Along with a number of required and elective courses, all schools offer subinternships, also called acting internships, with major responsibilities for patient care; the acting intern assumes the role of the intern as the primary hands-on clinician, treating the patient under the immediate guidance of the resident and with oversight from the attending physician faculty member.

The other purposes of the fourth year are to advance clinical skills, explore career options, and interview for residency programs. Flexible time for these activities is important, as is the opportunity to take additional clerkships in specialties that are not in the core clerkship sequence. The major challenge with this individually developed program of study is offering appropriate career advising services so that students make good course selections and career decisions. However, the elective nature of the fourth year presents an opportunity for students to individualize their curriculum and pursue areas of interest. It can also be a time for students to decompress, take time off, and enroll in less-demanding courses.

Schools have attempted to impose greater coherence on the primarily elective fourth year through a variety of mechanisms. For example, UCLA has developed a fourth-year college system around acute care, applied anatomy, medical science, primary care, a master's in business administration and a master's in public health, and the Drew Urban Underserved Program (Coates, Crooks, Slavin, Guiton, & Wilkerson, 2008). The domains tend to map onto particular specialty areas: acute care to emergency medicine and critical care, applied anatomy to surgery and the surgical specialties, and so on. College activities include an introductory course focused on advanced clinical skills and decision making, a monthly series of evening seminars, a longitudinal academic activity that can be either teaching or scholarship, and regular advisory meetings including feedback to students on their performance on the comprehensive clinical exam. Colleges are also encouraged to create electives that continue to connect clinical practice with advances in biomedical sciences.

Another approach is to encourage students to pursue an area of interest that is unrelated, or perhaps complementary, to their future specialty. For example, the University of California, San Francisco, developed Areas of Concentration, a program that is much like an academic minor at the undergraduate level. It imparts institutional structure for sustained inter-disciplinary projects in seven thematic areas throughout the four years of medical school. Students identify a project and work with faculty mentors to complete an academic and experiential program of prepa-ration and inquiry. Prior to graduation, students produce and present a legacy project, which may be in the form of a traditional scholarly paper but may also be an exhibit, performance, curriculum module, or patient registry. This has evolved into Pathways to Discovery, a pro-gram that emphasizes inquiry and discovery, cuts across undergraduate and graduate medical education, and includes other health profes-sional students and may include an optional master's degree. Pathways are offered in molecular medicine, clinical and translational research, health professions education, health and society, and global health sciences.

Some research-intensive medical schools, such as Duke University, Harvard Medical School and the Massachusetts Institute of Technology, Case Western Reserve University and Cleveland Clinic, and Stanford University, immerse their students in research with the aim of produc-ing physician-investigators committed to conducting medical research. Several universities, including the University of Washington; the Univer-sity of California, San Diego; Stanford University; and Yale University, dedicate time for scholarly projects throughout the curriculum with completion of the project in the fourth year. In some schools, students choose an additional year of research; at others, such as Duke, a year of research is achieved within the four years by compressing the basic science curriculum into one year.

Many schools afford their students the opportunity to pursue a joint degree. The nature of the degree programs varies with the university but typically includes such options as a master's degree in public health, public policy, global health, business, law, or clinical and translational research. Like fellowships in research, these dual degree programs offer students expanded education for future work in health care and are selected by a minority of students.

Curriculum Affects Pedagogy and Assessment

Although curricular models vary according to the level, we found that at the preclerkship level the majority of schools offer integrated block courses that are organized around organ systems, focal problems, or content themes. At the clerkship level, most schools offer a series of specialty-specific block rotations while a few offer longitudinal integrated clerkships or a mix of the two. How the curriculum is structured has a profound influence on the learning environment in which students find themselves, and, as we discuss in the next two sections of this chapter, on the dominant pedagogies they encounter, as well as on how their learning and performance is assessed.

The Pedagogies of Undergraduate Medical Education

The divide between the heavily formal-knowledge-oriented portion of the curriculum that is delivered primarily in the classroom and the practice-oriented portion that occurs primarily in a clinical setting is reflected in the dichotomy of the pedagogies used in each. In the classroom, the learning experience is more structured, controlled, and (with the exception of PBL) guided by the teacher. In clinical workplaces, the learning experience is largely guided by the actual patient care activities, and the teacher's role blends into her other roles—team leader, clinical supervisor, and primary physician of the patients. In this context, because students receive feedback from multiple sources—patients, residents, nurses, other health care staff—teaching can come from many sources. As a result, the pedagogies that are predominant in the preclerkship years tend to be quite different from those in clerkships and clinical training.

The case presentation and discussion is considered, to use Shulman's term, a "signature pedagogy," one of the profession's characteristic forms of teaching and learning (see, for example, Shulman, 2005b). In preclerkship, in courses introducing them to patient care, students typically learn a standard format for a case presentation. They practice preparing write-ups from a single encounter with a patient or from a simulated case and then presenting the write-up to fellow students and a faculty member. They receive feedback, usually about appropriate location of information, conventional terminology, the relative importance and level of detail expected, and the accuracy of their interpretation and synthesis of information. Although these activities help students develop important clinical reasoning skills such as integration and synthesis of information, they often fail to convey the larger purpose and context of the case presentation; it is a stylistically unique form of communication in which one professional transmits patient information to another. By experiencing the case presentation for such a limited pedagogical purpose, students often mistakenly perceive what is fundamentally a core part of communication in clinical settings as an academic exercise (Lingard, Schryer, Garwood, & Spafford, 2003).

For example, by the third year, this is how a medical student might present a case to the clinical teacher in clinic:

STUDENT: Ms. Flint is a thirty-four-year-old woman complaining of sharp, right-sided, nonexertional chest pain of four hours' duration. The pain came on suddenly and is exacerbated by deep breathing. She has a slight cough since the onset of pain. She denies fever. The examination is notable for a heart rate of 100 and respiratory rate of 20. She was afebrile. The lung exam was clear but with decreased breath sounds on the right compared to the left. Her cardiac and abdominal exams were normal.

I am concerned that this might be pneumonia or gallstones. She is the right age for gallstones and the pain is in the right location. But she doesn't have anything on examination to confirm this. I thought about kidney stones too, but she didn't have any hematuria or flank pain. I think she is too young for this to be cardiac. What else should I be thinking of?

PRECEPTOR: Well, you mentioned that she has an abnormal lung exam. Can you think of anything in the lungs that could cause this kind of pain?

STUDENT: I guess that pneumonia or a pneumothorax, or even a pulmonary embolus could present like this. Could she have something like that?

PRECEPTOR: I think those are all good thoughts. Based on the exam you described with decreased breath sounds, it seems like pneumothorax is the most likely possibility. Pneumonia can present with decreased breath sounds if a dense consolidation or pleural effusion is present, but crackles or rales are more common. Also, we would expect her to have a history of cough and fever preceding the pain. A pulmonary embolus, on the other hand, usually presents with a normal lung examination. Since these could be serious conditions, let's go see her right away and make a decision about what to do next.

In this example, the purpose of the activity is to present information in a very truncated, formulaic manner. The student is articulating his understanding of the case, seeking input and guidance, and potentially learning something new about the patient's illness to better help him select appropriate next steps. The interchange is thus a means of both telling a memorable and coherent story about the patient and inculcating the habits of mind needed to think like a physician. The challenge of learning is to understand how the presentation needs to change with the context and location (emergency room versus clinic), the complexity of the case, the purpose for sharing the information (seeking confirmation of a diagnosis or therapeutic option), the specialty, and the participants involved. However, because the contextual nature of this communication is rarely discussed with students, even during clerkship, it makes learning how to do it particularly, and perhaps unnecessarily, difficult (Lingard et al., 2003).

The case presentation is but one example of an activity in which patient care and pedagogical strategies are blended. Pedagogies that facilitate a situated, participatory learning process closely connected to patient care are the ideal for medical education at all levels. However, if goals such as scoring well on an exam or getting honors in a particular clerkship overtake patient-care goals, pedagogies can reflect a similar shift. This is perhaps why the pedagogical strategies around the case presentation in preclerkship years are so disconnected from the actual patient care purposes; at this stage students are largely focused on mastering facts, concepts, and skills so they can perform well on exams. They have no real patient care responsibilities, so the larger purpose and context is not salient to them unless teaching strategies are used that make them salient.

As we discuss the teaching strategies used in UME, we consider the goals of professional education: conceptual understanding, practice and performance, inquiry and improvement, and professional formation. Although pedagogies often promote development toward multiple goals, because they typically have a primary orientation we discuss them with respect to that primary focus. We also discuss important dimensions of pedagogies, such as how actively they tend to engage learners, the extent to which they strive for authenticity with respect to task and context, and a concern for learning that is progressive and developmental over time.

Pedagogies for Conceptual Understanding

We start by discussing less active and less authentic pedagogies and then move to those more active and authentic—those that orient learners toward use of concepts in a real clinical environment.

LECTURE. Lectures and other didactic sessions are the predominant form of teaching in the preclerkship curriculum and are used for a broad spectrum of formal content, from basic science concepts such as the Krebs cycle to behavioral concepts such as goal setting for weight management. Didactic instruction is also used in the clerkships and subsequent clinical training, but the student group size is usually smaller. Typically, lecture is the least authentic with respect to the context in which learning occurs and how learners engage with material and information. However, even in the clinical years where these connections seem more feasible, there tends to be little effort to connect the formal content covered in didactic sessions with the actual patients the students are seeing during rotation. Only recently have a few schools developed tutorial sessions on the basis of the actual patients for whom students are providing care. These sessions capitalize on opportunities to reinforce connections between theory and practice (Cohen, 2009).

Although lectures given by gifted teachers can inspire learning and present a coherent picture of the content to be learned, lecture tends to be a passive learning experience that can devolve into a litany of facts with little conceptual integration. We note that attendance at lectures is no longer mandatory at most schools; perhaps this signifies growing awareness that for many students other modes of instruction are more appealing and more effective. However, schools are beginning to use technologies such as audience response systems, podcasts, and web-based learning communities to make lectures more interactive and accessible both within and beyond the classroom.

SMALL GROUPS. Some schools restrict lectures to 50 percent of formal class time in the first two years of the curriculum, and some PBL schools ban lectures entirely. Small-group sessions are used instead of lectures to more actively engage learners and create a culture of interdependent learning where each person's contributions advance the discussion and understanding of the group (Shuell, 1996). Such sessions can enhance conceptual understanding through interactive case discussions, collective problem solving, peer-to-peer teaching, and guided discussion of complex topics. In small groups, students need to articulate what they know and do not know, challenge assumptions, wrestle with the limits of understanding (their own and their group's), determine what information is relevant to the solution of a problem or completion of the task at hand, and think about how to use and apply what they have learned to a clinical context. In doing so, these sessions more closely approximate the clinical learning process that will continue throughout physicians' careers than lectures do.

The experience of learning in small groups is generally superior to that of lectures (Springer, Stanne, & Donovan, 1999). However, careful consideration must be given to the goals and objectives of the small-group session, the group process (including the role of faculty members), the nature of the task or activity, the methods of monitoring performance, and the process of giving feedback to learners. In our site observations, we often encountered programs that use small groups but do not pay adequate attention to the objectives and elements of small-group learning that make it effective.

In light of the significant resources required for small-group teaching (such as space and facilitator time and skills), team-based learning has been introduced as a way of engaging students actively in learning during large-group sessions (Michaelsen, Knight, & Fink, 2004). This approach involves assigning readings in advance, beginning each class with a readiness assessment test, discussing the test, and later discussing an application case in small groups followed by large-group discussion. The process moves from individual testing to small-group discussion to total-group review. This instructional strategy is used in a minority of medical schools but is gaining popularity. It has been shown to increase learning and subsequent performance on the United States Medical Licensing Examination (USMLE) and is used in both preclerkship and clerkship instruction (Levine et al., 2004; Thompson et al., 2007).

TECHNOLOGY. Web-based modules can offer learners more flexible access to a range of concepts. The limited body of research on web-based learning in medical education suggests that adding these technologies and materials to a course usually (though not always) improves knowledge, can be more efficient than traditional courses (Bell, Krupat, Fazio, Roberts, & Schwartzstein, 2008), and is usually well received by learners, even though the materials are often used less frequently than educators would expect (Chumley-Jones, Dobbie, & Alford, 2002; Cook, 2006).

Furthermore, learners can cover the content at their own pace and explore in greater depth according to their interests and needs. Some studies indicate that students can master the same amount of content in a third less time using computer-assisted learning than in lectures (Bell, Fonarrow, Hays, & Mangione, 2000; Lyon et al., 1992). This is a surprising and intriguing finding. Although the social context is less rich, some schools have developed virtual learning environments so students can raise and respond to questions and engage in discussions of the content. Learners have indicated preferences for more interactive web-based learning (Chumley-Jones et al., 2002).

New web-based learning resources and delivery systems, flexible and technology-enhanced classrooms, and the ability to create networks of learners and teachers support more participative learning and can represent the distributed nature of clinical knowledge. Such technologies aid individualized learning and small group learning even if not in the same space at the same time.

Pedagogies that are intended to enhance conceptual understanding outside of real clinical settings are ones that allow knowledge and skills to be analyzed, deconstructed, practiced, and recombined without the pressure of the real clinical environment. Clearly there is an expectation that learners will draw on this new understanding when they are in clinical settings with real patients. However, as we describe in the next section, there are also pedagogies that are designed to target clinical reasoning and conceptual understanding in the midst of real patient care.

Pedagogies for Practice and Performance

Just as we see teaching approaches fostering opportunities for students to use concepts authentically, there has been a related trend toward more authentic ways of supporting development of students' clinical skills and performance. Pedagogies for practice and performance generally allow learners to practice clinical skills and procedures in more realistic situations, but with more time, less risk, better and more immediate feedback, and greater opportunity to incorporate feedback on the spot and try again. In the preclerkship years, these pedagogies are most commonly used in simulation centers or in small-group sessions that are part of courses such as doctoring or introduction to clinical medicine, which focus on history taking, physical exam, and communication skills.

Simulation experiences range from as basic as students practicing on each other to more sophisticated scenarios involving standardized patients and sophisticated technologies involving mannequin simulators. In undergraduate medical education, simulators are particularly useful for development of basic psychomotor skills in routine situations, for familiarizing learners with equipment and particular technologies, and for practicing communication skills and roles in interprofessional teams (Issenberg, McGaghie, Petrusa, Gordon, & Scalese, 2005; Kneebone, 2005; Robins et al., 2008; Stefanidis, Scerbo, Sechrist, Mostafavi, & Heniford, 2008). As students progress into clerkships, simulation can be an important opportunity for students to step back from the complexity and fast pace of a real clinical setting to revisit and refine skills that are rarely used or rarely observed directly by more advanced clinicians. Simulation is also a means by which learning experiences can be customized to match the needs of the learner in a way not typically available in most patient-care driven learning environments, particularly when efficiency and safety are top priorities.

Standardized patients are widely used for communication and interpersonal skills as well as for the clinical reasoning used in problem formulation, differential diagnosis, assessment, and treatment planning. Standardized patients can be trained not only to act out certain scenarios but also to observe students' behaviors, provide coaching, and offer specific feedback. In addition, taping these interactions allows students to review and assess their own performance as well as that of their peers and provide constructive feedback. Clinical teachers can review the videos with learners for guided reflection or to offer structured feedback. This approach makes practice and performance more visible to learners and thus yields material for a more evidence-based discussion of performance.

It is increasingly difficult for students to practice procedural skills on real patients in real time because of time constraints, safety considerations, and prioritization of the needs of other clinical learners over those of medical students. As a result, labs and simulation centers are now widely used as venues for students to practice such skills as suturing and knot tying, pelvic exams, and IV placement. Programs designed to enhance skill acquisition include such educational components as deliberate practice with feedback, clear learning objectives, rigorous outcome assessment, and high achievement standards (Wayne et al., 2006).

When working on ward teams or in clinics, students regularly have both formal and informal conversations with physicians, nurses, staff, and even patients and families that advance their conceptual understanding so as to improve focused history taking, differential diagnosis, management and treatment decisions, and communication of information. More formal techniques such as the One Minute Preceptor (Aagaard, Teherani, & Irby, 2004) or SNAPPS (Summarize the H and P; Narrow the differential diagnosis; Analyze the differential; Probe the preceptor; Plan patient management; Select a case-related issue for future learning) (Wolpaw,

Wolpaw, & Papp, 2003) suggest efficient techniques for quickly gauging the learner's level of understanding, providing positive and corrective feedback, teaching a general rule or principle, and stimulating reflection and self-directed learning.

A significant portion of what students learn, both early on during clinical immersion experiences and during clerkships, occurs through observation. Even after students begin contributing significantly to patient care, they continue to learn from the actions they observe on the part of faculty physicians, residents, and staff (Kenny, Mann, & MacLeod, 2003). In some situations, students evaluate approaches to patients, activities, and communication with colleagues and emulate the ones they evaluate favorably. At other times, students simply accept that how everyone else does things is how things should be done. With few exceptions, students have insufficient assistance in distinguishing between and reflecting on acceptable variations in practice patterns.

As their ability to participate in authentic clinical work progresses, students begin to engage meaningfully and substantively in patient care activities. Students take responsibility for specific tasks such as collecting and presenting lab results, contacting a subspecialist for a consult, looking up current treatment options, discussing a treatment plan with a patient and checking the patient's understanding of the plan, discussing the patient's home situation prior to hospitalization with a visiting nurse, or coordinating follow-up visits for a patient. Assigning specific tasks to learners that are appropriate for the learner's skills and abilities and that target specific areas of need are important in supporting improved performance of patient care. However, such pedagogies are longitudinal in focus and thus require reliable and valid ways for students to document their progress and longer-term relationships with faculty preceptors who observe students' performance over the course of several months. More often than not, the pedagogies used in clinical settings offer little sequencing, continuity, and guided support along a developmental trajectory, all of which are key parts of effective pedagogies to facilitate workplace learning.

Pedagogies for Inquiry, Innovation, and Improvement

Pedagogies for inquiry, innovation, and improvement facilitate learners' development of the habits of mind, motivation, and commitment to excellence that are essential parts of being a physician. The pedagogies associated with inquiry, innovation, and improvement are a relatively new focus for teaching and learning, particularly in medicine. They tend to incorporate principles related to metacognition and collaborative approaches to learning. In medical education, such pedagogies are represented in the design of problem-based learning, in mentoring relationships that engage and support students' involvement in research and other scholarly activities, in quality improvement projects, and in clinical conferences and teaching sessions that challenge students to explore multiple perspectives, push the limits of their understanding, and search for new possibilities or alternate approaches to a difficult or uncertain aspect of a patient's case. Typically these pedagogies are oriented toward individual learners rather than toward learning communities and cultures.

In preclerkship education, there are aspects of the curricular structure and embedded pedagogies that can facilitate development of these commitments to inquiry and improvement, such as small-group discussion sessions, problem-based learning, collaborative projects, and protected time for scholarship in an area of interest. The focus of these pedagogies in preclerkship education tends to involve efforts to help learners engage in critical thinking, self-directed or self-regulated learning, and reflection. When these activities are treated as skills, they are usually taught through structured activities such as review and critique of journal articles in small groups, analysis of cases in a problem-based learning format or facilitated case discussion, and writing assignments. The role and skills of the teacher or facilitator, the quality of the tasks, and the nature of group interactions have significant implications for how any of these influence students' habits of mind, motivation, and commitment to excellence. For example, small-group discussions or PBL sessions that are completely teacher-directed; reflective writing assignments that are never reviewed, discussed, or used to guide future learning; and projects that are not peer-reviewed or implemented will likely contribute little to students' development of inquiry, innovation, and improvement. During clerkships, students also experience pedagogies such as guided reflection through questions and discussion, clinical discussions with peers, quality improvement projects, and protected time for independent learning and scholarship—all of which can encourage inquiry, innovation, and improvement in daily activities.

Currently many schools incorporate small-group discussions on evidence-based medicine, legal and ethical issues related to clinical topics and cases, health care policy, and health care delivery systems. Authenticity in these activities is an issue; there is much variation in the extent to which faculty members design these sessions to challenge learners to connect the topics to some of their own clinical experiences and work independently or collaboratively with their peers to examine the problems and generate potential solutions. However, these are exactly the kinds of pedagogies that lead learners to incorporate such questions into their daily practice and to appreciate them as an expectation rather than just as a classroom activity. As students move on to clerkships and regularly encounter systems issues, practice variations, service gaps, and errors, there are numerous opportunities to take a few minutes on rounds to discuss issues and brainstorm improvements that can actually be implemented by a member of the team.

Regardless of the setting, it is of the utmost importance that learners identify and incorporate feedback on their performance. There are many possible sources of feedback on performance, though typically medical education focuses on feedback given to learners by residents and attending physicians or preceptors. Ideally, feedback focuses learners' attention on aspects of their practice and performance that can be improved, permits insight into how such improvement can be achieved, and motivates learners to invest the effort needed to improve. In light of evidence that learners are rarely directly observed during interactions with patients by attendings, preceptors, and residents (Holmboe, 2004), additional sources of feedback have been introduced in preclerkship and clerkship clinical experiences, such as patient or standardized patient ratings of communication and overall satisfaction with the interaction with a student, checklists and evaluation forms for nurses and other staff, peer ratings, video review of encounters with standardized patients, and reflective activities to encourage students to begin synthesizing various pieces of feedback received during a day or a rotation. Videos and portfolios offer additional ways for students to document and engage others in discussion of their work. Ideally, feedback should be part of every pedagogy, but it needs to be scaffolded, progressively shifting away from teacher-directed and motivated feedback for improvement toward learner-directed, intrinsically motivated feedback for improvement.

Although the goals of scholarly projects and concentrations, whether elective or required, are often aligned with inquiry, innovation, and improvement, such activities do not constitute pedagogy in and of themselves. In terms of pedagogy, the key for these scholarly projects is strong advising, guidance, mentoring, and feedback. Although most schools require a designated advisor, there are rarely any firm guidelines or standards for advisors and mentors to follow. A few schools have developed comprehensive pedagogies to support longitudinal scholarship through such vehicles as areas of concentration or scholarly projects. These programs include not only didactics and advising but also situated learning experiences in which students interact with the members of a community, be they health policy activists, research scientists, or aficionados of medicine and the arts whose interests connect to the student's project.

Where pedagogies for inquiry, innovation, and improvement tend to come up short is in attention to the community and culture of the learning environment, which is to say capitalizing on the social and participatory nature of learning. The term *social pedagogies* is appropriate to describe a set of strategies for creating educational environments in which learning occurs in the context of a community and in which learners engage in activities that involve representing knowledge to others. The focus of social pedagogies is on development of shared values, ethics, and reasoning among members of a group or community that support the ongoing quest for improvement in process, understanding, and outcome.

Pedagogies for Professional Formation

As we remark in closing Chapter One, we believe that professional formation, along with standardization and individualization, integration, and habits of inquiry and improvement, should be a central goal of medical education. We stress the importance of understanding professional formation, as we explain in Chapter Two, as "an ongoing, self-reflective *process* involving habits of thinking, feeling, and acting" (Wear & Castellani, 2000, p. 603). It is critical to medical education to understand that these habits of thought, feeling, and action ideally develop so as to allow students to demonstrate "*compassionate, communicative, and socially responsible physicianhood*" each in his or her unique way (Wear & Castellani, 2000, p. 603, italics in original).

In direct contrast to what we would hope, however, a number of studies suggest that students become less empathic and less altruistic as they progress through medical education, with the largest drop in empathy occurring between the beginning and the end of the first year and between the beginning and the end of the third year of medical school (Newton, Barber, Clardy, Cleveland, & O'Sullivan, 2008). Students' empathic identification with their patients often conflicts with that of hospital team members, who can appear unempathic and distant. Students report having great difficulty in adjusting to the culture of the hospital (Branch et al., 1998). Also, as students progress through the clerkships, moral development is often described as being arrested or regressing (Branch et al., 1993; Branch, 2000), and students may feel trapped between their moral principles and sensitivity to their patients and the desire and need to fit in with the norms, values, and actions of their team members (Branch, 2000).

Although there is no single explanation for these decrements in empathy, altruism, and moral development, multiple hypotheses arose from our interviews and observations: the pressures of a competitive learning environment in medical school; the corrosive effects of the informal and hidden curriculum in clinical settings, that is, unprofessional behaviors of team members observed by students; the unwillingness of medical schools and teaching hospitals to take action against unprofessional behavior on the part of faculty and staff who create a hostile work environment; the lack of opportunities for students to reflect on and learn from professionalism issues; and insufficient contact with positive role models who embody the highest values of the profession. In every context, students are looking for cues about appropriate behaviors and attitudes; unfortunately much of what they observe violates the highest values of the profession.

Professional formation is a synthetic process that occurs along with learning and development in all other domains: conceptual understanding, practice and performance, and inquiry, innovation, and improvement. This is not to say, however, that specific pedagogies to support professional formation are unnecessary. Instead, it is important that they be understood in the broader context of students' learning and experience. Creating caring, compassionate, resilient, and altruistic physicians in training is part of the process of medical education.

In the past, there was little explicit attention to ways of "teaching" professionalism, perhaps because there was little perceived need to do so. Immersion in clinical settings, apprenticeship to physicians and teams caring for patients, and identification of ideal models of behavior were all taken for granted as the best means for students to become professionals. However, because the last thirty years have seen so much change in the practice environment, greater calls for physician accountability, and growing awareness of the hidden curriculum and its potentially inimical effect on students' professional development, many efforts have been proposed and implemented to more directly teach for professional formation (Cruess & Cruess, 2006; Hafferty, 1998, 2006; Wear & Castellani, 2000; Wear & Zarconi, 2008).

The pedagogies that can be linked to professional formation span a range of areas, such as teaching formal knowledge related to ethics and professional standards or expectations, developing moral reasoning and reflective judgment as skills, modeling and encouraging a range of behaviors such as empathy and concern for patients or shared decision making about care, engaging learners in reflective practices, and supporting or reinforcing students' development of professional values.

As we noted with respect to formal scientific content knowledge, some approaches to professional formation suggest that students must first learn the formal moral and ethical principles underlying professional practice, then practice using this knowledge to reason through cases of progressively greater complexity or uncertainty, and then, once the cognitive processes are sufficiently developed, enter into real clinical settings where they will enact behaviors that are consistent with the moral and ethical principles they have learned to use. Many of the schools in our study use something akin to this approach. Students may participate in longitudinal small groups that focus on discussion of cases illustrating ethical or legal principles that have been covered in reading assignments or lectures. Faculty facilitators may frame the discussion, clarify or elaborate as needed, or lead the discussion to higher sophistication or complexity according to the group's readiness. The challenge in these sessions is situating them in a meaningful context matching the students' level of professional development. Many students have very limited clinical experience at the time these discussions occur and thus may not realistically be able to engage the knowledge and conceptual understanding so as to serve their professional formation. A more effective pedagogical strategy involves using examples from students' own experiences (clinical or not) early on in medical school. Ideally, this allows moral and ethical reasoning to progress through engagement with meaningful contexts. As students gain clinical experience, faculty facilitators can present more opportunity to incorporate them into the discussion. Also, clinical experiences are an important opportunity for students not only to employ cognitive skills but also to behave and act in a way that may or may not be consistent with their conceptual understanding of the principles. Reflection on their own behaviors and attitudes, as well as those observed among peers, residents, faculty, and staff in clinical settings, can generate rich material for discussion in facilitated small-group sessions.

Professional formation, however, involves much more than cultivating moral and ethical reasoning. There are additional skillful practices related to awareness of one's own beliefs, emotions, and values and how those values, emotions, and beliefs influence interpersonal interactions. With the capacity for awareness more fully developed, learners can then begin to more consciously focus these beliefs, emotions, and values to benefit patients or move them toward the professional stance they envision for themselves. Perhaps because this aspect of professional formation is more personal, the pedagogies are less clear and concrete. Several schools now have courses on professional development that span most of the undergraduate curriculum, or all of it. Students are often put in small groups that remain together for the whole course, with the rationale that being in the group will be an opportunity for students to establish meaningful relationships with colleagues that furnish a safe, supportive forum for discussing issues related to professional formation. In preclerkship years, discussion in small groups is often used to help students articulate some of their beliefs and assumptions about professional and unprofessional conduct, what it means to be a physician (such as different roles), or the meaning of the social contract between physicians and society, and to hear the perspectives of their peers. A key to the success of these pedagogies is keeping the content of the discussion relevant to the level and experience of the students (Cruess & Cruess, 2006). Through establishing collaborative and supportive peer and collegial communities students may also learn to set norms, boundaries, and expectations as well as to give feedback and open communication (Arnold et al., 2007).

Most medical schools now promote opportunities for students to interact with patients and work in real clinical settings in the preclerkship years. A number of teaching approaches enrich and focus these experiences: reflective writing assignments on the meaning of the experience; observations related to ethical, legal, or professional issues; or other connections to students' personal and professional development. During the actual experiences, faculty and staff may give students specific, authentic tasks to gain a sense of purpose, responsibility, and confidence in a focused aspect of the physician's work. Students can use this experience of assuming the stance of the physician to reflect on emotions that arose, new insights into patients' experiences that occurred, or opportunities to improve patients' experiences and how care is delivered. Second, some faculty members engage in explicit role modeling or involve students in discussion of valued behaviors and approaches, including patient-centeredness or relationship-centered care. Third, storytelling can open a powerful window on the experiences, wisdom, and expertise of physicians. Stories containing embedded case knowledge and important lessons learned have been widely described as making a lasting impression on novices, though their actual impact on behavior in practice is difficult to establish (Cox, 2001; Greenhalgh, 2001).

In clerkships, much of the pedagogy for professional formation continues to be implicit rather than explicit, with little attention to the situated nature of professional formation. Students refine their concepts of professional and unprofessional behavior on the basis of the examples they observe in practice and the kinds of thinking, feeling, and action they see rewarded or disparaged in practice. In the best situations, students are fortunate to work with residents and faculty who serve as positive role models; encourage and enrich students' developing areas of interest, inquiry, and commitment; and are able to articulate their own beliefs, perspectives, and intentions with respect to patients, colleagues, organizations, and the profession. In less desirable circumstances, students find themselves uncertain about the negative behaviors they observe in practice and have no opportunity to discuss their observations with others who might be able to offer greater insight into what happened. The key point is that without a more systematic and explicit focus on professional formation, there is little hope of ensuring that it is occurring in a desirable way.

In today's clinical settings, promoting a learning environment that optimally supports students' development as compassionate, communicative, and socially responsible physicians continues to be a challenge. In light of this reality, some schools have taken a symbolic approach as a starting point to a larger cultural change. Events such as white-coat ceremonies, honor societies, and other ceremonies acknowledge contributions to the profession through exemplary service, leadership, teaching, and research; they send important messages about institutional values. Including students on education, curriculum, quality improvement, and medical center committees and encouraging student participation in local, regional, and national professional organizations are other symbolic—yet practical—actions. Through appreciative inquiry, some schools, such as the University of Indiana, are identifying and sharing stories about exemplars of the highest ideals of the profession. Taking another approach, some schools have launched efforts to counteract undesirable messages conveyed by the hidden curriculum, setting explicit standards of professionalism and giving all individuals involved in patient care access to a system to report unprofessional or otherwise concerning behaviors or attitudes.

Assessment in UME

Assessment motivates and imparts direction for future learning. Therefore, assessment systems must be aligned with desired outcomes and designed to document progress with respect to professional competence using multiple measures. Epstein and Hundert (2002) define *professional competence* as "the habitual and judicious use of communication, knowledge, technical skills, clinical reasoning, emotions, values and reflection in daily practice for the benefit of the individual and community being served" (p. 226; see also Epstein, 2007). Two major goals of an assessment system are to give students formative feedback that enables them to create specific learning objectives for guiding their learning, and to conduct summative evaluation certifying that students have achieved the requisite level of performance to move to the next level of training or licensure.

Both of these assessment goals, formative and summative, can support learning in three core dimensions of medical practice—formal knowledge, clinical performance, and professional formation—and can be connected to the ACGME competencies: medical knowledge and clinical reasoning, patient care skills, communication abilities, professionalism, systems-based practice, and practice-based learning and improvement (Accreditation Council for Graduate Medical Education, 2007). By anchoring assessment in professional competencies, one can evaluate all areas of performance (Epstein, 2007). As medical schools continue to incorporate a variety of tools for assessment, several dimensions must be considered in selecting appropriate methods: authenticity of the setting in which assessment occurs (fidelity), the purpose of the assessment (formative, summative), the timing of the assessment and how it fits into the general picture of learners' development of professional competence, and the resources required to conduct the assessment. Assessment systems that are designed comprehensively, with these dimensions in mind, improve the evaluation process itself and advance professional development of students (van der Vleuten, 1996; van der Vleuten & Schuwirth, 2005). In Table 3.1, we summarize the various assessments used in UME, both those that students experience within the medical school program and those that are part of the external licensing system.

Assessment of Formal Knowledge

Medical knowledge is associated with both comprehension and reasoning abilities and is located within the cognitive domain. This domain has long been the primary focus of assessment throughout medical education and thus has been a guiding force in designing curriculum and instruction. Acquisition of formal knowledge is tested most often by written examinations that use a multiple-choice format. The virtue of multiple-choice (MCQ) items is that they can sample a large domain of knowledge in a relatively short period of time. The context of the question (for example, case information or clinical scenario) can add complexity in order to test conceptual understanding rather than just factual knowledge (Epstein, 2007).

Depending on the organization of the curriculum, these examinations may test knowledge along more or less disciplinary lines within the basic, clinical, social, and behavioral sciences. As students move through training, the exams typically test understanding of increasingly complex bodies of knowledge, rather than facts or recall of information. In U.S. medical schools, these exams tend to occur at discrete points in the curriculum (for example, at the end of a course) and do not necessarily or systematically assess the same content at multiple points in time. Consequently, there is little way to track changes in students' knowledge and

Table 3.1. Assessment Methods Used in Undergraduate Medical Education, Formative and Summative

	Year 1	Year 2	Year 3	Year 4
Assessment of formal knowledge:				
MCQ (multiple choice) exam	S	S	S	S
Licensing exams: USMLE steps 1 and 2		S		S
Assessment of clinical performance:				
Computer-based patient management exam			S	
Focused observation (mini-Clinical Evaluation exam or mini-CEX, Brief Structured Clinical Examination or BSCO)			F	
OSCE, Clinical Performance exam (CPX)	F	S	S	S
Write-up of complete history and physical exam with discussion of patient's problem	F	F and S	S	S
Critique of journal article	F and S	F and S	S	S
Global evaluations by faculty	S	S	S	S
Global evaluations by residents			S	S
Peer-to-peer evaluations	F	F	F and S	S
Staff evaluations of students	F	F	F and S	S
Patient logs			F	
Portfolios	F and S	F and S	F and S	S

Note: F = formative feedback for improvement;
S = summative assessment.

understanding of specific content over time. One important exception is the progress test, which is given twice a year to every medical student in the school. Individual student progress can be plotted over the four years, along with group performance and school performance (Muijt-jens, Schuwirth, Cohen-Schotanus, Thoben, & van der Vleuten, 2008). Though widely used in Canadian and Dutch medical schools, progress tests are rarely used in U.S. medical schools.

Formal knowledge is also assessed in the USMLE licensing examinations, which we describe in detail in Chapter Five. Many schools also purchase customized examinations for their basic science curriculum and specialty-specific exams for their clerkships from the NBME. The questions are high in quality and offer the school a national norm for comparison purposes.

Additional methods of formative assessment of medical knowledge and conceptual understanding are beginning to appear, notably concept mapping (Schmidt, 2004; Torre et al., 2007; West, Park, Pomeroy, & Sandoval, 2002) and assessment of knowledge in real time through high-fidelity computer simulation of actual patient encounters (Downing, 2002).

Assessment of Clinical Performance

To perform clinically, students must have both working medical knowledge at a basic level and the skills necessary to collect accurate and complete information from patients (Gruppen & Frohna, 2002; Holmboe, Lipner, & Greiner, 2008). Clinical performance requires understanding what to do, when, and why; and the ability to put that knowledge into action by caring for a particular patient either individually or as part of a team. This domain is now a significant component of student assessment. Given the breadth and complexity of this domain, multiple tools for assessment have been developed.

In the earliest stages of medical education, competence in patient care is typically broken down into component parts. Without such decomposition, the learner can become overwhelmed and distracted in trying to pay attention to the endless array of details and stimuli. At this level, competence involves performance of such discrete tasks as examining parts of the body (for example, the abdomen or neurological system), taking a focused history, or reviewing a chart. These are often practiced in a controlled or simulated environment with trained and standardized patients.

One standardized method of evaluating interpersonal communication, procedural skills, and clinical reasoning is through objective structured clinical exams (OSCE). This form of examination involves use of trained patients or standardized patients to represent a particular clinical presentation or problem. Students are sent into an exam room to see a patient and perform a focused task. For example, the student might be asked to communicate bad news to a patient, explain the results of a well-baby check-up to a mother, or interview and examine a patient complaining of acute abdominal pain or a severe headache. Student performance on these tasks is assessed with a checklist of specific behaviors, ratings of interpersonal qualities and communication skills, or direct or video observation. Videotaping is an opportunity for students to review their performance and receive additional formative feedback from faculty members. Typically ten stations or rooms, each with a set of patient care tasks and each lasting ten to twenty minutes, is recommended to achieve reliability and validity sufficient for summative assessment. This form of assessment can be tailored to specific educational goals (Petrusa, 2002; Tamblyn, 1998).

By the time students have more clinical experience, competence in patient care typically involves a more integrated set of clinical skills and reasoning processes such that the questions in a history reflect more sophisticated understanding of a problem and more efficient processes of working through a differential diagnosis. Assessing learners' performance summatively for tasks of this level of complexity—in other words, for tasks that are close approximations of real patient exams—is quite challenging. Much work remains to be done to establish the reliability and validity of this kind of performance assessment (Petrusa, 2002).

For specific procedural and technical skills such as knot tying, suturing, using a bag valve mask, or performing one's role in a trauma resuscitation or code, simulation centers have been added as a way of supporting both instruction in and assessment of procedural, communication, and teamwork skills.

When students enter a clerkship, they are evaluated by faculty and residents using global ratings of their performance. Unfortunately, faculty seldom observe students performing skills and so tend to base their assessment on the student's ability to give a coherent case presentation, work with the team, and get basic tasks completed. To encourage faculty to observe students performing a history and physical examination, a time-efficient observation system has been developed. This miniclinical evaluation exercise (mini-CEX) brings structure to a ten-minute faculty observation of a student with a patient. After the observation, the trainee is asked for a diagnosis and treatment plan, and then the faculty member offers feedback. The reliability of this measure is equivalent to an objective structured clinical examination in a clinical skills center when approximately ten observations are made (Norcini, Blank, Duffy, & Fortina, 2003). The brief structured clinical observation, called BSCO, is similar in intent, a quick observation in order to give specific feedback (Kuo, Irby, & Loeser, 2005).

Additional assessment techniques include peer assessment (Norcini, 2003), patient satisfaction ratings, and portfolios that capture student work, reflections, and projects (Carraccio & Englander, 2004). Because no one method will assess all areas of competence, multiple methods are needed.

Assessment of Professional Formation

By including professionalism and communication and interpersonal skills in the learning objectives for medical student education and in the core competencies for graduate medical education, the AAMC and the ACGME have taken the position that professional formation should be formally assessed. We, however, use the term *professional formation* rather than *professionalism* to emphasize the developmental and multifaceted nature of the construct. Arnold and Stern (2006) offer a framework that is aligned with our understanding of professional formation. They view clinical competence, communication skills, and ethical and legal understanding as foundational qualities that all learners must develop for basic professional competence at any given level. However, these alone are not enough. True professional formation involves additional aspirations in excellence, humanism, accountability, and altruism. Development in each is unique to the individual and thus difficult to reconcile with a competency-based framework (Wear & Castellani, 2000). Perhaps equally important in comparing learners to one another or to a standard is tracking their progress over time through a variety of methods and making sure that a discussion or narrative reflection with an advisor or mentor occurs.

Assessment of the foundational elements of professional formation is captured, in part, through the methods described earlier for formal knowledge and clinical performance. However, as Epstein and Hundert (2002) point out, professional competence is a synthetic, integrative construct that requires looking across domains (domain-independent) rather than within isolated domains. Thus, even though there are reasonably good ways of assessing a student's factual knowledge, problem solving, physical exam skills, technical skills, and communication skills, important domains that may matter more for professional competence and patient outcomes are less frequently assessed. This includes such things as clinical reasoning, patient-physician relationships, use of technology, and systems-based care. Several of these elements fit well with the aspirational dimensions of professionalism in Arnold and Stern's framework of humanism, excellence, altruism, and accountability (2006). We note three approaches to assessment of professional formation: making brief observations, or "snapshots"; using benchmarks of development; and monitoring the learning environment.

SNAPSHOTS.   Brief observations, or snapshots, of professional behavior target overt behaviors and implicit or explicit attitudes that fall short of minimal standards and expectations. Observation of communication and interpersonal skills such as delivering bad news, patient education and counseling, establishing rapport, and negotiating a plan that is agreeable to both the patient and the physician is one key way aspects of professionalism are assessed. This assessment often occurs in simulated scenarios with standardized patients, but tools have also been developed to facilitate focused assessment of students' behaviors during real clinical encounters. By means of standardized patient ratings of the patient-physician interaction, one can flag students with concerning behaviors or attitudes for future monitoring and potential remediation.

Attitudes as well as other observable behaviors such as reliability, honesty, and organization are often captured in written comments or on global assessments by residents, faculty members, or other health care professionals with whom students work. When egregious violations of acceptable standards of professional behavior occur, formal reporting systems are implemented in some institutions to document and deal with such instances (Papadakis et al., 1999, 2001; Papadakis & Loeser, 2006). Lastly, sessions in which faculty members, residents, and staff members who worked with a student over the course of a rotation come together to review and discuss their perception of the student's professional conduct were found to be a better method for capturing deficiencies in student professionalism than checklists or written evaluations (Hemmer, Hawkins, Jackson, & Pangaro, 2000).

In addition to snapshots of behaviors and attitudes, some argue that cognitive assessments are called for, ranging from factual knowledge of legal and ethical principles to use of knowledge and reasoning skills to think through complex cases. Such assessments are most often used in the preclerkship curriculum when the formal curriculum tends to cover such topics. Little has been done to systematically assess knowledge and use of this knowledge in authentic clinical situations.

BENCHMARKS OF DEVELOPMENT. The second approach is more developmentally oriented. This approach to assessment tends to be more formative than summative, although some efforts have been made to establish benchmarks for learners at different levels. Benchmarks may be appropriate for the foundational elements of professional development such as communication and interpersonal skills and moral and ethical understanding and judgment. The aspirational elements of professionalism do not fit easily into a generalized competency framework, although it is important to keep them in focus and reflect on them over time (Buyx, Maxwell, & Schone-Seifert, 2008). Students may be asked to reflect on their personal and professional development through reflective writing assignments, regular meetings with a mentor or trusted small group of peers, or a portfolio that documents events or activities the students believe to be a significant contribution to their professional development (Howe, 2002). Patient satisfaction surveys or more general feedback cards have been used to give students additional formative information, but these instruments rarely have enough sensitivity and specificity to be used for summative purposes. Their primary purpose is often positive reinforcement.

THE LEARNING ENVIRONMENT. The third approach monitors the learning environment rather than specific individuals. Although this is not directly a method of assessment, we know that the learning environment can be a powerful socializing agent and very influential in the student's professional development (Feudtner, Christakis, & Christakis, 1994; Hafferty, 1998). At present, there is one instrument for assessing the patient-centeredness of the learning environment from the students' perspective. The instrument captures students' perceptions of role modeling, experiences, and support for patient-centered behaviors. Tests of the psychometric properties of the instrument found very good to excellent internal consistency and reliability (Haidet, Kelly, Chou, & Communication, Curriculum, and Culture Study Group, 2005; Haidet et al., 2006). Institutionwide reporting systems have been part of a culture shift in some institutions. If appropriately explained, supported, and reinforced, such systems can bring attention to incidents that occur at any level in the institution (from administration to faculty, to nursing staff, to residents and students). Such systems can also be used to call attention to positive events that deserve acknowledgment.

In summary, assessment of clinical performance has advanced to the point of more comprehensively addressing the various competencies required of every physician. Even though the multiple-choice exam is still the norm for evaluating cognitive knowledge, many other forms of assessment are being added, among them progress tests; objective structured clinical exams, simulations; portfolios; self- and peer assessment; and ratings by faculty, residents, and sometimes patients. Some schools have created developmentally oriented assessment and mentoring processes that longitudinally advance the competence of each student, although most do not.

UME: The Work Ahead

There is work ahead for UME in the United States. The curricular models, pedagogical strategies, and assessment practices described here are perhaps best conceived as works endlessly in progress given the ever-changing nature of undergraduate medical education. Each model has sought to advance teaching and learning, and each has experienced challenges in doing so. However, as we view them through the contributions of the learning sciences and consider the premises that learning is progressive and developmental, participatory, and situated and distributed, we see that UME needs fundamental reform. Thus, although the seeds of the future already reside in the curricular models of today, these approaches require serious rethinking to address their shortcomings. At the most basic level, the overall structure of undergraduate medical education is still built on the Flexnerian model of two years of basic science instruction followed by two years of clinical clerkship experience; and it is still assumed that the proper progression in learning is to master scientific facts and reasoning and then apply them directly and seamlessly to patient care. However, clinical reasoning is based on both abstract knowledge and clinical experience. Progressive development of knowledge and skills is best achieved by going back and forth between general knowledge and particular patients. The process of pattern recognition, so characteristic of an expert's approach, is a product of extensive experience with patients overlaid on a formal knowledge structure. It takes both kinds of knowledge to achieve success, and experts use both (Norman, 2006).

Recognizing that clinical reasoning develops from formal and experiential knowledge has implications for the curriculum and suggests that learning in clinical and classroom settings should be more equally balanced throughout medical school. The current model of mastering huge amounts of abstract knowledge without clinical context leads to cramming and forgetting ("binge and purge" is a hallmark of the pre-clerkship learning process and the sequential block-style clerkship year). Progressive disclosure of knowledge (formal and experiential) with active pedagogies of engagement will facilitate connecting these two types of knowledge. Immersion in clinical settings early helps students acquire situated knowledge and recognize that knowledge is distributed in those environments. Assessment that includes formative feedback and guidance as well as summative certification of competence at each level of development will ensure successful completion of undergraduate medical education.

Thus, although a great deal of progress has been made in undergraduate medical education, much work has yet to be done. The progressive and developmental nature of learning calls for greater longitudinal connections to be made among teachers, learners, and patients. This is needed across the four years of medical school. The participatory aspect of medical education, long a major strength of medical education, is now being tested by the financial pressures on the clinical enterprises that are marginalizing teaching and learning, as we discuss in Chapter Five. New models for teaching, assessing, and financing clinical education must be found. Finally, the situated and distributed nature of learning suggests that there has to be a stronger connection between clinical learning in specific contexts and formal knowledge basic to the practice of medicine. This would suggest the importance of fostering early clinical immersion and continuous connection of formal knowledge to clinical experience. These issues have consequences for curriculum, pedagogy, and assessment at the graduate level of medical education, which we address in Chapter Four.

4

THE RESIDENT'S EXPERIENCE

GRADUATE MEDICAL EDUCATION

AS DRAMATIC as the transformation from medical school matriculant to graduate is, the growth from beginning intern to residency graduate is even more remarkable. Four weeks after graduating from medical school, interns ("PG1s," for first postgraduate year) begin residency training, often in a new hospital in a new city (or country), neophytes in their chosen specialty, unfamiliar with their peers and supervisors as well as their new medical center's physical environment, protocols, and systems. Three to six years later, they depart, ready for subspecialty training or for independent practice of their discipline. Residency training gives medical school graduates the knowledge and skills required for practice of a specialty and the experience to apply their knowledge and skills with judgment and discernment. In the course of graduate education, they become their teachers' colleagues—and sometimes even their physicians.

In this chapter, we describe residency training as it is currently conducted in the United States. After an overview of the resident experience and a brief discussion of residency in the larger context of financing and regulation, we address in detail curricular structures, pedagogical practices, and approaches to assessment. We close with a discussion of key issues that affect how residents are supported in capitalizing on patient care opportunities to advance their knowledge, skills, and professional development. Through descriptive analysis and illustrative vignettes, we present examples of innovative approaches to residency education that we encountered in our fieldwork and highlight problems common to residency programs. In describing innovation, we draw particular attention to programs and practices that recognize the progressive and participatory nature of clinical learning and the situated and distributed nature of clinical knowledge and skills, premises about learning that we discussed in detail in Chapter Two.

The Residency Experience

○

Megan O'Neale is a twenty-eight-year-old second-year resident in internal medicine at a community hospital affiliated with a nearby medical school. Now in the fourth month of her PG2 year, she is in her second month of inpatient medicine, having completed a month of CCU and a consultation rotation in endocrinology. It's 12:45 p.m., and, sandwich in hand, she has stepped out of noon conference (a presentation by a member of the infectious diseases division on initial selection of antibiotic treatment for patients with a variety of serious infections) to touch base with her two interns and one subintern before leaving the hospital for her weekly afternoon outpatient clinic. Over the remainder of her year, the middle of a three-year training in internal medicine, Megan will do three more months of general inpatient wards, a month in the emergency department, and an elective month in her community's Planned Parenthood clinic, learning contraceptive management. Today she will see six patients in clinic before returning to the hospital to evaluate the patients her team has admitted while she was gone. She will spend the night in the hospital and won't head back to her apartment until 1:00 or 2:00 p.m. tomorrow.

○

GME is a complex amalgam of experiential learning powered by grad-uated participation in patient care in a variety of clinical settings, informal one-on-one and group case discussions, and formal didactic instruction. Whereas medical school, particularly the first two years, emphasizes the-oretical knowledge, principles, and general concepts, residency training is focused on the particular, using the residents' care of individual patients to support development of a detailed, nuanced experience with diseases and important clinical situations within their specialty. In addition to each resident's individual experience, GME is structured to afford substantial vicarious experience; thus residents learn not only from the patients they take care of but from good and bad outcomes experienced by their fellow residents' patients. At its best, the learning of residents is participatory, developmental and progressive, and situated and distributed.

The Learning Trajectory

From barely functional intern stymied by unfamiliar conditions, protocols, and systems to competent residency graduate capable of independent patient care across most of his specialty, the trajectory of a resident's learning can be characterized as a journey through a series of questions. For example, PG1s, caring for patients under close supervision and largely executing care designed by more advanced clinicians, are learning the answers to *how* questions: How do we assess the severity of community-acquired pneumonia? How are liver transplant patients stabilized postoperatively? How is an open appendectomy performed? Advanced residents are focused on *when* and *whether* questions: When should a patient with a low but real possibility of giant cell arteritis undergo temporal artery biopsy? Does this patient with pyelonephritis require admission? Should this patient with bowel obstruction from colon cancer undergo surgical decompression? As residents reach the final year of their training, they should have become competent in the usual management of common problems within their specialty. However, they are still on a steep learning curve with respect to advanced and complex problems within their specialty (Ringsted, Skaarup, Henriksen, & Davis, 2006).

Just as the nature of the residents' primary learning changes over the course of graduate medical education, the issues that they struggle with shift as well. Interns labor to master their new environments and learn how to get things done and how to function efficiently (Sheehan, Wilkinson, & Billett, 2005). In the procedural specialties, residents tackle progressively more challenging bedside and operative procedures. The first three years of a five-year general surgery residency is largely devoted to this technical mastery; in the fourth and fifth years, while gaining experience with the most challenging surgeries of the specialty, the residents learn to design management plans that their subordinates execute; to make decisions, often under conditions of significant uncertainty; and to tackle the *when* and *whether* questions. Because the tasks are so different, a resident who may have performed well under direction as an efficient, get-it-done intern can encounter significant difficulty as a team leader (Yao & Wright, 2005).

The "progressivity" of resident learning in the nonprocedural disciplines, such as pediatrics and family medicine, derives primarily from the greater role and increased responsibility they play in the care of patients, not from the fact that they are seeing different clinical conditions and learning procedures that are more technically demanding. The content of their learning is, of course, progressively more specialized as well, and the residents learn this primarily through consultation rotations in the subspecialties of their fields and through their exposure to the allied specialties of medicine. Like their surgical colleagues, advanced residents in nonprocedural fields are challenged to make decisions under conditions of uncertainty. Equally, delegation and team management may prove difficult for residents who performed well as interns. In both the procedural and nonprocedural fields, it is likely that individuals destined to arrive at the end of residency training well prepared to care independently for patients within their discipline follow divergent trajectories in arriving at that state of competence.

International Medical Graduates

It is important to keep in mind that a significant proportion of GME trainees face additional challenges to learning during residency. As we noted in Chapter One, every year about 27 percent of the PG1s graduate from non-U.S. medical schools (Hart et al., 2007), most arriving in the United States solely to pursue graduate medical education. In addition to the challenges of a new working environment and responsibilities, international medical graduates may struggle to adapt to U.S. mores, acquire the language skills necessary to comprehend regional accents and appreciate subtleties in discussion of treatment choices, and make sense of the U.S. health care system.

Regulation and Financing: Implications for GME

In Chapter Five, we describe regulation and financing of GME in the larger context of regulation of medical education, but we comment on both throughout this chapter because of the implications for the resident learning experience. Until recently, unlike UME, residency education has seen very little experimentation and innovation, reflecting, we believe, an inherent characteristic of the system: it is conservative on a number of levels and actively resists change. For example, the residency review committees that define the content of GME for every specialty are typically composed of physicians who have served, or are serving, as program directors and who may find it difficult to imagine radical reorganization of residency training within their specialty. Also, because residents are engaged in a significant amount of patient care, medical center administrators tend to assign them where the patients are, regardless of educational priorities. Of course, advances in medical science and the advent of new diseases have changed the epidemiology of inpatient medicine, but residency remains largely a hospital-based clinical experience in which residents see and care for whoever happens to be hospitalized.

Emphasis on Inpatient Care

Because the central activity of residency is direct patient care, resident participation in the care of patients extends and builds on the PBL learning cycle described in Chapter Three. However, rather than teachers devising paper, video, or standardized-patient cases to raise learning issues deemed appropriate for students at a given point in their education, assignment of residents to settings where patients with particular conditions or disease processes of a certain severity are diagnosed and treated is (or should be) what creates the learning opportunities the program intends. In this way, Megan O'Neale will learn about contraceptive management because she has chosen to do a month at Planned Parenthood. However, residents are not always assigned to clinical settings that have the greatest educational value. Tradition and time-honored agreements between departments and among clinical units are influential. Even more dominant in most residency training programs is the medical center; because the dollars associated with GME flow through the medical center, not the residency training programs, the medical center director can (and typically does) deploy the residents where there is the greatest need, not where the residents' education will be best served. For this reason, Megan will complete residency with stronger inpatient skills than outpatient abilities because, as do almost all residency programs, hers requires spending the significant majority of her time in hospital settings.

The few changes that transpired before the mid-1990s primarily concerned the length of training in a specialty: the pyramidal structure of residency training, especially in surgery, has been abandoned and young physicians embarking on a residency can now expect to complete a requisite number of years, assuming they are academically and professionally capable. Similarly, "short tracking," or truncating the internal medicine residency from three years to two and allowing early entry into subspecialty training such as cardiology or endocrinology, has been largely abolished, except for those planning careers in biomedical research who short-track into physician-scientist training programs where the two years of residency and four of research add up to the same six years of a conventional three-year residency and three-year fellowship.

However, over the past ten years, the ACGME has become increasingly activist. A transformation in the approach to assessment of residents, shifting the metrics from so-called time-and-process measures, in which satisfactory completion of residency is determined by counting the number of months a resident spent on various rotations, to a competency orientation is having profound effects on assessment programs and even on the structure and organization of residency training. Regulations governing shift length and mandating days off are likewise forcing reorganization of resident clinical assignments and creating an urgent need to make the graduate medical educational process more efficient. Meanwhile, concern is developing in some quarters about the absolute length of training, because it results in delayed delivery of surgeons to unsupervised practice (Coverdill et al., 2006) and of physician-investigators to independent researcher status (Zemlo, Garrison, Partridge, & Ley, 2000). This issue, combined with sharper focus on decreasing variability of approaches to common clinical problems and intense concentration on patient safety, is bringing significant external pressures to bear on the conduct of residency training. With this context in mind, we turn to the curriculum, pedagogy, and assessment of residency education.

The Residency Curriculum

As with the third and fourth years of medical school, but to an even greater degree, the patients seen and the clinical care delivered by residents constitute the curriculum. Repeated exposure to common and important conditions and participation in management afforded over the course of residency amounts to a structural form of "deliberate practice" (Ericsson, 2004) and results in a deep reservoir of tacit knowledge (Norman, 2006) that underlies clinical judgment (Mylopoulos & Regehr, 2007). Here we look at the residency curricula: the rotations and formal and informal teaching and learning activities.

Clinical Rotations

The basic unit of the residency calendar is the rotation or clinical assignment. Although most rotations last one month, residents may be assigned to core experiences such as inpatient internal medicine on a particular hospital unit for two months, and some ancillary or adjunctive rotations may be as short as two weeks (for example, an internal medicine resident might have a very brief clinical experience in dermatology or office gynecology). During a hospital rotation, residents are typically assigned to a team or service, caring for all the patients or a subset of the patients on that team. As patients are admitted from the emergency department or the clinic, they are assigned to services according to a schedule designed to moderate and balance the workflow across all the admitting residents in the specialty. The resident and his or her team care for the patient until discharge. Some residency training programs, most prominently in surgery, assign residents to faculty members rather than to geographical units or services. These three-to-six-month assignments, considered "apprenticeships," are intended to increase the resident's understanding of preadmission assessment and postoperative outpatient care, enhance the resident's understanding of the day-to-day professional life of a working surgeon, and facilitate establishment of a strong relationship between the resident surgeon and a faculty mentor. Although we did not encounter residency-level apprenticeship systems outside of surgery, it is likely that they exist, particularly in family medicine and in rural settings.

CONTINUITY CLINIC AND OUTPATIENT BLOCKS.   Residents also have responsibility for care of outpatients. For surgery and many subspecialty rotations in internal medicine and pediatrics, these outpatient experiences are integrated into inpatient-based rotations. For example, a PG3 in pediatrics doing a pediatric rheumatology rotation at a referral hospital might spend the bulk of her time caring for inpatients hospitalized on the rheumatology service and doing consultations on other hospitalized patients, but also see patients in rheumatology clinic two half-days a week. Similarly, an orthopedics resident doing two months on spine surgery would spend most of his time in the operating room and much of the remainder caring for hospitalized postoperative patients, but likely would see outpatients with back problems in clinic as well. Although surgery is a hospital-based specialty, outpatient experience is critical to surgical training, as residents must learn to make a surgical diagnosis, select the operative plan, and care for the patient preoperatively and postoperatively. A variety of factors, including the increasing importance of outpatient surgery and duty-hour limitation, are making it increasingly difficult for surgical residents to participate continuously over an episode of surgical illness (Melck, Weber, & Sidhu, 2007).

Continuity clinic is a key part of the education of residents in the generalist disciplines, whether or not they will ultimately specialize. Residents in internal medicine, pediatrics, family medicine, and often neurology and obstetrics and gynecology have a panel of patients whom they care for over time. Continuity clinics may be longitudinally arranged, with the resident seeing outpatients the same half-day, week in and week out, or arranged in blocks of a month. Many programs, particularly those emphasizing primary care, use both designs. Some programs take this even farther, organizing pairs or teams of residents in a shared practice (Sharif & Ozuah, 2001). In this model, a pair or small team of residents shares care for a panel of patients. The residents' schedules are coordinated so that when one resident or half the team is doing an intense inpatient rotation, the partners have an outpatient block and can care seamlessly for their colleagues' patients.

Resident continuity clinics are administratively challenging and often do not achieve the intended continuity or the desired connection among trainees, patients, and their families over time (Melck et al., 2007; Smith, Morris, Hill, Francovich, & Christiano, 2006; Smith, Morris, Francovich, Hill, & Gieselman, 2004). The patient no-show rate can be high, and many appointment slots are taken by other physicians' patients needing drop-in care. Continuity clinics have been additionally compromised by the mandates of duty-hour reduction. For example, the stipulation that a resident who has worked twenty-four hours overnight in the hospital not work more than six hours the next day prohibits an afternoon clinic following a night on call. Although this discontinuity compromises the ability of residents in outpatient settings to observe illness unfolding over time and the course of convalescence (neither of which is easily appreciated from the perspective of an inpatient unit), it does yield opportunities to strengthen skills in collaboration and team care. Unfortunately, because of limited resources for outpatient education, most residency programs have not capitalized on this opportunity.

Our observations suggest that training in ambulatory care needs increased attention across GME, from the outpatient-based generalist specialties to the subspecialties of surgery. Many of the deficits we observed reflect the intrinsic difficulty of the work: the short visits and time pressures, lack of clinical definition of many problems seen in the outpatient setting, and intermittent patient availability for reassessment. Further, because no education funds are associated with resident education in outpatient settings, the teaching faculty are often attempting to see their own patients while supervising residents. Moreover, medical education's commitment to outpatient education has been limited. Although medical students, and likely the public, tend to regard inpatient medicine as particularly intense, complex, and challenging, the demands of outpatient medicine with its high-stakes distinctions that must be made between potentially very ill and not-so-sick patients should not be underestimated or underrepresented in residency training.

SKILLS, RESEARCH, AND OTHER ROTATIONS.   Residency programs are increasingly providing options for residents beyond clinical care in their home program. Rotations may be designed to accomplish specific goals in clinical skills development, often without direct patient care involved. For example, Atlantic Health's procedural skills block for PG1s allows interns to learn and practice procedures fundamental to inpatient medicine—venipuncture, IV insertion, placement of a Foley catheter, lumbar puncture, arterial blood gas sampling, and so on—under the supervision of phlebotomists, nurses, and physicians. Once the intern can perform the procedure at an appropriate level of proficiency, either on a fellow intern volunteer or in a simulation setting, she is credentialed to perform it on patients under her care. Likewise telemedicine rotations, where residents learn skills in telephone management and distance consultation, augment the skills residents learn in face-to-face care of patients.

To meet the ACGME requirement that all residents learn the methods of scholarship; gain experience collecting, analyzing, and presenting medical information; and contribute to the field, residencies offer research blocks for advanced residents. In large academic surgery departments, for example, residents are often required to do a year of research. Work abroad is increasingly popular as well, and many large academic programs offer opportunities in global health.

Curriculum Didactics: Meetings and Conferences

---
o

It is 7:00 a.m. and a small group has gathered in the hospital cafeteria. Dr. Paul Starker is meeting with two surgery interns at Morristown Hospital, part of Atlantic Health. Over coffee and muffins, Dr. Starker guides a discussion of repair of inguinal hernias. Using a gentle Socratic approach, he explores the interns' understanding of methods of repair, their pros and cons, and the history of various technical approaches. Taking a piece of paper, he makes informal diagrams to reinforce his teaching points. At 7:45 a.m., the three head off to clinic.

---
o

The formal and informal activities that contribute to the residency curriculum range from frequent attending rounds to monthly departmental meetings. Several times a day, for example, residents meet with their faculty supervisor to discuss the patients on their service. They may sit down together in a conference room, or the resident and faculty member, with or without the other members of the team, may move from room to room, checking on patients and reviewing the diagnostic thinking and next steps for care. These daily scheduled meetings, called attending rounds, allow the faculty physician to probe the knowledge base and understanding of the students and residents on the team, observe the teaching and leadership of the most senior resident on the team, and offer direct teaching.

In the cognitive specialties (internal medicine, pediatrics, neurology), the residents assigned to the inpatient service meet daily with a senior physician, perhaps the chief of the service, or several senior physicians to discuss newly admitted patients and those who present interesting, instructive, or difficult diagnostic or management problems. This meeting, called residents' report or morning report, is organized by a chief resident selected to do an extra year on the basis of exceptional clinical and teaching skills. Residents' report allows peer teaching (Smith et al., 2009), as well as the input of the near-peer chief residents and the senior faculty physicians. At USCF, the chief residents in medicine prepare one-page written summaries of complicated or unfamiliar issues discussed in residents' reports. These summaries are posted on the department's website. Morning report is typically the teaching conference that residents most highly value (Gross, Donnelly, Reisman, Sepkowitz, & Callahan, 1999). However, its dynamics require careful attention to achieve appropriate rigor while avoiding an excessively competitive or intimidating environment. Although the morning report is most characteristic of the cognitive specialties, some surgical residencies have experimented successfully with it (Stiles et al., 2006).

Much teaching at the resident level occurs as informal clinical discussions. As was previously noted, residents typically take advantage of the fact that their entire team is assembled in the hospital on admitting days to go over a common issue in the discipline or teach about a topic they have recently reviewed in response to a patient problem. Faculty do much the same thing: an attending on a medicine service, discovering that the previous evening of admissions has brought two patients whose serum sodium is low though for different reasons, may spend fifteen minutes in attending rounds leading the PG1s in interactive discussion of the differential diagnosis and initial evaluation of hyponatremia. Expecting that the topic is comfortable for the PG2, the attending may offer the resident the opportunity to correct a misunderstanding on the part of one of the interns, thus assessing both the resident's knowledge and her approach to teaching. Likewise, except when a technical challenge or an untoward development commands everyone's full attention, much time in the operating room is spent in clinical discussion.

Of course, there are many scheduled teaching conferences as well, such as the noon conference Megan O'Neale attended on empiric use of antibiotics. The ACGME demands that every residency program have a formal curriculum and document how it is delivered to the trainees. Traditionally, this "delivery" has been accomplished through early morning, lunchtime, or preclinic conferences, but some residency programs are now devoting a half-day to resident education. Arrangements are often made for residents to pass off their pagers so that the educational sessions are not interrupted by clinical chores. At Henry Ford Hospital, the education half-day for the surgery house staff begins with an hourlong session attended by all. The group then splits up by year of training for didactics appropriate to each level. Residency programs with a strong component of longitudinal outpatient experience typically have a thirty-minute clinic conference preceding or following clinic and covering common problems in ambulatory care in the discipline or featuring a challenging diagnostic or management problem. In an effort to ensure the consistency of coverage of content, regardless of which faculty member is supervising, and to accommodate residents who are unable to attend conferences because of schedule conflicts, core content is now being made available to residents online. This kind of asynchronous teaching is effective if the faculty are engaged and hold their residents responsible for the web modules (Maddaus, Chipman, Whitson, Groth, & Schmitz, 2008).

Grand rounds is the most venerable of the traditional teaching conferences. Originally, this was a clinical discussion, often with the patient present. A resident, or perhaps a community physician, would present the patient's history and then a professor would call attention to important features of the history and physical examination and conduct a learned discussion of the condition at hand. Now more commonly it is a weekly fifty-minute formal conference, emphasizing recent research or review of a clinical topic. The educational value of this exercise has been questioned (Hebert & Wright, 2003; Mueller, Segovis, Litin, Habermann, & Thomas, 2006).

Departments hold a morbidity and mortality (M and M) conference weekly to monthly. This systematic review of complications that have occurred on every clinical service is a requirement of the Joint Commission (until 2007, the Joint Commission on the Accreditation of Health Care) but is also an important occasion for teaching. Historically, residents regarded M and M with trepidation because they were often pilloried for complications and poor patient outcomes, sometimes despite executing care specifically directed by a faculty member. Increasingly, discussions in M and M are being structured so that the focus is less on individual culpability, or "blame and shame," and instead more on system failings (Bates, Shore, Gibson, & Bosk, 2003; Gore, 2006; Kravet, Howell, & Wright, 2006; Prince et al., 2007). Through these conferences, residents see faculty modeling responses to error and learn skills such as root-cause analysis.

During our fieldwork, we observed some conferences where residents were present but the educational potential of the moment was underused. Discharge planning rounds is one such conference (Mistiaen, Francke, & Poot, 2007) that we consider a missed opportunity. This multidisciplinary conference, attended by nurses, social workers, at least one member of the physician team, and often others, focuses on making arrangements for patients whose hospital discharge is likely to be complicated by a poor home situation, complex medical needs, cognitive challenges, behavioral difficulties, or some combination of these and other problems. Discharge planning rounds seemed to be regarded by the residents as a clinical administrative chore, a sort of necessary evil and not a learning opportunity—a perception perhaps reinforced by the faculty supervisor rarely being part of the discharge planning group. This is, however, an important opportunity to observe residents collaborating with nonphysician members of the health care team and engaging in systems-based practice. We found no descriptions of GME-level programs focused on the discharge planning process, corroborating our sense that this is an overlooked but promising forum for interprofessional education. Perhaps the escalating attention to quality and publicity about the startling readmission rate for Medicare patients will raise the stature of this exercise.

Stimulated, Directed, and Self-Directed Learning

In the process of delivering supervised care, the experience with patients, either as individuals or collectively, raises questions in the mind of the resident or causes her to recognize knowledge or skill gaps. These questions and gaps should stimulate learning, encouraged and guided as needed by faculty and other supervisors and participants in care. In fact, given the distributed nature of information in the clinical environment, something as simple as a discussion about a patient with his nurse or with a medical student who was a physical therapist before enrolling in medical school may result in learning. However it occurs, the obligation to provide high-quality care should lead to recursive assessment of the match between the resident's knowledge and skills, the capabilities of the care team, and the needs of the patient (Croskerry, 2003; Kuiper & Pesut, 2004). If the patient needs more than the team can deliver, it is the responsibility of the resident, with the support of the supervising faculty member, to correct the mismatch.

Reading is the primary method by which residents address knowledge gaps. However, surprisingly little is known about how much residents read and what their sources of information are (Lai et al., 2006). Furthermore, there have been obvious, widespread, and profound changes in how medical learners, and residents in particular, relate to the medical knowledge base. A generation ago, third-year students used simple textbooks; interns relied heavily on spiral-bound manuals, and residents tackled the key textbooks of their specialty, leavened as their graduate training progressed, by the reading of original papers. Many of these references are now available online, but more has changed than the method of access; there is now a vast array of just-in-time information sources, the market leader being UpToDate (http://www.uptodate.com). Investigators at the Mayo Clinic exploited the fact that the software tracks use (the time during which a topic is open, and whether a topic is printed) to evaluate the association among accessing the electronic resource, attendance at clinical conferences, and year-over-year improvement on the In-Training Examination (ITE). Adjusted for demographics and prior achievement, self-directed use of the electronic resource twenty minutes or more a day was associated with a 4.5 percent improvement in the ITE score, comparable to the 5.1 percent improvement associated with an additional year of residency education (McDonald, Zeger, & Kolars, 2007). However, some faculty members told us they are concerned that, given the easy availability of authoritative information from sources such as UpToDate and the stipulations of duty-hour reduction, residents are not investing in reading to build their fund of knowledge and deepen understanding as they did in the past. Perhaps paradoxically, individuals in residency programs with a less strong academic history may actually be reading more, with their reading monitored by faculty members, in an effort to attain or maintain an acceptable board passage rate (de Virgilio, Chan, Kaji, & Miller, 2008).

JOURNAL CLUB. Residents conduct many formal didactic sessions, including talks expected as part of consultation and elective rotations, resident-led clinic conferences, capstone presentations given by graduating residents and chief residents, and journal club. Journal club is typically a monthly exercise that is intended to be a forum for discussion of recent papers in the specialty as well as a mechanism for residents to learn how to assess the quality and import of clinical research papers; residents are expected to select an original research paper, not a review (Alguire, 1998). The critique of the investigative methods is as important as the clinical conclusion; the presenting resident is expected to lead a discussion that culminates with the question, "Will this study change my practice?" Both procedurally oriented specialties and cognitive specialties such as internal medicine hold journal clubs. However, because large randomized clinical trials are less common in disciplines such as surgery, in those areas the research literature tends to focus on developing and testing innovative technical approaches. Some journal clubs are more broadly focused, emphasizing, for example, the perspective and experience of the patient (Cave & Clandinin, 2007).

TEACHING BY RESIDENTS. Residents also teach subordinates. In addition to formal exercises, such as presentation of a topic review during a consult month or leading a discussion of a paper at journal club, residents conduct impromptu teaching sessions and teach almost continuously in the course of supervising the patient care given by their juniors. Both the resident teachers and their team members benefit from this teaching, the junior members for the usual reasons and the residents because they often must further their own understanding in order to articulate concepts and approaches to beginners and are sometimes required to research a topic to adequately respond to a student's questions (Boud, Cohen, & Sampson, 2001; Sobral, 2002; Tang, Hernandez, & Adams, 2004).

Even first-year residents, neophytes themselves, are expected to support the learning of their juniors, the medical students on the service. These teaching responsibilities expand as residents progress; a fifth-year surgery resident will assist his third-year resident in learning surgical approaches of moderate complexity as well as beginning to address the *when* and *whether* questions of surgical management. He will also oversee the third-year resident's teaching and supervision of the interns and students on the service. Likewise, a third-year pediatrics resident doing an inpatient rotation at a large teaching hospital will oversee several PG1s, a third-year student, a fourth-year subintern, and perhaps a pharmacy student or nurse practitioner. Admitting days offer a particularly rich stimulus for learning and teaching, both because newly admitted patients bring new conditions and problems to consider and because there is frequently some downtime in the interval between admissions.

Pedagogies for Residency Education

What a resident learns in the course of her residency education is not the result of random patient care experiences. It is purposeful and developmental and reflects—or should reflect—a careful structuring, sequencing, and progression of roles, activities, and responsibilities to support learning. When an activity is at the boundary of a resident's competence, the attending will create an opportunity for low-stakes practice by asking the resident to describe the care he intends to administer ("Tell me what you make of this and what you are planning to do") or having the resident perform the care under direct observation, or both. On Megan O'Neale's team, for example, the resident has a similar relationship with the intern, and the intern has a comparable relationship with the third-year student. This highly structured set of relationships, characterized by layers of delegation and supervision, operates to allow clinical learners at various points in training to focus on practicing tasks they have just learned and on pushing the boundaries of their skills and understanding to the next level while avoiding undue risk to patients

(Carraccio, Benson, Nixon, & Derstine, 2008; ten Cate & Scheele, 2007).

Whereas medical students' interactions with patients often feature just one element (taking a history, examining the heart, placing a Foley catheter), residents' interactions engage patient care more holistically. Correspondingly, although those who supervise residents may use decomposition, breaking down of tasks or concepts, and other approaches to simplify the learning task (Grossman et al., 2009), pedagogies at the graduate level tend to be multipurpose. Thus two distinctive features of clinical teaching at the residency level are (1) the dominance of peer- and near-peer teaching and (2) the complex role of the faculty supervisor, who serves as the teacher, the supervisor of care and guarantor of quality, the team leader (a role shared with the senior-most resident), and in some cases the patient's own long-term physician.

Although contemporary conceptions from the learning sciences focus on the student, the teacher is nonetheless important. The relationships that attendings establish with residents on a clinical rotation powerfully affect those residents' estimation of the learning value of that rotation (Kendrick, Simmons, Richards, & Roberge, 1993). The distributed sources of teaching make the environment for learning at the residency level rich and stimulating. Because of the complexity, any discussion of how teaching occurs at the resident level must necessarily simplify quite dramatically. For example, our discussion focuses on physician-to-physician teaching, though there are of course others in the environment who have significant expertise but no explicit teaching role (most important, nurses).

In contrast to the powerful teaching that happens in the course of patient care, the planned teaching sessions on preset topics and other formal didactic settings that we observed were largely unadventurous. We saw many examples of resident conferences with chairs arranged in rows, Microsoft PowerPoint presentations, minimal interaction between the presenter and the residents, and no peer-to-peer discussion intended or encouraged. In general, UME educators are more actively experimenting with novel pedagogies, such as team-based learning, to promote learning in large-group and formal settings than are their GME colleagues.

Pedagogies for Conceptual Understanding

As in UME, case discussion is GME's signature pedagogy. However, the primary point is no longer mastery of the form, as it is for medical students, but exploration of the presenter's underlying understanding and creation of opportunities to invite the participation of other learners.

Usually, the case is used in clinical discussions about patients that the team is responsible for, but skilled teachers use it to good effect in formal settings as well.

○

Forty-some general surgery residents of various levels are gathered in a well-appointed small amphitheater for their educational half-day. The teacher is an energetic young radiologist; the topic for the session is Interesting Abdominal CT Scans. The faculty radiologist has brought several of her learners, radiology residents doing an interventional radiology rotation, with her. She projects a CT image, provides a thumbnail clinical sketch, and gives the group a minute to study the scan. Then she poses a question: "What do you see?" Remarkably, she seems to know the names of most of the surgery residents. Calling on one of the PG2s, she asks for a description of the salient findings. She then turns to a PG3 for the differential diagnosis and asks one of the radiology residents to refine the surgeon's suggestions. At one point, she asks the radiology residents to discuss how the information that the surgeon puts on the requisition assists them in the reading room. The atmosphere is lively and friendly, but many of the patients presented are gravely ill. The stakes are clear, and all the residents are quiet, engaged, and attentive.

○

Case discussions involve considerable to and fro. How they are perceived by learners and their effectiveness as a teaching strategy depends on the atmosphere established by the teacher. If the questions asked are low-level (Wilen, 1991), with a definite right answer and involving an obscure point of factual knowledge, learners will hesitate to participate, particularly in teaching situations where multiple levels of learners are present, for fear that a more advanced learner (or even worse, a less advanced learner) knows the answer to a question that the person called on cannot answer correctly. However, skillfully managed large-group case discussions are an engaging and efficient approach to teaching (Barnes, 1994). Some work has been done with resident learners that demonstrates how learning can be potentiated through use of audience response systems (ARS); residents had modestly greater learning gains at the conclusion of the teaching session and much better retention three months later when small-group case-based teaching was augmented by ARS (Pradhan, Sparano, & Ananth, 2005; Schackow, Chavez, Loya, & Friedman, 2004). Questioning is a particularly characteristic approach to teaching in the operating room. Again, quizzing, or, as it is commonly called, "pimping," can either make learners afraid to take risks or, if the appropriate level of challenge and support is given, energize and excite learners (Brancati, 1989; Detsky, 2009).

A central function of the case discussion is to make visible the reasoning underlying the clinical formulation and management strategy for a particular patient. The teacher may interrupt a case presentation to create progressive disclosure and give other members on the team an opportunity to participate. We saw many examples of attendings pausing one intern's presentation to ask a second intern, "What would you be thinking of at this point? What would concern you most?" These high-level questions present learning opportunities at no risk to the patient. As learners practice case formulation and propose approaches to management, the faculty physician and more senior residents gain insights into the developing sophistication of their junior colleagues. Residents greatly appreciate the invitation to propose management strategies. As one surgical resident remarked, "The best question an attending can ask is, 'What do you think we should do?'" Rather than having residents, who are of course relatively advanced learners, simply execute the management strategies of their attendings, posing such questions allows the teacher to build a strong sense of the resident's fund of knowledge, attention to key findings, and ability to prioritize. Any ensuing negotiation of the care plan is an opportunity for the resident to notice where her plan did not match the attending's and where she may have a knowledge gap.

The numerous occasions of resident teaching are also an opportunity for residents to reflect on and improve their approaches to instruction (Busari & Scherpbier, 2004). Work rounds, the daily or twice-daily bedside visit conducted as a team, with the acting intern or intern presenting an update to the team on patients' changes in clinical status and diagnostic test results, afford rich opportunities for residents to explore their subordinates' understanding of patients' conditions.

Pedagogies for Practice and Performance

Clinical medicine is a practice and is learned through experience. Asking how clinical medicine might be taught and learned in a way that is safe and respectful for patients and learners alike (Berry, 2008; Kennedy, Regehr, Baker, & Lingard, 2005) is a complex question. The attitudes embodied in the approaches to resident learning express the professional values of the field and affect, potentially significantly, the capabilities of new residency graduates. In other words, even though it might seem desirable to have residents practice under conditions of quite constrained independence, to the extent that they do not exercise their own decision-making capabilities and do not undertake challenging procedures while they are in an educational environment, with support and supervision, they will presumably have to learn to make those same decisions and do those same procedures as independent practitioners. Having decisions made and procedures performed by the most experienced physician available is not a bad thing, but it comes at a cost.

The trend over the past three decades has been to more closely supervise residents; it is accelerated by concerns about patient safety, despite evidence that teaching hospitals provide safer and higher-quality care than do hospitals that do not host graduate medical education (Allison et al., 2000; Ayanian & Weissman, 2002). This trend is combined with an absolute and dramatic increase in what residents have to learn as a result of development of new techniques and advances in medical science and a 24 percent decrease in the average resident work week as a consequence of duty-hour reduction mandates. Residents and their teachers are concerned that there simply is not enough time in residency training to become competent and prepared for independent patient care at the completion of residency training. This concern is particularly acute in the procedural fields, where practicing motor skills is essential to achieving acceptable performance (Grady, Batjer, & Dacey, 2009).

Thus, in all residencies attendings are available twenty-four hours a day to hear cases and advise regarding management. The rules governing when the resident must discuss care with the attending vary from program to program and within resident-attending pairs. Some faculty members ask to be called for every new admission; others, believing that one of the key things residents should be learning is when they need help, allow more latitude (Stewart, 2008). Typically, however, the faculty supervisor would expect to be notified in real time of significant changes in clinical status (raising the possibility of transfer to the intensive care unit, for example) and patients needing imminent surgery.

SIMULATION. The opportunity to practice decision making and procedural intervention in settings where the well-being of actual patients is not at stake is now recognized as one way to address some of these important practical and ethical challenges (Wayne et al., 2006). Simulation is generally associated with high- or low-fidelity facsimiles of physical environments, mannequins, and procedures. However, as we suggested earlier in discussing teaching through cases, it is important to recognize that teachers who ask questions of the *what-if* type are creating intellectual simulations. For example, a skilled teacher in a nonprocedural field, faced with a routine admission, will put a twist on the question to allow learners to practice at a higher level of challenge than the patient at hand actually affords.

One of the strengths of simulation is the opportunity it creates for residents to isolate the elements of complex procedures, such as surgery, and practice them in a progressive sequence. This breaking down, or decomposition, of complexity can make it easier for learners to appreciate and master the component steps. For example, computer science students at the University of Washington, in collaboration with faculty in the department of surgery, have developed computer programs in which the steps of such common surgeries as herniorrhaphy, appendectomy, and cholecystectomy are represented on a computer screen as images of the operative field (see http://www.isis.washington.edu/classes.html#T1). The trainee's task is to select, in proper sequence, the correct instrument from a tray also shown on the computer screen and touch the appropriate place in the "operative field" with the virtual instrument. Certainly, this has nothing to do with the ability to operate on live patients or even to correctly maneuver real surgical instruments, but it does require that the surgery intern learn the steps of the operation and the associated instruments and proceed through the surgery in the correct sequence. Only then does the intern move on to using the actual instruments in a box trainer.

Some residents believe that simulations are better suited to familiarization with surgical instruments than actually learning how to perform procedures because mannequins and models do not display the anatomical variation found in nature and because it is difficult to represent the "feel" of handling living tissue (or haptics) persuasively. Conversely, very low-fidelity simulations can be a powerful learning experience if the learner engages with the premises of the simulation and takes the experience as real (Hamstra, Dubrowski, & Backstein, 2006).

Simulations also afford an important opportunity for doing and redoing complex care under conditions of pressure, or even crisis. The leaders of the simulation center at the University of Washington stress the importance of designing simulation exercises that are ambitious enough to create the opportunity to learn in multiple domains in one exercise. As an example, the director described being approached by a faculty member in urology who wanted a simulation on the placement of a suprapubic bladder catheter for his residents. The director persuaded the faculty member to think more broadly, and the result was an emergency-room simulation involving nursing students, a medical resident, and a urology resident. The "patient" presents with symptoms the nursing students should recognize as likely bladder outlet obstruction. The nursing students and medical resident work together to pass a Foley catheter but have difficulty. Together, they are expected to recognize when they need the assistance of a subspecialty colleague. Finally, the urology resident, also unable to pass the Foley catheter, does the suprapubic procedure. The simulation was broadened beyond a simple technical skill to cover inter-professional communication, assessment, judgment, consultative skills, and patient reassurance.

Similarly, simulations can be organized so that they benefit a broader group than just those with a role to play. At the University of Florida campus in Jacksonville, we observed a mixed group of internal medicine residents, emergency medicine residents, and nursing students working on a severe asthma simulation. An emergency medicine faculty member initially played the agitated, dyspneic patient until intubation was required; the patient role was then taken by a mannequin. Although there were only three or four active roles, the simulation was attentively observed by a group of about twenty, taking notes on a structured form. When it came time to debrief (a critical element in effective simulation), the observers were as much a part as those who had been hands-on participants.

FROM LEARNING SKILLS TO PRACTICING PROCEDURES. Eventually, of course, learners must apply their growing skills to the care of real patients. Creating systems and strategies to allow residents to acquire and practice skills, gain experience and develop judgment, and feel the weight of responsibility for the well-being of their patients is at the heart of clinical teaching. Despite their obvious contrasts, both procedural and nonprocedural disciplines approach this similarly: by making careful assessments of a resident's capabilities and offering him or her opportunities, under supervision, just beyond the limit of those capabilities. Aspects of care that the faculty supervisor is confident the resident can address unaided are delegated to the trainee to be performed independently, although the faculty member remains responsible. The attending or another more senior physician takes on the elements of care that the resident has not mastered, often with the resident assisting or observing.

To offer challenging learning opportunities for residents who are working toward competence as independent practitioners, while ensuring that patients receive care of the same quality they would receive were trainees not involved, at least three conditions must be met (Kennedy, Lingard, Baker, Kitchen, & Regehr, 2007). First, physician teachers must be able to correctly gauge the capabilities of their juniors, specifically the decisions and procedures they can undertake without direct supervision. If attendings are not able to do this accurately, quality of care may be compromised as residents make decisions or perform procedures with insufficient knowledge and skill. Likewise, resident learning will be compromised if the person is oversupervised and micromanaged in performing elements of care that she is capable of on her own. Second, residents must be able to identify when a situation is beyond their abilities or experience (Berry, 2008; Stewart, 2008); of course, this is a necessity for all physicians, not just those in training. Third, having identified the resident's "learning edge," faculty must be able to construct opportunities that provide challenge and allow the trainee to build skills and gain experience without hazarding patient safety.

In the cognitive specialties, in which nuanced judgment is paramount, the developmental progression stems not so much from having residents engage with progressively more challenging diagnoses over their graduate medical education but from playing a more central and responsible role. Thus an intern in internal medicine will perform a history and physical examination of a newly admitted patient with community-acquired pneumonia. She would be expected to be able to generate an appropriate list of diagnostic possibilities to account for the patient's symptoms, physical findings, and laboratory abnormalities, but not to act on her diagnostic impressions. At the PG1 level, this experience with management decisions would be acquired largely through verbal practice. Only after more junior residents have repeatedly rehearsed complex care do they begin to take on components of it, under supervision.

In the case of specialties in which procedural and technical competence is central, developmental educational progression is achieved by having residents learn and practice first the simple parts of simple procedures, then the more complex parts, and then the entire procedure. They proceed to the simpler parts of more demanding procedures, and so on. In surgery, for example, residents progress from observing to assisting with minor components of a surgery, to the role of first assistant. The first assistant stands on the opposite side of the table from the surgeon and essentially "co-operates." This requires detailed knowledge of the surgical procedure, the ability to adjust to anatomical variations and unexpected developments, and familiarity with the operating surgeon's procedures and preferences. Then, initially with more straightforward procedures and ultimately with complex operations, the resident takes the role of the operating surgeon and the faculty member serves as the first assistant. The attending surgeon thus cedes "motor control" but retains visual and overall control; if he believes that the resident is going off track he may try to guide indirectly, perhaps by suggesting another exposure. Failing that, he may provide direct instruction, or in more extreme circumstances resume motor control (Moulton, 2010).

In this manner a surgical resident progresses from doing an incision and drainage under direct supervision while still an intern, to performing a hemicolectomy as a late third-year resident, and then executing a complex vascular procedure such as an abdominal aortic aneurysmectomy as a fifth-year resident nearing completion of training.

Of course, faculty surgeons vary in their willingness to entrust the role of operating surgeon to a resident; this can be a particular challenge for more junior faculty who may lack confidence in their ability to assess a resident's skill level, prevent a misadventure, or recover from a resident error. Some surgery departments, including the Department of Surgery at Northwestern University, have faculty development programs intended to assist younger faculty members in learning supervisory styles that decrease their need to take over the case. At the Mayo Clinic, where surgery residents spend several months at a time in an apprenticeship pairing with a faculty surgeon, the pairings are based largely on the faculty member's pattern of practice. A surgery teacher, regardless of seniority or stature, who is quite reluctant to cede the operating surgeon's position to a resident, would be paired with a PG1 or PG2, for whom the observer or assistant role is appropriate, whereas a surgeon just starting his career would be partnered with a PG4 or PG5 if he is able to work confidently from the first assistant position.

How well can attending physicians judge the ability of residents? A study at the University of Washington assessed the psychomotor skills of surgical residents at a low-fidelity task trainer for minimally invasive surgery. Beginning residents performed far less well than faculty physicians in terms of fluency and economy of motion and avoidance of excessive force. Residents made modest gains over years one and two of residency, associated with opportunities to learn and practice simple procedures. The second and more substantial gain in psychomotor skills was seen over the fourth and particularly over the fifth year of residency, as the surgical residents tackled (under supervision) more demanding procedures, including advanced laparoscopic procedures. Perhaps more important, in the second phase of the same study faculty surgeons were asked to review the videotapes of the task trainer performance. They were able, with only brief observation, to identify the level of the trainee simply by watching him or her move the instruments (Rosen, Hannaford, Richards, & Sinanan, 2001).

At its best, supervision is unobtrusive, but this unobtrusiveness does not mean the resident is functioning autonomously. Good teachers construct a "learning space" for residents, setting an appropriate level of challenge while ensuring that the care the patient receives is equivalent to the care he would have received if the faculty physician were treating him directly.

Midlevel and advanced residents contribute some elements of care without direct observation by an attending, reflecting the faculty physician's determination that the resident's skill level is adequate to the complexity usually encountered in the setting and the attending's confidence that the resident recognizes the bounds of her capabilities (Teunissen, Boor, et al., 2007). In this situation, there is regular communication between the attending and the resident, and the attending is available to come to the bedside when needed. This progressive delegation is important for the maturation of the resident, who needs to be ready to practice independently at completion of the residency.

Pedagogies for Inquiry, Innovation, and Improvement

Residency education, like medical education in general, is overwhelmingly focused on bringing learners up to speed with the current state of the art. However, pedagogies that concentrate on conveying today's knowledge and skills may fail to prepare residents to unlearn today's practices and learn new concepts and approaches. More important, teaching approaches that treat today's understandings and methods as the end goal of education represent medical knowledge as static and fail to recruit residents as field builders in medicine.

Done effectively, an evidence-based approach to discussion of diagnostic testing strategies and treatment selection can serve to highlight areas in which field building is needed. Residents who are expected to justify their proposed diagnostic or therapeutic approach will need to develop an awareness of the state of their specialty. For a particular clinical situation, is the proposed treatment solidly established as preferred by virtue of multiple clinical trials, rigorously compiled as a systematic review, supported only by a consensus of experts, or merely endorsed by local custom? Evidence-based medicine is sometimes regarded as inimical to intellectual approaches more based in fundamental mechanisms and hence linked to the sciences underlying medicine, but this is a false dichotomy (Timmermans & Angell, 2001). "Basic science thinking" generates hypotheses that can, and should, be tested in clinical trials; conversely, empiric observations can generate ideas about possible basic mechanisms to be explored in the laboratory. Thus pedagogies that support learners in preparing for productive inquiry use an orientation to evidence-based medicine that holds residents responsible not only for knowing what to do but also for the level of evidence that a particular approach is better. In addition, where the basis for preference for one treatment over another is weak, residents should be encouraged to think about what better evidence would look like and how it might be acquired.

Ideally, when feasible, residents should be encouraged to proceed to implement the studies they devise; the Goldman Cardiac Risk Index (Goldman et al., 1978) is an example of a study conceived and undertaken collaboratively by residents at a single institution, to the benefit of patients and an entire specialty. Teachers should press residents to consider what a clinical trial might mean with respect to pathogenic mechanisms and to generate testable hypotheses. The resident who knows that, as of 2009, many clinical studies have not demonstrated a benefit of tight glucose control in preventing cardiovascular events in patients with diabetes should be encouraged not to stop there but to wonder why this might be, in terms of fundamental mechanisms.

Pedagogies for field building must constantly focus the attention of learners not just on what they do not yet know but on where medicine's gaps are (Bereiter & Scardamalia, 1993). These are not *how* questions; they are not even *whether* or *when* questions. They are *what next* questions: What do we need to understand better to deliver effective care to patients? Sometimes these are basic science questions: What do we need to understand better about the pathogenesis of this condition? Residency programs, particularly in the large training programs based in schools of medicine, have traditionally aspired to train future academics and have recruited medical school graduates who already possess a track record of participating in research. Many GME programs make it possible for residents to participate at least modestly in a research investigation during residency; most academic surgery programs expect residents to take one to two years during residency to work in a lab. However, not all important questions in medicine have to do with fundamental mechanisms, for the answers to very practical questions can be field builders as well (How can the treatments that we know benefit patients be more effectively delivered?) In fact, very few of the sixteen thousand students who graduate from U.S. medical schools every year will engage in basic science or clinical research, but all practitioners can engage with questions of designing their own practice to improve the effectiveness of the care they provide and improving the health of their community.

Increasingly, residents are undertaking mentored quality-improvement projects (Krajewski, Siewert, Yam, Kressel, & Kruskal, 2007; Philibert, 2008), like the one in the internal medicine residency at the University of Pennsylvania that we describe later in this chapter. Many projects of this type conceptualize the resident's work environment, whether an inpatient unit or an outpatient clinic, as a microsystem (Nelson et al., 2002). Residents, along with other participants and stakeholders, are empowered to study the microsystems in which they find themselves, identify their shortcomings, develop improvement plans, actually make changes in the processes of care, and then restudy the system to ascertain if the desired effects have been achieved (Tess et al., 2009).

Teaching approaches that support development of skills in system redesign involve both the interactions of individual faculty members with residents and, even more important, creation of possibilities within residency programs and the medical settings that house them. Residency training programs must leave more time for trainees to engage seriously with this set of competencies, and medical center and hospital administrators must invite residents into the venues in which important operational and management decisions are made. In addition to the benefit that could accrue to the systems on which residents focus their attention, this type of work allows residents to acquire a broader knowledge base, develop skills in interdisciplinary collaboration and teamwork, and cultivate the professional attributes required to do difficult work in systems change. Rather than excluding residents, medical centers should include their trainees, and use their intimate and detailed experience with what works well and what does not to improve processes of care.

Because this is unfamiliar territory for faculty and trainees alike, it is ill suited for formal didactic teaching methods; role modeling and coaching are likely to work better. However, there is formal knowledge associated with domains that residents will encounter when they begin to undertake work in systems redesign and community engagement; collaborative exploration of new literatures, such as that found in organizational development (Madsen, Desai, Roberts, & Wong, 2006), change management, accounting and financial controls, quality improvement methodologies, and teamwork, will be useful. Helping residents access this knowledge in palatable forms and furnishing tools so that early ventures have some reasonable prospect of success is important in minimizing frustration with this often messy work. Emphasizing the iterative nature of learning through cycles of experience undertaking change, reflection, and a next attempt, such as the plan-do-study-act (PDSA) cycle, is an important teaching strategy, as is building in the understanding that doing the work of patient care and improving the work are two interdependent pieces of the physician's role. The experience of residents caring for patients can be used to engage their interest not just in how health care is delivered in the medical systems in which they work but in how it is organized and financed regionally, statewide, and nationally (Jacobsohn et al., 2008).

Of course, the most familiar field-building work undertaken at the GME level is research. In many ways, wet lab research conducted by residents illustrates what we believe should be more broadly available across the domains of inquiry, innovation, and improvement. The resident is welcomed as a legitimate junior partner in the laboratory or clinical research environment, one who undertakes initially simple but necessary elements of the program of investigation. As his sophistication and capabilities grow, he is allowed, and expected, to tackle more demanding activities. The entire endeavor is based on the premise that a fundamental goal is to create physicians who are capable of, and intent on, generating new knowledge. Why should it be any different for residents whose interests incline them toward designing improved systems of health care delivery or working at the policy level to create a health care system that is more accountable, effective, and just?

A number of medical schools have developed programs at the undergraduate level to encourage, and in some cases require, medical students to engage in field building across the broad range of inquiry and improvement activities that physicians engage in. Examples are the Areas of Concentration program at the University of Pittsburgh and the Scholarly Concentration program at Stanford University School of Medicine. However, in part because residency programs have tended to exist in departmental silos and because medical center administrators and department chairs have been reluctant to assign residents to settings and activities that are not explicitly linked to direct medical education funding (DME) and indirect medical education (IME) funding, GME has lagged significantly. This is beginning to change, albeit slowly. UCSF has developed Pathways to Discovery, a program conceived as a complement to the clinical curriculum of medical students, residents, and fellows. Participants will choose one of five pathways: molecular medicine (wet lab basic science), clinical and translational science, global health, health and society (policy studies and advocacy, community engagement, humanities and medicine) or health professions education. While completing their clinical training, they will do master's-level work combining didactic course work and original scholarship.

Pedagogies for Professional Formation

○

It is a Tuesday afternoon and internal medicine residents, PG2s and PG3s, are gathered in a conference room in their outpatient practice. One of the residents has brought a patient to the group. The topic for the session is poor adherence. The resident and her patient review for the group the difficulties that the patient has had with weight loss and smoking cessation, both essential elements in management of her diabetes. After this introduction, the faculty teacher for the session takes over and begins working with the patient, using the principles of motivational interviewing. The conversation with the patient lasts ten minutes or so; before excusing her, the teacher asks the patient if she has any questions. She asks several of the observing residents where they are from and what their plans are, and she wishes the entire group well. Once the patient has gone, the faculty member facilitates a discussion of "difficult patients." One of the residents comments, "It's not the patients who are difficult; it's our response to them." This leads to a candid and supportive exploration of patient care experiences that they have found challenging.

○

Residency education is holistic; it is therefore difficult to isolate pedagogies that are dedicated to supporting professional formation, that is, the dimension of becoming a physician that has less to do with fund of knowledge and technical skills and more to do with the character, disposition, and automatic choices, the moral compass, of the trainee. The simplest and most easily discerned elements concern the knowledge that practicing physicians require about ethical standards and legal requirements (Arnold & Stern, 2006). Many residency programs have a regular conference devoted to this material; at UCSF, this content is addressed in the Healthcare Ethics, Law, and Policy series. The conferences mix didactics, covering, for example, the change in California law requiring written informed consent for HIV testing, and case discussion. Likely more powerful, however, is the lived-out example—how faculty members and the program treat challenges that residents deal with as they care for patients, interact with fellow physicians and nonphysician members of the health care team, and take on leadership roles in clinical services and in nonclinical arenas, if they have this opportunity.

Ordinary clinical work regularly poses extraordinary challenges and can be associated with significant psychological morbidity (Golub, Weiss, Ramesh, Ossoff, & Johns, 2007). Making decisions under conditions of uncertainty, being called on by patients and families for advice when the stakes could not be higher, making the wrong choice and being forgiven (or not), being entrusted with intimate confidences never before shared, and being a witness to the beginning of life and its end are all part of the daily experience of residents. Mistakes and bad clinical outcomes are part of the territory of clinical medicine and hence of residency training. These untoward occurrences are part of the curriculum of graduate medical education. Much formation of professional character arises as residents learn to deal with these inherent difficulties, accepting responsibility and reflecting on achieving better results in the future, but avoiding paralyzing self-doubt (Paget, 2004). As a program director observed,

"When mistakes happen, residents have to learn to be appropriately self-critical. One size does not fit all." Teachers often help trainees negotiate this difficult terrain; good listening skills, strong empathic capacity, willingness to be appropriately self-disclosing, and the ability to promote reflection characterize effective teaching in this domain.

Some residency programs have regular, scheduled sessions intended to help residents process the challenges of clinical work in a supportive atmosphere, minimizing isolation and offering guidance on dealing with patient death, interpersonal conflict in clinical settings, and errors (Bragard et al., 2006). Sometimes called "stress rounds," these are often thought of as being more appropriate for the junior house staff and are less commonly available for residents in the later years. Not surprisingly, residency programs with a culture of rugged individualism are often skeptical of what they consider touchy-feely sessions. Across the board, these programs require a charismatic faculty champion to lend credibility, establish ground rules, facilitate productive discussion among the residents, and demonstrate through his or her own participation how to reflect on and cope with the inherent difficulties of practice.

Among the purposes of many advising systems is to create one-on-one relationships that residents can use ad hoc, as they encounter not just career decisions, academic hardships, or personal difficulties but challenges to their professionalism. Just the commitment of program resources to an advising system sends an important symbolic message; however, approaches that rely exclusively on assigned pairings organized centrally are typically compromised by weak and ineffective relationships when personal chemistry is lacking. Henry Ford Hospital uses a hybrid approach: PG1s work with an assigned advisor, and in subsequent years residents choose their advisor on the basis of shared interests and personal compatibility. An effective advising system that is capable of moving beyond counseling about fellowship options is likely to be especially important in large academic training programs, where a single GME program may have scores of residents and most faculty members spend only a small portion of their time teaching.

A final point bears emphasis: we regard ethical comportment and aspiration to the highest goals of the profession of medicine as being situated and distributed in the clinical environment. How their peers, their program, and the culture in which they are working, learning, and living treat these challenges and residents' responses to them can either inspire trainees or breed cynicism. The contextual and cultural factors that support or impede residents' becoming the physicians their programs want them to be—and their patients need them to be—have just recently attracted much attention. Just as knowledge and technical know-how is situated and distributed, so professionalism is as much a feature of context and the culture of the specific environment as it is an individual asset (Goldstein et al., 2006; Humphrey et al., 2007; Viggiano, Pawlina, Lindor, Olsen, & Cortese, 2007). Residency training programs, and more broadly the clinical settings in which residents are placed, must hold themselves much more accountable for the environments they foster. The macro environment and microsystems in which residents work and learn may call forth the best from them, because a high sense of purpose pervades the setting; others in the environment reliably demonstrate integrity, respect, and humility; and conflict is managed openly and collegially. Or residents may be held to one set of professional values, while the context in which they are working is entirely otherwise. At the very least, residents who are required to hold to the highest standards of professional behavior but expected to work in an environment where faculty are tardy, give inadequate supervision, and verbally abuse house staff and each other will become cynical about their professionalism expectations. Worse, they may begin to emulate the behavior they see around them.

Unfortunately, the microsystems, and in some settings the entire macro environment, in which residents learn are not always conducive to proper professional formation. Furthermore, we believe that complex issues relating to the number of hours residents have been expected to work have become confused with the quality and meaning of their work experience. Assuredly, residents have been exploited in the past by their residency programs and medical centers. However, simply decreasing the number of hours of a poor-quality experience does not make it more salutary. Conversely, even though this is not intended to encourage residency programs to flout duty-hour reduction requirements, residents may miss profoundly important patient care experiences, the ones physicians remember at thirty years' remove as having forged a part of their identity as a healer, if they slavishly depart the bedside of a dying patient at 2:00 p.m. or leave a surgery with forty-five minutes to go because of the twenty-four-plus-six rule. Without argument, residency programs have needed the discipline of formal duty-hour reduction rules, with significant sanctions for noncompliance, but the process has had unintended and deleterious consequences. One of the saddest may be a shift in how residents regard investigating their patients' condition, acquiring new understandings stimulated by a desire to take outstanding care of a patient on the service, or developing a teaching aid to help a third-year student on the team understand a fine point of localization of a neurologic lesion or some subtlety of renal physiology. Duty-hour reduction has led some residents to regard all patient care activities as having a dimension of burden from which they need to be protected. This connotation can contaminate not just residents' bedside activities but how they regard reading and researching clinical topics at home. Residents have been heard to say that once they are off they should not have to invest personal time in learning about their patients, even though the ACGME states explicitly that "duty hours do *not* include reading and preparation time spent away from the duty site" (Accreditation Council for Graduate Medical Education, 2001).

These challenges notwithstanding, most residents see among their peers, students, and teachers many outstanding examples of compassion, commitment, dedication, and excellence and choose wisely which examples to follow and which to regard as cautionary. Perhaps the best example of a culture relentlessly calling for and supporting dedication and service to patients that we encountered in our fieldwork is the Mayo Clinic. When asked for an example of professionalism, an internal medicine resident at the clinic told a story about a peer. The resident colleague was caring for a patient with widely metastatic cancer. The patient had come from a European Union country, having been told by his physicians there that his cancer could not be cured. The patient arrived in Rochester, confident that the prognosis would be different if the treatment were designed and delivered by Mayo physicians, but was told again that the best medical science could not cure his malignancy. The narrator described his friend, caring for a patient who was thousands of miles from home, who had to communicate with his physicians in a nonnative language, and who lacked the money and perhaps the physical strength to make the return trip, as well as the resident's intense desire to do something for his lonely, frightened patient. He discovered the patient's favorite beer, spent his afternoon off looking for it, and smuggled it into the inpatient unit so that his dying patient could have a simple pleasure that reminded him of home. Although recognizing that the action was quite possibly a violation of hospital policy, we, like our narrator, regard this as a wonderful example of professionalism. This story was told to us in 2005 as contemporaneous. By chance, one of the authors ran across a recounting by the protagonist that was published in 2009. The author was contacted and reported that the incident occurred in the late 1980s. Either it has become part of the lore of the Mayo Clinic or it has happened more than once (Peter Ubel, M.D., Professor of Medicine, University of Michigan, personal communication July 2009).

Residency programs often do a good job as well in celebrating residents who consistently display qualities of character and the devotion to patients that are hallmarks of the "true physician." Many programs honor an intern of the year; typically, these recognitions reflect outstanding character and ethical comportment in addition to well-developed clinical abilities. In the cognitive specialties, it is an honor to be invited to do an additional year as a resident, the "chief resident" (not to be confused with the chief resident year in surgery, which reflects a level of responsibility that must be attained by all residents in order to complete the training program). In residencies that have such an honor as a chief resident year or awards such as intern of the year, the professionalism of the candidate is a key factor in selection.

Assessment in Residency Education

In Chapter Five we outline external assessment of residents' skills and knowledge as part of the profession's licensing and certification process. Here we discuss assessment within residency programs, which has traditionally combined in various proportions formal knowledge assessment through periodic testing, direct observation of the resident's care of patients, and indirect inferences based on residents' discussion of clinical problems in settings such as residents' report and M and M, and more formal discussion of clinical topics, journal club articles, and research projects. More recently, patient logs are being used, particularly in the procedural specialties, to yield an inventory of the resident's technical experience, while global assessments capture domains such as professionalism and interpersonal skills. The limitations of contemporary assessment include poor compliance with the performance assessment system on the part of faculty members (Littlefield et al., 2005), overweighting of knowledge, highly variable direct observation of performance from specialty to specialty and across residency programs (Holmboe, 2004; Williams, Klamen, & McGaghie, 2003), and insufficient and poorly accepted formative feedback.

Assessment of Knowledge

Assessment of knowledge is, in general, accomplished well in residency training. Programs use standardized in-training examinations to assess resident progress, anticipate performance on the end-of-residency board certification exams, and evaluate their own success in giving trainees productive clinical experiences and useful didactics (Babbott, Beasley, Hinchey, Blotzer, & Holmboe, 2007). Because residency programs are assessed in part by the pass rate of their graduates on the specialty board certification examination, and because medical school graduates understandably favor programs with demonstrated success in preparing their residents for the specialty certification process, less-competitive residency programs often devote more attention explicitly to preparing residents for the exams and use the in-training exams extensively, both as practice and to detect residents likely to have problems (de Virgilio et al., 2008).

Assessment of Procedural Skills

Procedural skills are assessed by direct observation, and increasingly in the simulation lab. Medicine and surgery training are an interesting contrast in this area, for a number of reasons. First, residents in medicine and many other procedurally oriented specialties simply do far fewer procedures than a generation ago. Subspecialty fellows perform liver biopsies and bone marrow biopsy and aspiration; intensivists and surgeons perform central line placement and thoracentesis; many simpler procedures such as paracentesis are performed in the radiology suite, with ultrasound guidance, and quite often by the radiologist. Even the procedures that are performed by the resident are often done in the absence of a faculty member because, in the nonprocedural specialties, most resident-faculty contact time occurs away from the bedside in conference settings such as attending rounds. Therefore supervising teachers typically have little opportunity to assess residents' aptness in performance of procedures. This is generally true in such specialties as internal medicine, but the growing use of hospitalists as supervisors of residents doing inpatient rotations in medicine and pediatrics may result in more opportunities for observation. Hospitalists are presumably more adept at inpatient procedures and more available for supervision than the multiply committed university faculty member or community attending. The situation is quite the opposite in surgery, where faculty members spend many hours across the operating table from their residents. As we noted earlier, there is empirical support for the contention that attending surgeons can gauge a resident's technical competence and assess its appropriateness for his or her level of training by direct observation. However, some surgery residencies are compromised by very large size. In these large academic training programs, because the PG4s and PG5s supervise and observe the PG1s, PG2s, and PG3s, a resident may become a PG4 before the faculty become aware of significant, and perhaps irremediable, technical deficiencies. Teachers at several large programs we visited spoke poignantly of the challenges of counseling an inept resident who has already devoted three or more years to the rigors of surgery training.

Because of problems of this type, residency programs, especially surgical programs, are becoming much more systematic about procedural skills assessment. Skills verification programs in which residents must request faculty observation of the performance of level-appropriate technical interventions are more prevalent than ever. Southern Illinois University (SIU) has developed the Objective Structured Assessment of Technical Skills (OSATS). However, it has not been widely accepted because it is time-intensive for faculty members and results in reduced operating room time for interns compared to programs where interns are allowed to participate in simple operative procedures without prior demonstration of a threshold level of technical competence. Asynchronous review of resident videotapes by faculty is being explored in an effort to make the OSATS more feasible for widespread use. SIU, a leader in surgical education and in assessment in particular, also uses an explicit operative performance rating system (OPRS). Recognizing that the exact clinical exposure of an individual resident cannot be entirely controlled or predicted, the OPRS identifies two "sentinel" operative procedures per year of training that residents are certain to have the opportunity to participate in and that call on skills expected at that level of training. Residents must be observed and formally assessed on several occasions per year on each of that year's OPRS surgeries.

Taking the lead from this kind of program, it would not be difficult for residency programs in the nonprocedural specialties to select sentinel skills that they regard as critical in development of competence and then mandate observation and formal assessment. These skills might or might not be procedural. For example, a residency program in internal medicine might require observation early in the PG1 year of interns giving hospitalized patients discharge instructions, or examining a patient with acute dyspnea in the role of the cross-covering PG1. Midway through the year, the sentinel skills in intravenous line placement, arterial blood sampling, and catheterization of the bladder could be assessed; this observation and assessment could be delegated to residents with proper training on performance standards and feedback. Late in the PG1 year, the assessment might focus on development of an appropriate assessment and management plan for a patient with a cardinal symptom such as abdominal pain or altered mental status. PG2 residents might be observed and assessed conducting a "do not resuscitate" discussion and developing an assessment and management plan for a patient with a complex presentation, selected from a list of presentations seen with some frequency at that medical center. PG3 residents might be observed and assessed in a consultation role and working with a teamwork challenge, such as an interservice conflict or a problematic subordinate, or simply developing an effective relationship with the nurses and other nonphysician health professionals in an inpatient or outpatient setting. Initial work along these lines has been described (Torbeck & Wrightson, 2005).

Assessment of Professional Formation

As we emphasize throughout this book, we prefer the term *professional formation* to *professionalism* to underline the continuous, dynamic, multifaceted, and profound nature of the construct. Building on an essential foundation of clinical competence, communication and interpersonal skills, and ethical and legal understanding, professional formation necessarily extends to aspirational goals in performance excellence, accountability, humanism, and altruism (Arnold & Stern, 2006). It is especially important to acknowledge the contrast with "mere" competence at the level of graduate medical education, though the current, useful emphasis on competency standards has the potential to obscure the distinction (Brooks, 2009). In developing the competency framework, the ACGME quite deliberately chose the midpoint of the Dreyfus skills-attainment continuum of novice, advanced beginner, competent, proficient, expert (Batalden, Leach, Swing, Dreyfus, & Dreyfus, 2002; Carraccio & Englander, 2004). This choice reflects the belief that the public deserves, at a minimum, competent clinicians, and that the level of practical experience and clinically driven learning required to achieve true expertise cannot be attained within the time envelope of the most efficient residency training program. However, in addition to their obligation to produce competent graduates, GME programs must ensure that their residents develop the personal characteristics to ensure lifelong commitment to the aspirational goals of excellence, accountability, humanism, altruism, and continued progress toward expertise after completion of training.

Because it is a complex construct, dimensions of professional formation often appear in assessments designed to focus on knowledge or procedural skills. During one of our site visits, a teacher of obstetrics and gynecology showed us a videotape of a resident responding to a relatively low-fidelity simulation of a delivery complicated by shoulder dystocia. The resident capably performed the required maneuvers and expeditiously accomplished the delivery but was visibly stressed, which she acknowledged. When asked about this response, the faculty member, extensively experienced in simulations for residents, said that it was usual; residents with desirable professional attributes "willingly suspend disbelief" while residents who refuse to believe the simulations quite frequently had other attitudinal difficulties. He has not tested the idea, but he speculated that, although the simulation was designed to primarily assess residents' ability to manage this obstetric emergency and secondarily to communicate with and reassure the frightened mother, it could be used as a marker for problems in professional formation. Other simulation experts have made the same suggestion (Hamstra et al., 2006).

In addition to formal assessments, there is much information about residents' professional attributes distributed in the environment within which they work. Unfortunately, this rich source of potentially valuable feedback to residents is incompletely captured, largely because potential informants, such as nurses, are not included in the evaluation process or because other residents are reluctant to share what they know. Because of its complexity, professional formation is best evaluated in authentic contexts, and those who work most closely with residents are in the best position to contribute (Norcini, 2003); indeed, even though their contributions are important, supervising faculty may have relatively little high-quality information on which to base their assessment of residents in this domain. Residents certainly know who within their peer group they would trust with the care of a family member; the key is creating a nonpunitive culture in which residents will share such knowledge of their colleagues. At Atlantic Health, residents nominate peers who they believe know their work well; the program director may add names to the list of resident evaluators. Are the evaluations truly candid? Some potential cross-checks exist: chief residents are typically close to resident scuttlebutt and could verify whether formal comments are concordant or discordant. Also, it is generally well known which residents are popular supervisors of more junior trainees and, in residency programs associated with schools of medicine, medical students. Although this popularity reflects sense of humor, enthusiasm for teaching, and other attributes that are not strictly components of professional formation, subordinates do tend to seek out supervisors who strive for excellence, are compassionate and gentle with patients and their families, and are otherwise admirable role models (Kenny et al., 2003).

The fundamental prerequisite for successful collection of this type of distributed information about resident professional formation is a culture that creates a shared understanding of its legitimacy and importance (Maudsley, 2001; Viggiano et al., 2007). If residents believe that their program will use insights they furnish to punish or disadvantage a peer, they generally will not share the information, even if they have significant concerns. However, if the purpose is to help every resident take better care of patients and residents have available appropriate and effective assistance, programs may be able to obtain forthright assessment from residents.

The perspective of nurses is similarly valued or discounted, depending on the culture of the program. Although most programs have mechanisms through which nurses may complain about individual residents, surprisingly few systematically collect feedback from nursing staff. To some extent, this may reflect structural challenges. In large teaching hospitals, a resident may care for patients scattered over four or five units. When this is the case, there may be insufficient contact for nurses to form an opinion and for residents to take their comments seriously. A geographic organization of resident teams would likely promote development of more engaged and functional interprofessional relationships and facilitate participation of nurses in assessing residents.

Some programs have experimented with standardized patients in a "mystery shopper" format. With adequate authenticity, these can be powerful assessment tools. However, it is expensive, and for this reason repeated sampling is not feasible. Like other simulations, fidelity seems to become an increasing issue as the residents progress in experience; advanced residents indicate that working with real patients is more useful to their learning.

Self-Assessment, Reflection, and Portfolios

A number of assessment methodologies are being recommended to address ACGME competencies underrepresented by formal testing and episodic direct observation. It is hoped as well that some of these approaches will become habits of mind for trainees and thus support continued professional development after completion of residency training. Clinically driven learning is premised on the assumption that physicians can identify gaps in their capabilities, knowledge, or skills and are motivated to correct them, once identified. It has been shown that practicing physicians do not accurately self-assess (Colthart et al., 2008; Eva & Regehr, 2005), but beginning students in PBL programs have no problem identifying topics to learn about, stimulated by a paper case. Why this ability erodes over the course of training is not clear, although it may be that educational programs misrepresent the goal of medical training as production of physicians who have mastered a knowledge and skill base and are thus competent. The object instead is to nurture and challenge medical learners and inculcate the aspirational goal of lifelong learning. Extension and refinement of the skills addressed at a basic level in PBL through explicit attention to residents' skill at identification of new learning goals and use of appropriate and effective approaches to self-learning might mitigate the observed deterioration in accuracy of self-assessment. As has been discussed with respect to other dimensions of professional formation, this has a clear cultural aspect. Settings in which residents, and physicians in general, are celebrated and rewarded for what they know, or claim to know, will not promote acknowledgment of deficits that are learning opportunities. This type of environment may be exactly the influence that leads physicians to overestimate their capability to avoid the dissonance associated with admitting a gap.

By contrast, learning and practice environments in which it is understood that all physicians practice imperfectly and that the best physicians actively seek out evidence that they have a performance gap (whether the evidence is a trifling intuition of insufficient knowledge, unsatisfactory patient outcome data, or results from a more formal self-assessment program) and work to address these gaps once discovered could support maintenance of skills in reflection and self-assessment. Pedagogies involving reflection are intended to make visible this process of physician self-assessment (Branch & Paranjape, 2002); reflective exercises in which residents review and critique their performance and make plans for next steps to improve are a growing part of assessment of complex competencies such as practice-based learning and improvement and systems-based practice. As in UME, interest in portfolio assessment has grown in parallel with the desire to assess medical learners in a broader range of domains than clinical knowledge and the belief that learners benefit from the process of reflecting on their work and selecting products and accomplishments to showcase (Driessen, 2009; Driessen, van Tartwijk, van der Vleuten, & Wass, 2007). Work in inquiry and improvement, such as a clinic-based quality improvement project or advocacy efforts on behalf of a vulnerable or underserved population, is particularly amenable to portfolio presentation. Aspects of professional formation can also be highlighted in a portfolio.

GME: The Work Ahead

The many strengths of U.S. residency education are derived primarily from the intellectual ability and motivation on the part of the learners and the stimulation and challenge of the learning environment. That residency education is remarkably impervious to change is evinced by fundamental curricular structures, instructional approaches, and assessment techniques, many of which have been in place since its inception. Its many long-standing weaknesses, or fault lines, have been exacerbated by the dramatic changes in how health care is delivered in the United States. It is worth noting that this stasis in GME has had important implications for UME, as much of the clinical education of medical students is accomplished by assigning them to resident teams. For this reason, until the past ten years much of the change effort in UME focused on the first two years of medical school.

Pedagogy in resident education needs attention at two levels. First, faculty preparation for teaching should be significantly enhanced. Many faculty members could use assistance in using institutional resources for the benefit of their learners. However, residency programs are strikingly "siloed," even in a single university or medical center. In contrast to UME, teaching improvement efforts, to the extent that they are undertaken at all, are small-scale efforts within a department. Faculty members need support for development of their skills. As with all teaching, clinical teaching is challenging, and every teacher can benefit from opportunities to advance pedagogical content knowledge, observe good teaching and be observed, and reflect (Gruppen, Frohna, Anderson, & Lowe, 2003; Steinert et al., 2006). Formal faculty development programs focused on the important skills of clinical teaching, such as diagnosing problems in clinical reasoning, are extremely important. Perhaps equally critical is creation of a "teaching commons" where ideas about teaching are shared and built on (Huber & Hutchings, 2005).

Our other critique of pedagogy at the residency level concerns emphasis on current factual knowledge. A strong grounding in the contemporary knowledge base is absolutely necessary, but far from sufficient. Although much lip service is accorded "lifelong learning," most medical teaching occurs from an "authoritative expert" stance. Such a stance leads to difficulties: faculty members may feel anxious when confronted by a teaching situation for which they are not entirely in command of the medical knowledge base, and it also creates unreasonable expectations for learners in terms of their own growth and development. Those moments when physicians—whether faculty or residents—notice that they cannot adopt the authoritative expert stance are an opportunity, not a failing. It can be difficult, in a culture that celebrates expertise, to relish not knowing, but of course this is where continued learning comes from. Collegial pursuit of a good question should be a fundamental element of teaching at the residency level.

The scope of assessment in GME needs to be broadened and the methods diversified. Current approaches overemphasize current factual knowledge and underemphasize knowledge seeking and skill building. The relative paucity of assessment methodologies is related to overemphasis on factual knowledge, although whether GME educators have restricted the scope of resident assessment because they place less priority on nonknowledge domains or have overweighted knowledge because it is relatively easy to measure is not clear. Even though all residency programs have learning objectives for each resident rotation, a system for assessing whether residents have actually met those objectives is commonly lacking, as are mechanisms for alternative rotations or doing the assigned block at a more advanced level for residents who have achieved the basic objectives of a particular rotation. Developing and testing approaches to remediation of residents whose performance is not meeting goals is required as well (Torbeck & Canal, 2009).

Omitted and Neglected Content

As important as these comments about instructional approaches and assessment are, the principal deterrent to change in GME is that the residents' curriculum—what they spend their time doing rather than their formal didactic program—has been determined primarily by the needs of hospitals to have residents help with busy inpatient services rather than focused on what individual residents and cohorts of residents need, from an educational perspective. Along with a system of assessment that has focused on time spent in specified activities rather than exhibited competence and departmental "siloing" retarding the spread of curricular strengths from one department to another, this has inhibited educational innovation and resulted in numerous curricular deficiencies.

In virtually all residencies and across all specialties, graduate medical education is dominated by attention to highly practical, even concrete issues: how to accomplish what absolutely must be accomplished in the hospital and then discharge the patient. Discharge becomes the highest goal. Most residency programs, across specialties, devote excessive time to inpatient settings, and despite the increasing severity and complexity of conditions encountered in outpatient medicine, they subject residents to poorly organized, educationally unproductive ambulatory care experiences. Residency education privileges learning settings in which all participants are physicians and fails to explicitly address the distributed nature of clinical intelligence and the critical importance of effective interactions with nonphysician members of the health care team. Largely because of the pace of the clinical environment, residency affords insufficient time for reflection, study, and consideration of the connections between a patient's situation and the foundational sciences. This decreases (if not eliminates) the opportunities for residents to speculate on where their field is going next and what questions need to be addressed to improve patient outcomes. As a consequence, a great range of content is underrepresented in the residency experiences, from underlying basic science to the social purpose of medicine.

BASIC SCIENCE.   In Chapter Three, we argued that medical students need clinical experience to put their "high science" learning in an appropriately patient-centered context. The situation in graduate medical education is the reverse; residents need the opportunity to step away from the practical exigencies of patient care to connect their developing know-how with the cutting edge of their field, to address the *whether* and *why* questions. We believe that medical learners should not regard basic sciences simply as prerequisites for clinical learning but rather as the living foundation of practice in residency training and through a life of practice.

Why does a practice-bound resident need to stay conversant with basic science concepts and the growing edge of the field of medicine? What does science actually have to do with clinical medicine? A strong foundation in both the traditional basic sciences and the behavioral sciences established in medical school and further developed and expanded during a lifetime of practice permits the intellectual flexibility on which adaptive expertise depends. It is not enough to have time-proven and reliable approaches to routine problems; every physician requires a depth of understanding that allows him or her to respond to unusual clinical problems with original rather than habitual approaches (Bereiter & Scardamalia, 1993; Bransford et al., 1999; Hatano & Oura, 2003; Linn, 2007). It is, in fact, this ability that should distinguish physicians from non-M.D. clinicians. A second significant benefit of continued attention to the scientific foundations of medical practice is the relative ease of incorporating new discoveries. A clinician who depends on lists and who practices in an algorithmic manner must entirely abandon the list or algorithm whenever a new discovery disrupts it. By contrast, a physician who has remained connected to science, who has been following, for example, the story of interfering RNAs or the working out of genetic determinants of drug metabolism, is ready to incorporate discoveries into practice as what was cutting-edge science becomes a new insight into pathogenesis or an addition to the therapeutic armamentarium.

Thus medical educators need to be concerned by evidence that once medical students complete the "science phase" of their education, science rarely makes an encore appearance, and when it does it is isolated from clinical content in a research block (Kanna et al., 2006). Although they have merit, research blocks do not address the broader question of how to encourage all residents to update their basic science knowledge base and participate, even if they intend to be full-time clinicians, in field building by playing their own part in "translation," that is, helping to identify important questions for scientists to address. The question of how much of the basic science that physicians learned in the early phase of medical school is actually retained into residency and beyond has been contentious (Custers, 2008), but there is no debate that, given the accelerating rate of medical discovery, physicians need to stay abreast of the relevant foundational sciences. However, experiments in bringing basic scientists to attending rounds have been, by and large, unsuccessful. The imperative in the clinical environment is efficient patient management and swift disposition of problems; this task-focused environment is inhospitable to exploration of areas of emerging science, even those relating to the patients at hand. Still with the correct support and with enough time, residents and medical students alike can be encouraged to consider such questions as "What do we need to discover next or understand better to have more impact on this patient's condition?" and "What do fields like neuroscience or medical genetics offer in terms of increasing our understanding of this problem?" Innovative programs demonstrate that residents and fellows appreciate engagingly presented basic science that is highly relevant to their clinical work (Clark & Simpson, 2008; Hammond, Taylor, Obermair, & McMenamin, 2004).

Identifying the appropriate teachers is challenging as well. Even in large academic health centers, laboratory scientists have had little enthusiasm for teaching in a clinical environment. It is typically difficult to find a patient whose problem plays directly to the very narrow expertise of a particular laboratory researcher, and most wet lab investigators are not particularly comfortable at the bedside. Additionally, a significant majority of the seven thousand residency programs in this country are not based at academic health centers and thus do not have easy access to scientists. The clinical teachers supervising residents in their patient care and providing clinical teaching are not experts, either. However, it may be that the model is wrong. Perhaps what is needed is not a science expert at the bedside, the person with the answers, but a culture that values productive questions. The solution to this problem may lie less in bringing the expert with the answer to the resident and more in encouraging the resident and his or her teacher to ask the questions. Residency educators must become more creative in approaches to bringing concepts in the foundational sciences to the bedside, without relying on wet lab scientists to do all the teaching in this area.

UNDEREMPHASIZED CLINICAL CONTENT. Because residents (and, indeed, all clinicians) learn by caring for patients, what they learn depends on what they see. Residency programs are insufficiently deliberate and intentional in organizing resident rotations to ensure that trainees encounter the clinical problems they will manage as independent clinicians, in the settings in which they will see those problems. This discrepancy is particularly problematic for such specialties as internal medicine, pediatrics, and neurology (Arora, Guardiano, Donaldson, Storch, & Hemstreet, 2005). For hospital-based specialties such as surgery and radiology, residency training better approximates how practitioners spend their time. Because they emphasize outpatient care in their training programs, family medicine and psychiatry also achieve a reasonable facsimile of the independent clinician's work.

It has been rationalized that it is appropriate for trainees to spend more time in inpatient settings than they will after completion of residency because hospitalized patients represent the severe-illness end of the clinical spectrum; so, it is argued, a physician who is capable of caring for hospitalized patients is prepared for anything. However, this argument fails on several counts. First, even very ill patients are now cared for entirely as outpatients more than ever. Keeping in mind the premise that learning is highly situated, it follows that what one learns about caring for a patient with a particular condition—say, a markedly elevated blood sugar—in the hospital will have limited pertinence when trying to treat an outpatient with the same condition. In many ways, outpatient care is more demanding, because the patient is not continuously available for reassessment and adjustment of treatment strategies. Second, there are a large number of important conditions for which patients are never hospitalized. When residency training overemphasizes inpatient settings relative to what practicing clinicians do, residents leave their programs underprepared to care for people whose problems are largely addressed in an ambulatory setting.

We do not intend to suggest that the inpatient setting lacks merit as a teaching site. Inpatients tend to have more physical findings and are, of course, more available for repeat visits for teaching with learners of different levels. The gravity of much inpatient illness affords opportunities for teaching about bad news, negotiating changes in the stance of care, and working with families under stress. The routines of inpatient care allow the attending physician to observe residents at the bedside and assist residents in advancing their team management and teaching skills. However, it must be acknowledged that outpatients are not merely less ill than inpatients; they are situated in different conditions, and different skills are required for their care.

CLINICAL REASONING AND JUDGMENT. Medical teachers, of course, believe they are teaching clinical reasoning (Montgomery, 2006). Most educators have, however, only an intuitive sense of what clinical reasoning and judgment are and very little understanding of how to teach them; in fact, the constructs themselves are poorly defined (Moulton et al., 2006). One might recognize the trainee who is endowed with strong abilities and the resident with deficits, but most clinician-teachers do not follow the learning sciences and have not kept up with advances in the field of medical decision making. In addition, some educational cultures, both specialty-based and institutional, may promote residents' acquiescence to authority, thereby inhibiting development of judgment and advanced reasoning skills. In the course of our fieldwork, we heard, particularly in our conversations with surgical house staff, that some faculty members were resistant to appeals for evidence, and more generally to house staff skepticism, insisting that the attending's preferred course of action be followed simply "because" (Bhandari et al., 2003). Evidence-based medicine may be something of a culprit in its own right; physicians need the ability to access information; assess its quality; decide if it is pertinent to the patient at hand; reason from first principles; and gather and weigh a variety of technical, sociocultural, and value-laden considerations and perspectives to meld them, with the patient, into a plan or approach, often under circumstances of considerable uncertainty, where time is of the essence (Timmermans & Angell, 2001).

PRACTICAL SYSTEMS ISSUES.   Residents learn and care for patients in a system they cannot significantly influence, much less manage. As a consequence, a universe of skills and knowledge related to running a practice is omitted from most residency education (family medicine is an exception to the critique); setting up a practice, personnel management, payer and insurer issues, and regulatory compliance are common orphan topics. We occasionally saw some of these issues being addressed in didactic settings; examples include sessions on medico-legal concerns and an interactive conference for fourth-year surgery residents on billing and coding, but because residents are isolated from management of the clinics, inpatient units, and medical centers where they are being educated, these issues are not compelling for them. This is an important problem, not only because residents (at least those who plan to proceed into practice at completion of their graduate medical education) need to gain an understanding of these issues but because, immersed as they are in the clinical environment, residents have important insights into care delivery and systems operation that the administrators and executives in their clinic settings would be wise to capture and learn from.

Even more basic systems-based practice issues are often overlooked in GME. Although expected to skillfully manage a team composed of medical learners at various levels, and perhaps a podiatry student and a pharmacy student; and to coordinate care of patients by collaborating with nurses, occupational therapists, and nutritionists, residents are given little or no instruction in the basics of team management or time management (Stanley, Khan, Hussain, & Tweed, 2006). Even worse, residents practice in an environment where their faculty role models are characteristically dissociated from the rest of the care team. "Interestingly, physicians tend to be the weakest link in the coordination of both surgical care and medical care. Physicians' relational coordination with the rest of the care provider team tends to be systematically weaker than it is for any other care provider discipline despite the fact that physicians play a central role in delivering patient care" (Gittell, 2009, p. 21). At virtually every site visit, residents reported that their greatest challenge was learning to delegate and manage and that the most common form of interprofessional conflict was with nurses. This situation seems likely to perpetuate itself indefinitely if not confronted and corrected.

SYSTEMS IMPROVEMENT METHODOLOGIES. The current focus on patient safety and quality improvement is beginning to be reflected to a modest degree in residency programs (Batalden & Davidoff, 2007; Tess et al., 2009). However, much more ambitious efforts are required if graduate medical education is to produce physicians who are, across the board, capable of engaging the problems of our health care delivery system, making patient care more reliable, and producing better outcomes for patients. The problem, in general, is that residents are not empowered in their medical centers as agents of change. Whenever they are, improvements happen. At the University of Pennsylvania, PG1s in internal medicine do a clinic-based quality improvement project; a sampling of projects that made things better for patients is selected for presentation at grand rounds the subsequent year. At Northwestern University, PG4 surgery residents developed a system for identifying and analyzing "near miss" errors on surgical services; discussion of these near misses is now a valuable part of every M and M conference (Bilimoria, 2009). Programs that authentically engage residents in addressing gaps in the delivery of quality care and supply tools for their exploration and correction (Jacobsohn et al., 2008), such as use of PDSA cycles, should become universal in residency training.

Leadership is another underdeveloped area, despite every resident having repeated opportunities to serve as the leader of a team over the course of her education (Horwitz et al., 2008). Fortunately, many residents' prior experiences have offered considerable opportunities to experiment with approaches to leadership and deal with challenges associated with building a sense of common purpose, establishing group norms, and dealing with conflict. However, leadership and team management can be areas in which residents whose fund of knowledge and clinical skills are strong struggle, and even residents whose leadership skills are strong often desire to further their development in this arena.

THE SOCIAL PURPOSES OF MEDICINE AND THE FUTURE OF THE PROFES-SION. Residency training is relentlessly focused on the concrete and the present. Of course, GME would be failing the trainees as well as their current and future patients if there were not an unshakable commitment to ensuring that residents complete their training capable of providing high-quality care for the patients they see. However, as one member of our team observed about a top-tier university training program, "learning the skills of the trade so dominates that there is no time to consider the profession and where it is going." This is a time of enormous change and great possibility for medicine in the United States. Residents are the postdoctoral fellows and the future of the profession; as they develop advanced knowledge and skills in their specialty, they should also be grappling with what Bereiter and Scardamalia (1993) call the "constitutive problems of the field." Making them so busy that they are disinclined or incapable of doing so is an educational failure.

A Clearly Defined Core

Just as in medical school, selection and sequencing of clinical rotations for residents is a key curricular decision. However, although all residency programs have learning objectives for every resident rotation, a system for assessing whether residents have actually met those objectives is commonly lacking. A related curricular challenge has been inadequate definition of core content as a platform for lifelong learning in an ever-changing field. Instead, an anxious desire to include everything has led, and continues to lead, to an ever-lengthening duration of training. Given the dramatic increase in busyness of clinical settings, both inpatient and outpatient, and the proliferation of things to be learned, how does a residency program (or at the level of board certification, a specialty board) make it all fit? From an educational perspective, it is important that residencies commit to an appropriate core in order that residents see a sufficient number of examples and variants to develop elaborated conceptual frameworks and to practice psychomotor and other skills. Finally, we see inculcation of the values of medicine as one of the critical goals of medical teaching. Serious attention must be accorded the hidden curriculum because it is at least as important a force for learning as the formal curriculum, and it often works against what the residents' educational program states it is trying to teach (Hundert, Hafferty, & Christakis, 1996).

Efficiency and Individualization of Progress

Any careful review uncovers these and a number of other opportunities to improve residency education (diFrancesco, Pistoria, Auerbach, Nardino, & Holmboe, 2005). We are not suggesting, however, adding time to the residency period. We are suggesting instead that the efficiency of residency education be improved so that learners—and their patients—are guaranteed that a three-to-five-year training program offers the experience to prepare graduating residents to competently care for the majority of patients whose conditions fall within their specialty, the skills to enlist assistance when needed, and the discernment to identify those situations in which help is needed. Clearly, graduate medical education must arm residents with insight, humility, and deep commitment to patients to ensure this.

We are confident that there is time within the current envelope of residency training across the specialties to educate residents both more broadly and more deeply. Educational inefficiency is always problematic, but it cannot be tolerated at a time when the medical knowledge base is burgeoning, attending physicians are raising concerns that their residency graduates may not be ready for independent practice, educational debt is perverting career choice among young doctors, and physician-scientists are in their early forties before they achieve independent grant funding. It is thus imperative that residents have clinical responsibilities that support their learning rather than assignments that meet the needs of the medical center or hospital hosting their training. Further, residency training must become significantly more flexible so that programs are both efficient and individualized.

In many programs, residents, especially at the more junior levels, spend significant time doing clerical work. Eliminating time spent on clerical activities (Boex & Leahy, 2003) and allowing residents to move on to more challenging learning issues once they have achieved an acceptable level of performance for their stage in training (Long, 2000) would yield time to tackle new domains and higher levels of achievement. Elimination or minimization of this nonphysician work, combined with competency-based assessment and individualization of progress through residency experiences, holds the promise of freeing resident time and allowing significantly more substantive education to occur within the current time envelope of residency across specialties.

Residency programs require the ability to construct curricula that meet the needs of trainees in the field in general and of individual residents. Good-faith selection of clinical settings and experiences for GME trainees should be determined by what residents need to learn, not where medical centers need clinical labor. The clinical experiences of residents, their rotations, must be selected on the basis of what independent practitioners in that specialty should be capable of handling, not units that the medical center wants covered. This inevitably means that not every patient admitted to a teaching hospital will be cared for by a resident team. Furthermore, in nearly all specialties much more resident education should occur in outpatient settings, as fresh graduates across the specialties must be capable of working effectively in these environments and to diagnose and treat the conditions seen there. Similarly, for the benefit of both residents and medical students, new formats and venues, both clinical and nonclinical, should be developed, allowing residents to work with medical students outside the traditional inpatient disciplinary clerkship.

Moreover, residency education must develop mechanisms for providing alternative rotations, or, for residents who have achieved the basic objectives of a particular rotation, doing the assigned block at a more advanced level. Faculty members and program directors in particular have considerable difficulty in envisioning how such individualization of residency training might be accomplished. Of course, it would not be practical to allow a supervising resident to depart a clinical placement, leaving behind her intern and students, the day she demonstrates that she has met the core competency requirements of that rotation. However, residency training currently affords insufficient opportunity for mentored resident participation in activities representing the inquiry, innovation, and improvement activities of physicians. One option would be to more closely connect or integrate innovation, improvement, and inquiry activities to the residents' clinical settings, rather than treating them as entirely different (an issue we explore in greater depth in Chapter Seven). Improvement in pedagogy would also foster greater individualization. Anxious clinical teachers who dictate management strategies retard acquisition of critical competence, especially in more advanced learners. Teachers must become skilled at assessing resident capabilities and in constructing a space for learning in which the resident is acquiring new knowledge and skills and practicing recently acquired ones. A resident educational program that allows motivated and capable learners to proceed at their own pace and engage the constitutive problems of the field will require commitment to the core obligatory competencies and the means to verify that residents have achieved them.

A Commitment to Excellence

Perhaps most disturbing is the simple persistence of the recognized problems with GME. Given that little of what we have identified constitutes novel insight, we infer that there is inadequate commitment to correcting the deficits in residency education. The reasons for this are evident. Residency education is, at its heart, experiential learning; residents learn about the clinical work in which they participate. There are significant vested interests that control the choices about the clinical settings in which residents find themselves. Thus the current stresses in the health care system threaten many of the positive attributes we observed. We are especially concerned about the limited time that faculty members are able to commit to teaching, because of the increasing pressures of the medical marketplace. Thoughtful teaching takes time, as Ludmerer has so compellingly observed (Ludmerer, 1999, 2000). It is critical that faculty members with an inclination and aptitude for teaching not be forced to choose between preparing the next generation of physicians and activities that support their practice and their family. As we discuss in Chapter Five, too often the income stream associated with GME is captured by the hospital and does not make its way to the clinicians who are actually teaching. In addition, as has been repeatedly observed, the structure of IME and DME locks the residents into inpatient training (Iglehart, 2008; Rich et al., 2002). The sustained connection with faculty members that is so important to effective resident education is not possible without significant reorganization of the financing of medical education; accordingly, the recommendations that we propose in Chapter Eight address some of the disincentives to change.

PART THREE

EXTERNAL PRESSURES AND INTERNAL FORCES FOR CHANGE

5

REGULATING AND FINANCING MEDICAL EDUCATION

MEDICAL EDUCATION IS AFFECTED by strong external forces, from the organizations within which medical schools operate to the larger health care industry and federal agencies. Moreover, although each entity associated with medical education—medical schools; teaching hospitals; accrediting, certifying, and licensing agencies; financing bodies—strives to ensure quality, there is no overall coordination or oversight for all of medical education. Each of the various entities has a vested interest in ensuring the highest quality of medical education, yet most work separately to promote innovation, and this lack of coordination sometimes has the opposite effect. If transformational change is to occur within medical education, a companion revolution must occur in its external relationships, particularly regulation and financing.

In this chapter, after discussion of the implications of medical education's location within larger academic and health care organizations, we focus on how it is regulated and financed. Traditionally, medical schools and teaching hospitals have been amply financed through multiple mechanisms and have used revenue generated from one mission to cross-subsidize another, thus enabling all three missions (teaching, research, and patient care) to thrive. When resources were abundant, this process worked well. However, the margins for the research and clinical missions have decreased sharply, making such cost transfers no longer feasible and in some instances not allowable. However, where resources are aligned with mission and allocations are made in a fair and transparent manner, medical education flourishes, and to demonstrate this we close the chapter with four examples of institutions whose innovative approaches to financing support excellence.

Competing Missions, Competing Pressures

We begin this discussion with matters of definition. There are a number of interpretations of the terms *academic medical centers* and *academic health centers*, but we use these terms to indicate medical schools with their *university teaching hospitals*. The 130 LCME-accredited medical schools in the United States do not all have teaching hospitals. Thus, currently, according to the AAMC and the Commonwealth Fund, there are 126 recognized academic health centers in the United States, institutions that have an allopathic medical school, faculty practice plan, and affiliated or owned teaching hospital(s). The Association of Academic Health Centers (2009) defines *academic health center* slightly differently: "an accredited, degree-granting institution of higher education" that "consists of an allopathic or osteopathic medical school, one or more other health professions schools or programs (such as allied health sciences, dentistry, graduate studies, pharmacy, public health, veterinary medicine), and one or more owned or affiliated teaching hospitals, health systems or other organized health care services" (http://www.aahcdc.org/about/members/php; http://www.aahcdc.org/about). By this definition, there are more academic health centers because they include osteopathic programs, which, as noted in the Introduction, were not included in our study.

Working at the intersection of universities and teaching hospitals (academic health centers), then, those responsible for medical education must collaborate with both entities and be responsive to the larger context of health care financing and regulation. In this web of dynamic relationships, university and teaching hospital values and organizational structures, financial incentives, and regulations sometimes overlap and at other times diverge. Some medical schools and teaching hospitals have collaboratively supported and advanced undergraduate and graduate medical education, while others have not.

Both medical schools and university teaching hospitals share common social missions: to educate future health professionals, conduct biomedical research, care for the nation's poor and uninsured, provide general and specialized clinical care to some of the most severely ill and injured (often referred to as *tertiary care*), and develop leadership to improve the health care system. Medical schools and their teaching hospitals unite around these common missions and work together to achieve these ends (Commonwealth Fund, 2003; Committee on the Roles of Academic Health Centers in the 21st Century, 2003). However, the relative value attached to each mission varies with the organization, and often within an institution. In addition, freestanding teaching hospitals, not affiliated with medical schools, sponsor graduate medical education programs and often train medical students as well; these community hospitals, which typically provide less referral care than do university teaching hospitals and conduct little to no research, are the site of approximately two-thirds of the residency programs in the United States.

As we note in Chapter One, among the legacies of the Flexner Report is the location of medical schools within universities. Thus medical schools, like other university-based professional schools, are shaped by the values and structures of the university. In a university the research mission, the creation of new knowledge, which brings prestige and resources to the university, has primacy. Teaching of that knowledge is also an important mission and is particularly highly valued in community-based medical schools; it may be less highly valued in some research-intensive medical schools.

Patient care, the other major mission of medical schools, is the primary mission of community and teaching hospitals. The challenge for teaching hospitals is to balance the need to survive financially by investing in the latest technologies and patient-care services, especially those that entail high reimbursement, with the need to provide appropriate learning opportunities for trainees. These needs are often at variance and create constant tensions between medical school and hospital leaders. In the nineteen community-based U.S. medical schools that depend on community hospitals for educational experiences for their students and residents, training needs sometimes take a lower priority than service demands.

In addition to the influence of universities and teaching hospitals, medical education is shaped by powerful external forces, notably for-profit health care companies, Medicare and Medicaid, private insurance companies and purchasers of health care, state and federal governments, and regulatory agencies. In the 1980s and 1990s, for example, as a response to increasing health care costs, hospitals had to take major steps to reduce costs and operate more efficiently. Teaching hospitals were particularly hard hit because of the higher cost of their teaching, research, and charity missions. In a price-competitive market economy, teaching hospitals focused on containing medical costs in order to survive, intensifying a latent tension between the patient care and teaching missions (Ludmerer, 1999). "Most pernicious of all from the standpoint of education," according to Ludmerer, "house officers [residents] to a considerable extent were reduced to work-up machines and disposition-arrangers: admitting patients and planning their discharge, one after another, with much less time than before to examine them, confer with attending physicians, teach medical students, attend conferences, read the literature, and reflect and wonder. They were also deprived of much of the opportunity to follow the course of disease since patients would be so quickly discharged" (p. 359).

These financial pressures, combined with dramatic increases in the complexity, breadth, and power of new technologies, diagnostic, and therapeutic treatments, have made the clinical environment a challenging place in which to learn. Common illnesses, for example, are seen less frequently at teaching hospitals than they have been in the past.

Regulation: Accreditation, Licensure, and Certification

On the national level, there is no formal oversight of the whole process of accreditation, licensure, and certification across all levels of medical education. All of the organizational bodies work semiautonomously and sometimes at odds, which, as the following discussion suggests, is a major problem for medical education (Ludmerer, 1999; Committee on the Health Professions Education Summit, 2003).

Accreditation: UME

Education of medical students is guided by accreditation standards established by the LCME, which is chartered by the U.S. Department of Education to accredit medical schools and ensure high-quality medical education; it is jointly operated by the AMA and the AAMC. The accreditation process requires medical schools to undertake a self-study every seven or eight years, followed by a site visit by an accreditation team of volunteer peers. To remain accredited, a medical school must meet 125 "essentials," or standards.

The direct consequence of this process is uniformly high standards of medical education nationally: "The accreditation process requires educational programs to provide assurances that their graduates exhibit general professional competencies that are appropriate for entry to the next stage of their training, and that serve as the foundation for lifelong learning and proficient medical care. While recognizing the existence and appropriateness of diverse institutional missions and educational objectives, the LCME subscribes to the proposition that local circumstances do not justify accreditation of a substandard program of medical education leading to the M.D. degree" (Liaison Committee on Medical Education, 2008, p. ii).

Accreditation of GME

Accreditation of GME, illustrated in Figure 5.1, occurs at both the institutional level and individual residency program level. The ACGME—comprised of representatives from AAMC, AMA, American Board of

Figure 5.1. Accreditation Agencies for Graduate Medical Education

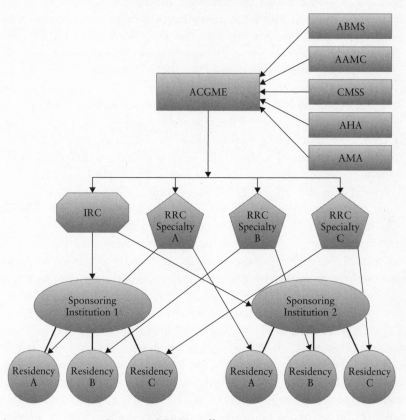

Source: ACGME staff communication.

Medical Specialties (ABMS), American Hospital Association (AHA), Council of Medical Specialty Societies (CMSS)—and its twenty-seven residency review committees (RRCs), and the American Board of Medical Specialties (ABMS) and its twenty-four constituent specialty boards oversee GME. Residency programs are accredited through ACGME; individuals are certified to practice in their specialty by ABMS. The specialty boards participate in both processes in two important ways: by (1) influencing the content of trainees' educational experience by determining the requirements for accreditation, and (2) assessing the graduates' knowledge and increasingly their performance through the certification examination.

Medical schools and teaching hospitals are accredited by the ACGME as institutions that sponsor residency and fellowship programs. Residency training qualifies graduates to sit for their first specialty boards; more specialized training, called fellowships, requires completion of additional training and qualifies the graduate to sit for a subspecialty board examination. Thus pediatric residency qualifies the graduate to take the pediatric board examination; subsequently, she may pursue fellowship training in pediatric cardiology. Likewise, an orthopedic surgeon (first board examination) may do a fellowship in hand surgery. The institutional accreditation focuses on educational quality and resident well-being across all residency programs in the institution, and the ACGME establishes common program requirements, spanning programs and specialties, such as the characteristics of the clinical sites for resident education, the level of faculty staffing supporting the program, resident duty hours, and the general goals or competencies to be achieved (Accreditation Council for Graduate Medical Education, 2007). ACGME accredits eighty-four hundred residency programs in the United States (in 126 specialties and subspecialties) that educate 107,000 residents.

Accreditation at the program level is through the specialty-specific RRCs, which set educational standards for the specialty and subspecialties. Each of the twenty-seven RRCs defines the content of GME for its specialty, specifying such experiences as the number of continuity clinics each internal medicine resident must have or, say, the minimum number of cholecystectomies a general surgery resident should have performed over the course of her residency, as well as the maximum time allowable in specific rotations to ensure that all residents are afforded a balanced and comprehensive educational program. Each RRC is composed of specialists who are nominated by the American Board of Medical Specialties, the American Medical Association, and the specialty professional society. These nominees are appointed by the ACGME, and the RRC's fiduciary responsibility is only to the ACGME. Although the institution reviews each residency program as part of its ACGME responsibility, residency program development and management occurs primarily at the department level.

In an attempt to increase and maintain the quality of all residency and fellowship programs, the RRCs have developed tightly prescribed program requirements. Although well intentioned, these requirements can inadvertently inhibit educational innovation. For example, a residency program director might want to increase resident time in ambulatory clinics but be unable to do so because of the prescribed number of weeks for inpatient rotations in that specialty. Therefore residents may spend an inordinate amount of time on inpatient clinical services, with no opportunity for rotations or clinics that would offer better learning experiences. Recognizing this problem, the ACGME and the Internal Medicine RRC have developed Educational Innovation Programs (EIP), designed to stimulate innovation and excellence. Residency programs may apply for an EIP if they have consistently met accreditation standards and can offer an innovative educational program proposal. If more widely adopted, such models would encourage innovation in GME.

Licensure and Certification

Physicians are trusted agents of the public's health and medical care. As a safeguard for the public, licensing and certification systems ensure that all practicing physicians demonstrate an appropriate level of knowledge and proficiency at various points in training and practice. Thus, when designing curricula, medical schools and residency programs must not only meet all of the accreditation standards but also take into account how the curriculum relates to the medical licensing requirements and certifying examinations, which are summarized in Table 5.1.

Table 5.1. Licensure and Certification Examinations for Physicians

	Agency Responsible	Examination	Timing
Licensure as a medical doctor (M.D.)	National Board of Medical Examiners Federation of State Medical Boards State medical licensing boards	United States Medical Licensing Examination (USMLE): Step 1: basic science knowledge Step 2: clinical knowledge or CK Step 2: clinical skills or CS Step 3: clinical knowledge	Step 1: end of second year of medical school Step 2: (CK and CS) in fourth year Step 3: during intern year
Certification as specialist	American Board of Medical Specialties and the Council of Medical Specialty Societies; individual specialty boards	Knowledge and clinical reasoning examination	At end of residency or fellowship training; sometimes after one or more years of practice
Recertification in specialty	Specialty boards	Knowledge and clinical reasoning examination	In some specialties every five to ten years

LICENSURE.   Awarding medical licenses is a state prerogative; the fundamental requirements are graduation from an accredited medical school and completion of some postgraduate training, generally one year for graduates of U.S. schools, and passage of all three steps of the USMLE, the medical licensing examination series. Some states have two levels of licensure: a limited license for supervised practice during residency training and a full license at the completion of GME. Other states award a full license once the fundamental requirements are met. USMLE is prepared by the NBME and co-owned and cosponsored by the NBME and the Federation of State Medical Boards (FSMB). NBME administers the Step 1 and Step 2 examinations; the FSMB administers Step 3.

As Table 5.1 indicates, students work through the three levels of the USMLE during medical school and residency. Students take Step 1, a multiple-choice exam testing basic science knowledge and clinical application, at the end of the second year of medical school. USMLE Step 1 assesses understanding and application of the scientific principles and concepts that are the foundation of medical practice. Emphasis is placed on principles and mechanisms relevant to health, disease, and modes of therapy.

In the fourth year, students take USMLE Step 2, which assesses application of clinical knowledge and skills to patient care scenarios, with emphasis on health promotion and disease prevention. Step 2 was originally only a multiple-choice examination testing clinical knowledge and reasoning, but in 2005 a performance component was added, focusing on the skills of taking histories, performing physical exams, and communication with patients, as well as professionalism; these are conducted at several national testing centers and use trained, standardized patients. Step 2 is the only portion of the licensing requirements that includes a performance component. The addition of this component acknowledges the distinction between cognitive skills and clinical and communication skills and recognizes the need to assess both in order to ensure readiness for supervised medical practice. Satisfactory completion of Step 1 and Step 2 is required for graduation from most medical schools.

Most residents training in the United States take Step 3, an assessment of clinical reasoning, typically taken at the end of the internship year. The USMLE Step 3 is "a final assessment of physicians assuming independent responsibility for delivering general medical care" (United States Medical Licensing Examination, 2009). The multiple-choice exam assesses knowledge and issues across medical specialties, understanding of biomedical and clinical science knowledge, and application of this knowledge to medical practice.

Because the mission of medical schools is to prepare students for practice and licensure, the faculty must be concerned about the content and timing of USMLE examinations. Some schools find the current timing an impediment to radical reorganization of the curriculum. For example, if a medical school wanted to create a new curriculum that integrated basic, clinical, and social sciences across all four years rather than covering the basic sciences in the first two years, this would make it difficult for students to pass Step 1 at the end of the second year because they would not yet have encountered all of the basic science curriculum. As we observed in Chapter Three, students in the second year often become excessively focused on Step 1 and may stop coming to class in order to spend more time studying for this exam, thus distorting their educational experience in the second year. The anxiety generated by this exam is fueled by the high-stakes nature of the assessment and by its inappropriate use in screening applicants for residency. Highly competitive residency programs do this despite poor correlation between USMLE Step 1 scores and supervisor ratings during residency ($r = 0.22$; 95 percent CI 0.13–0.30; see Hamdy et al., 2006). Increasingly, scores from both parts of Step 2 are being required by residency program directors as part of the residency application process.

Recent attention to the core competencies necessary for medical practice has sparked efforts to rethink the examinations required for licensure although it is unclear what, if any, changes will occur.

CERTIFICATION. Only after a resident or fellow has completed an accredited residency program may she be certified within her specialty. After completing an ACGME residency program in good standing and being vouched for by their residency programs as having the appropriate character and professional attributes of a physician, residency graduates may take their board examinations. The certifying exams are developed and administered by the specialty boards as described just above. The twenty-four members of the ABMS are a mixture of "first board" specialties, such as pediatrics and general surgery, and "secondary board" subspecialties, such as allergy and immunology and colorectal surgery. The specialty boards administer certifying examinations at the end of residency (first boards) and fellowship (second boards).

Individuals who pass the board examination are referred to as *board-certified*; those who completed an accredited residency but do not take or do not pass the board examination are referred to as *board-eligible*, although this is not a term that the specialty boards endorse. Approximately 75–80 percent of residency graduates take the initial board certification examination (Jeffe et al. 2006). We note that overall, the percentage of graduates of U.S. medical schools who plan to become board-certified appears to be declining (Davis & Ringsted, 2006). This may be due to the expense of the examination or its difficulty.

Increasingly, the specialty boards are requiring that practitioners recertify to describe themselves as board-certified; however, there are no systematic penalties for failing to certify. State licensing boards do not require initial or maintained specialty certification. In areas where the physician supply is adequate, insurance plans may expect specialty certification for their panel physicians, and hospitals and medical centers may require certification as part of the credentialing process. Physicians who have never been certified and who have not completed accredited residencies are more common in rural areas and underserved inner city populations, which may have difficulty attracting board-certified physicians.

Financing

The revenue for medical education comes from a variety of sources. Revenue for UME, for example, comes to the medical school from student tuition, state appropriations, parent university resources, endowment income, gifts from alumni and others interested in promoting medical education, grants, and medical school resources. From this mix of revenue, the school must cover faculty salaries, central administration and support services, technology, facilities, libraries, and scholarships. In contrast, a major contributor to funding GME is the federal government, through appropriations to Medicare and, in many states, Medicaid, which pays its fair share of the direct and indirect cost of medical education.

Revenues for medical schools have continued to climb over the past three decades, increasing most dramatically in the 1980s and 1990s with the influx of Medicare revenues and funding for biomedical research from the NIH. Although the size of the faculty, research, and clinical enterprises rose significantly during this period, medical student class sizes remained relatively constant, illustrating the growing commitment of faculty to activities other than education, as represented in Figure 5.2.

It is striking that today the largest revenue sources for medical schools, summarized in Figure 5.3, are the faculty practice (39 percent) and federal research grants and contracts (20 percent); these revenue streams correlate with faculty effort. As a result of expansion of faculty practice and grant revenues, the proportion of revenue that medical schools derive from their parent universities and state and local governments

Figure 5.2.   Growth in Medical School Faculty, Students, and Revenue, FY 1961–FY 2008

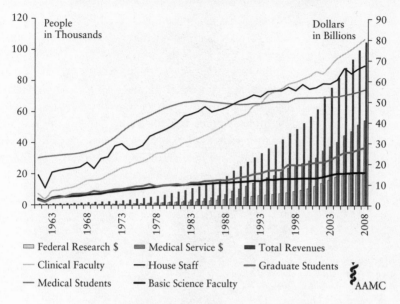

Source: AAMC staff, LCME Part I-A, Annual
Financial Questionnaire and LCME Part II, FY
1961–2008. ©2009 Association of American Medical
Colleges. All rights reserved. Reproduced with
permission.

has diminished to 6 percent on average, 11.6 percent in public and 0.5 percent in private medical schools.

Medical student education in state schools is typically funded on the basis of the number of students enrolled in the M.D. program. In some states, this comes to the school as a per-student allocation, and in other states it is based on a student-to-faculty ratio. For example, the University of California has historically funded medical school enrollment growth by providing for faculty salaries using a ratio of 3.5 full-time equivalent (FTE) medical students to one FTE faculty member, and seven residents to one faculty member. In public medical schools, the state and parent university portion of medical schools' revenues ranges from 1 percent to more than 35 percent as a percentage of total revenue based on figures reported on the AAMC's FY 2007 LCME Part I-A Annual Financial Questionnaire. As enrollments increase, new faculty FTEs are allocated to departments for use in their multiple missions of research, teaching, and patient care. Because most departments at research-intensive

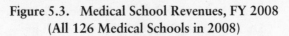

**Figure 5.3. Medical School Revenues, FY 2008
(All 126 Medical Schools in 2008)**

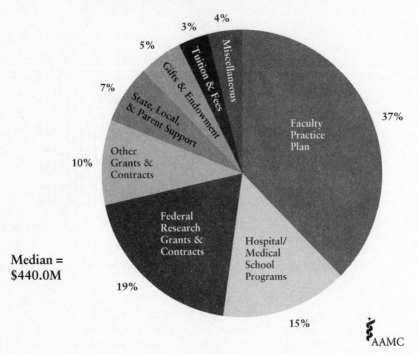

4%

3%

5%

7%

Miscellaneous

Tuition & Fees

Gifts & Endowment

State, Local, & Parent Support

Faculty
Practice
Plan   37%

Other
Grants &
Contracts   10%

Federal
Research
Grants &
Contracts

Hospital/
Medical
School
Programs

Median =
$440.0M

19%

15%

AAMC

Source: AAMC staff, LCME Part I-A, Annual
Financial Questionnaire, FY2008, Figure 1.1. ©2009
Association of American Medical Colleges. All rights
reserved. Reproduced with permission.

medical schools use faculty FTEs to recruit distinguished researchers, this leaves the teaching mission to be cross-subsidized by other departmental revenues such as clinical practice and philanthropy. There are slight variations in the sources of funding between public and private medical schools.

Table 5.2 portrays the similarities and differences between public and private medical schools in terms of funding. In addition to the public-private dichotomy, medical schools can be characterized in terms of the primary focus or governance structure of the school, such as research-intensive, community-based, and private freestanding. The twenty most research-intensive schools in the United States are among the largest institutions and are heavily invested in the research and clinical missions. The nineteen community-based schools use community

Table 5.2. Revenue Supporting Programs and
Activities at 126 Accredited U.S. Medical
Schools, Public vs. Private, FY2008
($ in Millions)

Revenue Source	76 Public Schools			50 Private Schools		
	All Revenue	% of Total	Mean	All Revenue	% of Total	Mean
Practice plans	$12,598	33.3	$166	$17,036	41.6	$341
Hospital purchased services and support	$ 5,874	15.5	$ 77	$ 5,683	13.9	$114
Federal appropriations	$ 215	0.6	$ 3	$ 27	0.1	$ 1
State and local govt. and parent university support	$ 4,710	12.4	$ 62	$ 247	0.6	$ 5
Tuition and fees	$ 1,173	3.1	$ 15	$ 1,523	3.7	$ 30
Endowment	$ 462	1.2	$ 6	$ 1,356	3.3	$ 27
Gifts	$ 773	2	$ 10	$ 1,328	3.2	$ 27
Miscellaneous sources	$ 1,633	4.3	$ 21	$ 1,482	3.6	$ 30
Total grants and contracts	$10,436	27.6	$137	$12,301	30	$246
Total revenues	$37,875	100.0	$498	$40,983	100.0	$820

physicians and community hospitals to conduct their clinical teaching programs; these predominantly small institutions derive a larger share of revenues from state and local appropriations and produce a high number of generalist physicians. The thirteen private freestanding medical schools in the United States do not have a parent university structure and receive little support from the government, relying more heavily on faculty practice revenue, tuition, and support from their affiliated teaching hospital(s). Figures 5.4 and 5.5 illustrate the differences between research-intensive and community-based schools.

In recent years, state, local, and parent-university support for public medical schools has decreased as a percentage of total medical school funding while grants and contracts, faculty practices, and tuition have all increased.

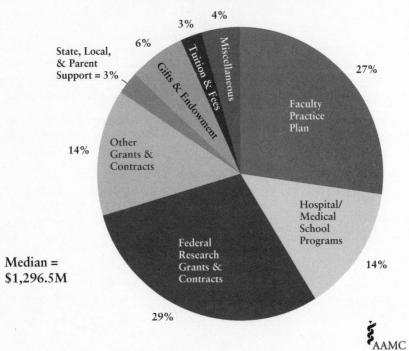

Figure 5.4. Medical School Revenues, FY 2008
(Top 20 Research-Intensive Medical Schools)

The Cost of Educating Medical Students

The literature on how much it costs to educate medical students and
residents is surprisingly sparse and based on a number of research
methodologies. One study collected time and activity data from students
during their clerkships at fifteen-minute intervals (Weinberg, O'Sullivan,
Boll, & Nelson, 1994). In a study conducted in 1992, the direct and indirect costs of educating a typical third-year medical student in the hospital
setting were calculated at $31,776, excluding the teaching contributions
of residents. Others have collected information from faculty self-reports,
teaching databases, and department teaching assignments. The instructional cost of adding medical students to a setting that already has
graduate medical education, research, and patient care, when adjusted to

Figure 5.5. Medical School Revenues, FY 2008
(19 Community-based Medical Schools)

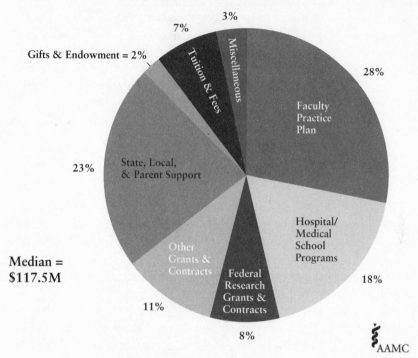

Median =
$117.5M

the base year of 1996, averages $40,000–$50,000 per student per year. The total cost of developing and managing a medical education program is estimated to be $71,000–$93,000 per student per year (Jones & Korn, 1997). Adjusting these figures to account for a decade of inflation (27 percent between 1997 and 2007) reveals that the total cost of educating a medical student ranges from $90,000 to $118,000 annually.

The presence of medical students in a practice, mostly studied in ambulatory settings, decreases physician productivity by 30 to 40 percent (Garg, Boero, Christiansen, & Booher, 1991; Vinson & Paden, 1994). In another study, the operating costs of ambulatory clinics with medical students and residents increased costs by 24 to 36 percent (Boex et al., 2000). When students were present in a nonacademic family physician's offices, the amount of time physicians spent working increased by

52 minutes per day, and their patient productivity decreased from 3.9 to 3.3 patients per hour (Vinson, Paden, & Devera-Sales, 1996). Thus, even if physicians are not being paid for supervising students and residents, there is a significant cost to the organization or practice in terms of lost productivity.

Similar results were found for the costs of training residents in general internal medicine ambulatory clinics. Teaching sites were found to have 36 percent higher operating costs than their nonteaching counterparts; 38 percent of these higher costs were due to infrastructure differences and 62 percent were the direct costs of teaching (Hogan, Franzini, & Boex, 2000).

Financial Burden on Students

Because the population benefits from having a stable workforce and appropriate distribution of physicians, state funding for medical student education has been strong in public schools. However, in the past decade, as state support for medical education has tended to decline in relative terms, student tuition has risen dramatically, resulting in higher student debt.

The AAMC reports that in 2007 88 percent of medical students received financial aid and 80 percent of that aid was in the form of student loans. In 2007, the average student debt was $129,800 for indebted graduates of public medical schools and $156,800 for indebted graduates of private medical schools. This is a dramatic increase from 1998, when it was $72,700 for public and $103,600 for private medical school indebted graduates (Association of American Medical Colleges, 2008). This growing debt, combined with lower salaries for generalist physicians, may contribute to graduates not selecting primary care specialties and not choosing to practice in underserved communities, thus exacerbating physician shortages in these areas.

Funding for Graduate Medical Education

Revenue for graduate medical education comes from multiple funders. As noted earlier, Medicare and Medicaid are the primary sources, but private insurers also recognize the higher cost of teaching hospitals. Additional funds come from federal training grants for residents and fellows, from patient-care revenue generated by fellows, and from medical school resources.

In 1965, Congress amended the Social Security Act and passed Medicare legislation that provided for a federally administered health insurance program for people sixty-five or older and certain disabled persons; it explicitly recognized the incremental costs of training physicians and other health personnel by supplementing payments for health care services. Medicare is the single largest payer of graduate medical education, contributing almost $8 billion to teaching hospitals in 2004. This funding comes in two segments. First is direct medical education (commonly referred to as DME) reimbursement of approximately $2.6 billion in 2004 to support Medicare's share of the stipends for residents, the cost of resident supervision, and other direct costs of the teaching program. Reimbursement is based on the number of residents in training and the percentage of Medicare patients at that hospital. The per-resident amount is updated annually from the base year (typically 1984) using the Consumer Price Index. Direct funding to teaching hospitals is then reduced for residents and fellows who have passed their first board certification (for example, residency training completed in internal medicine, first board certification) but are pursuing training in a specialty fellowship such as cardiology, second board certification (Knapp, 2002).

The second form of Medicare reimbursement to teaching hospitals is indirect medical education (called IME), $5.3 billion in 2004. This reimbursement covers the additional expenses the hospital incurs for educating trainees, such as more laboratory tests ordered by residents and supplemental expenses associated with having residents in the facility. Reimbursement is calculated from a legislatively determined multiplier and the resident-to-bed ratio of the hospital, which serve as proxies for all the additional costs to the institution of educating residents and the added cost of the highly specialized patient care services in these institutions. States are not required to contribute to GME but most do so through a federal-state partnership (Knapp, 2002).

Spending on GME has gone up every year since 1984, when GME payments were incorporated into the Medicare prospective payment system. None of these resources can be used to support medical student education, and most other third-party payers, including Medicaid, prohibit billing for educating medical students. Because these funds flow to the hospital, they may be blended with other sources of hospital income to support hospital services. They are used to cover resident salaries but may or may not be used to offset mandated indirect costs of resident education, such as an office of graduate medical education and departmental residency program administration.

Nonuniversity teaching hospitals host approximately two-thirds of all residency training programs nationally and educate a significant number of third- and fourth-year medical students. These teaching hospitals value their affiliation with medical schools because they believe it helps them recruit medical students into their residency programs, recruit and retain better medical staff, and improve patient care. Medical schools value these affiliated hospitals because they bring much needed and diverse training experiences for their students, residents, and fellows. Rarely do medical schools or state agencies pay these affiliated hospitals to train medical students.

Hospitals that treat a significant percentage of poor or uninsured patients also receive disproportionate share (DSH or "dish") funding from the federal government through an adjustment to Medicare reimbursement rates. DSH funding is not specifically dedicated to GME, but it is additional revenue that teaching hospitals need because they provide a large proportion of uncompensated care. The nation's 130 Veteran's Affairs (VA) medical centers have affiliation agreements with 105 medical schools. Approximately thirty-two thousand residents annually receive some training in these facilities, and the VA hosts about 9 percent of the nation's residency programs, accounting for approximately eighty-nine hundred residency positions. Some funding for GME also comes from the Department of Defense and the NIH. The total amount of GME funding from these sources could be in the range of $1 billion to $2 billion (Anderson, Greenberg, & Wynn, 2001).

Other third-party payers, such as managed care plans and private insurers, have historically supported GME through higher payments to teaching hospitals; however, in a competitive marketplace they have become less willing to do so. Though it is difficult to estimate how much this accounts for, it may represent 5–10 percent higher payments to teaching hospitals than to nonteaching hospitals (Anderson et al., 2001).

THE COSTS OF GME.   The costs of residency training have been studied in a variety of ways. The total cost of educating a family practice resident per year (excluding malpractice expense and Medicaid GME revenue) was $44,812 in 2003 (Pauwels & Oliveira, 2006). The cost of graduate medical education on inpatient service has also been examined; using hospital accounting systems to determine the costs of cases associated with residents and those without, teaching cases added 4.4 percent to the total direct and variable costs of inpatient admissions (Kane et al., 2005).

Another approach to studying the cost of graduate medical education is to examine all departmental expenses associated with the teaching and administration of residency programs. Administrative costs, such as staffing and coordinating residency programs and space rental, when figured on a per capita or per resident basis vary inversely with the size of the program (Nasca et al., 2001). In 2003, the training costs were $34,000 for a resident and $17,500 for a fellow per year

(Zeidel et al., 2005). The VA allocates $43,000 per year to its hospitals to cover education-related expenses in addition to the salary and fringe benefits for each physician in training (Department of Veterans Affairs, 2004).

Another form of analysis is to compare the costs of university teaching hospitals, nonuniversity teaching hospitals, and nonteaching hospitals. In 1993, urban academic health center costs per case were 83 percent higher than those for urban nonteaching hospitals. Nonuniversity teaching hospitals, those that train medical students and residents but are not closely affiliated with a medical school, had 23 percent higher costs than did nonteaching hospitals. After adjusting for case mix, wage levels, and direct GME costs, one finds that university teaching hospitals were 44 percent more expensive than nonuniversity teaching hospitals, which were in turn 14 percent more costly than nonteaching hospitals (Mechanic, Coleman, & Dobson, 1998).

Funding Issues

Funding of medical education has long been a topic of debate among medical educators and in Congress. Conflicts arise over the appropriateness of funding GME through Medicare and how to deal with the widening gap between reimbursement rates for primary and specialty care physician services. Finally, funding sources create incentives and disincentives to medical education, and aligning financing to mission is an important issue for institutions of all types.

A TOPIC OF POLICY DEBATE.   An intense policy debate has consistently swirled around funding for both DME and IME through Medicare. The focus of this debate has been on who should receive the funding (teaching hospital, outpatient clinics, medical schools, providers, or residents), whether the allocation formula is appropriate, and whether the federal government should be paying for GME at all (Anderson et al., 2001). Should funds be paid as they currently are to the hospital, or to the medical school (Anderson et al., 2001)? There are also concerns about wide variation in the amounts paid to teaching hospitals under the existing, historic formulas (Iglehart, 1999). The per-resident reimbursement rates for hospitals in New York, Massachusetts, and Illinois, for example, are high in comparison to hospitals in Texas and California thanks to inclusion of faculty teaching costs in some states and not in others. There are many in Congress who assert that GME should not be funded through patient-care expenditures associated with Medicare and Medicaid. The larger issue, however, is whether medical education is a public good to be supported by public funds or a market good that produces high-earning physicians who should pay the full cost of their own education (Gbadebo & Reinhardt, 2001).

THE WIDENING REIMBURSEMENT GAP.   There is an additional factor that affects funding of both UME and GME: the widening gap in reimbursement for primary care and specialty care. The salaries of general internists, pediatricians, and family practitioners are approximately half those of all other medical and surgical specialists (Bodenheimer, Berenson, & Rudolf, 2007). In addition to their importance to a well-functioning delivery system, primary care clinics are an important venue for learning initial clinical skills in medical school. Primary care faculty members also are responsible for a disproportionate amount of teaching in the medical student curriculum because their clinical activities support the general professional education of beginning physicians. However, they are also the ones who can no longer make their salaries from professional practice revenue because of low reimbursements and must be subsidized by the hospital, other specialty services, or the larger organization.

ALIGNING FINANCES WITH THE EDUCATIONAL MISSION.   Although most would argue that there are ample funds available to support the educational mission, the challenge is ensuring that the funds allocated to medical education actually are used for this purpose. A common refrain of university medical faculty members is "I don't get paid to teach," meaning they must fund their own salaries from patient care revenue or grants. It is unusual for faculty members to be paid directly to teach; it is assumed that each faculty member will contribute time to teaching as a volunteer.

To change this situation, it is necessary to identify revenue sources and connect them to faculty contributions to teaching, research, and patient care, aligning them where possible. For most faculty members and some department chairs, the relationship between revenue sources and faculty salaries is not well understood. Clearly identified revenue streams have been difficult to isolate, and cross-subsidization has been common. Over the past several decades, medical schools have worked to understand the costs and revenues associated with their multiple missions, align departmental expectations with accountability and outcomes, share transparent data, and make effective management decisions on the basis of this information (Mallon, 2009). This process is often referred to as "mission-based management" or "mission-based budgeting," a management approach that embraces open books, peer accountability, and collaboration. The first requirement is an integrated financial statement, and the second is a series of productivity reports that are based on quantitative assessments of the enterprise. Without such a system, strategic decisions are made in a vacuum and educational contributions of faculty members go undocumented and typically unfunded.

A number of schools document educational revenues and expenses and allocate funds specifically to the multiple missions according to faculty contributions and quality (Nutter et al., 2000; Sloan, Kaye, Allen, Magness, & Wartman, 2005; Stites, Vansaghi, Pingleton, Cox, & Paolo, 2005; Watson & Romrell, 1999). To make this work, deans and department chairs establish clear policies, metrics, and measurement systems to monitor and reward faculty contributions to education, research, patient care, and service. Most systems use "relative value units" (RVUs) to measure faculty effort. Educational activities, such as lecturing, facilitating small group learning, laboratory teaching, clinical teaching, developing educational products, creating an examination, advising and mentoring, educational leadership, research in medical education, and service on editorial boards, are enumerated. Then each activity is assigned a unit or value. For example, a lecture in the first two years of the medical school curriculum might be worth the amount of face time with the students plus five hours for preparation, mentoring, and testing (Jarrell, Mallot, Peartree, & Calia, 2002). Inpatient attending responsibilities might be valued at two hours per day (Watson & Romrell, 1999). Or a residency program director might receive 0.30 FTE and a clerkship director 0.20 (Stites et al., 2005). In addition to quantity, some systems also assess the quality of teaching contributions. These systems allow deans and department chairs to connect faculty contributions of teaching, research, and patient care to institutional expectations and resources.

Those schools that have used mission-based management report a significant shift in resource allocations on the basis of mission-related expenditure, with support for education typically increasing. If the metric is easily understandable, easy to implement, and fairly applied, faculty perceive a more equitable alignment of teaching effort and funding (Ruedy, MacDonald, & MacDougall, 2003; Stites et al., 2005). If not, faculty members criticize it for being overly complex and burdensome, difficult to implement, inequitable, and focused on quantifiable rather than important measures of success (Mallon, 2009). In 2003–04, thirty-five schools (28 percent of medical schools) implemented systems that distributed funding to departments and faculty members according to their contributions to education and another forty schools (32 percent) were developing such systems (Barzansky & Etzel, 2004). The popularity of this approach comes from its ability to align faculty activity with the appropriate mission so that resources are transparently matched with faculty effort and management decisions can be based on accurate information.

Innovations in Financing Medical Education

In the course of the study, we came across several promising approaches to funding medical education. By way of example, here we describe four such collaborations between medical schools and their teaching hospitals: the University of Florida, the Mayo Clinic, the University of Michigan, and the University of Pennsylvania.

University of Florida

The university's College of Medicine adopted mission-based management early. In 1994, the college created a three-step process of financial planning, assessment, and allocation: (1) revenues were prospectively identified for each mission and aligned with intended purposes, (2) faculty productivity (quantity and quality) were measured for each mission, and (3) productivity was linked to the prospective budget for each mission (Watson & Romrell, 1999). The dean defined the revenues for the educational mission and a committee recommended that 70 percent of unrestricted state funds be designated for the educational mission; by the time of this study, the dean had increased the allocation to 85 percent. Of these funds, 15 percent were allocated to general educational administration in the dean's office and 85 percent were distributed for departmental educational administrative costs and in recognition of the quantity and the quality of departmental teaching contributions.

Faculty productivity is determined across all missions using relative value units. Educational activities are tracked centrally for direct faculty contact hours, and faculty members are given two hours of preparation credit for each hour of direct contact as well as credit for directing a course or serving on an education committee. In the clinical setting, teaching on an inpatient service is counted as two hours of instruction per day; teaching in an ambulatory clinic is allocated 1.2 hours per half-day. Quality of teaching is assessed by student evaluations of faculty and courses, course directors' annual reports, student performance on both external examinations and the fourth-year comprehensive objective structured clinical examination, and finally on the quality of assessments used to evaluate student performance. From all these data, a committee annually assigns a quality factor to each course and clerkship; departments then receive their portion of the quality allocation for the educational mission. On the basis of these faculty and departmental productivity data, a number of standard reports are generated and data-driven decisions can be made about faculty assignments, rewards, and alignment of resources and missions.

In 2004, the College of Medicine and its affiliate, Shands Teaching Hospital and Clinics, entered into an Academic and Quality Support Agreement that defines the funds flow from Shands to the College of Medicine. Annually, a management committee consisting of the dean, the CEO of the hospital, and the university senior vice president of health affairs approves proposals for this funding stream in two categories: base support and board-designated funds support. The annual base support consists of the base support given in the preceding fiscal year and can be increased if Shands met certain financial performance targets and the College of Medicine met certain quality performance indicators in that prior fiscal year. Base support is paid out each month in advance and through invoices from the College of Medicine for costs incurred. The former amounts to $16.4 million or 61 percent of the total annual support funding, and the latter amounts to $4.3 million or 15.9 percent of the total annual support funding. The board-designated funding for specific approved projects amounts to $6.2 million or 23.1 percent of the total support funding.

Mayo Clinic College of Medicine

This is one of the smallest medical schools in the United States, with 41 first-year medical students and a total of 164 enrolled medical students. The major focus of education at Mayo is on graduate medical education with its 1,400 residents and fellows. It is unique in being embedded in a large health care system rather than a university, with locations in Rochester, Minnesota (1,550 salaried physicians); Scottsdale, Arizona (315 salaried physicians); and Jacksonville, Florida (300 salaried physicians). Mayo Clinic is the largest private group practice in the United States and is a nonprofit organization. The mission of Mayo Clinic and its College of Medicine is "to provide the best care to every patient every day through integrated clinical practice, education and research" (Mayo Clinic, 2009). This strong value of doing the best for the patient every time imbues the culture with a strong commitment to quality improvement, collaboration, teaching, and research.

Combined revenues from the Mayo Foundation sustain the practice. Education and research are supported by extramural funding, philanthropy, and other Mayo funds. In 2005, educational expenses totaled $129.3 million, of which $105.1 million went to graduate medical education and $3.6 million to medical student education. Thus graduate medical education is by far the largest educational program in terms of expense, as well as size.

All physicians at Mayo are salaried and may choose the missions in which they invest their time and energy. For those who choose to teach, there is a reduction in workload as appropriate to accommodate teaching responsibilities. Mayo has implemented a comprehensive, role-related, competency-based faculty development program. There are workshops to enhance skills in teaching, curriculum development, mentoring, assessment of learners and programs, applying for funding, and writing and publishing, as well as programs for personal and leadership development. Mayo funds programs for educational innovation and research, and it rewards scholarly contributions in education with advancement in academic rank.

University of Michigan

In 2002, the University of Michigan Medical School embarked on a new financial management approach (Elger, 2006). The leadership sought to create a new management system that would more closely align the school's mission, vision, and values with its financial resources and expenditures and allow faculty to better understand the choices that were being made in the course of managing a $1 billion operation. Through extensive discussion within the school, a series of key performance indicators were agreed on, among them the school's and departments' financial and management performance, the educational ranking of students, patient satisfaction and access to care, and faculty clinical work performance. This has developed into a multiyear database that can be queried and used to make timely strategic decisions. Although not universally appreciated by the faculty, it has created a more transparent financial system and improved the ability to connect resources with the appropriate mission.

In 2005, the School of Medicine moved beyond internal financial restructuring to negotiate an agreement with the University of Michigan Medical Center to transfer $15 million of the existing central GME funds into a fund functioning as an endowment. Over the first five years, the interest generated from these funds was put aside as designated funds to support capital expenses in the Clinical Simulation Center. Subsequently, the annual interest will be used to fund GME innovations as described in the next paragraph. It is anticipated that this will make approximately $750,000 available annually.

The Graduate Medical Education Innovations Program establishes a mechanism that faculty use to fund innovative educational initiatives in GME. During the first year, through a merit-based proposal process, $1 million was committed. The subsequent four years saw about $500,000 disbursed annually. In addition, a number of programs and initiatives were funded: resident mental health program, minority recruitment and development, contingency funds, internal review compensation, and faculty support. Once the central obligations were fulfilled, the funds remaining were disbursed to departments in proportion to the number of residents they trained and in relation to their compliance with reporting requirements.

University of Pennsylvania

Like other medical schools, the University of Pennsylvania draws on a variety of funding sources to support medical education. The dean of the medical school, the hospital administrator, and the head of the faculty practice plan determine allocations of medical education resources derived from the medical center. This integrated structure brings together the three largest stakeholders in the medical education enterprise to disburse $20 million, guided by the teaching efforts of the faculty as measured by Penn's RVU system and the quality of instruction.

Funds-flow principles were determined prior to distributing funds for teaching: align commitments with strategic plans, make it fair and transparent, match revenue with expenses, provide appropriate incentives, and measure performance over time. From these principles, the committee recommended that support should be given to the departments for didactic and small-group medical student teaching, for faculty time supervising residents and medical students, and for departmental administrative support for teaching programs. Teaching support was also extended for course directors and other administrative teaching duties. Funds for resident supervision were allocated according to the number of residents within a department and the average faculty salaries for those departments, using a ratio of one resident supervisor for six residents in the cognitive specialties and one resident supervisor for ten residents in the procedural specialties. Program director support was based on the number of residents within a program and adjusted according to specialty-specific ACGME requirements. In the absence of specialty specific requirements, programs with up to fifteen residents received 0.125 FTE of GME program director support, and this increased in gradations up to 1.0 FTE for more than seventy-five residents in a program.

In terms of the mission-specific funding from fiscal year 2005 to FY 2007, teaching support increased 300 percent from $7.6 million to $23.9 million, and defined research support increased from $11.1 million to

$33.0 million. In contrast, support for the clinical mission remained essentially stable.

Regulation and Financing: The Work Ahead

Medical education exists within a web of regulatory and financial relationships that both support and challenge educational excellence. Each relationship needs to be examined, strengthened, and aligned. The innovations of individual institutions and programs, although important, are not sufficient to effect reform of U.S. medical education; significant reform of medical education can be realized only with significant improvements in the national systems of licensing, accreditation, and certification. To this end, in Chapter Eight we propose a set of policy recommendations that would promote the conditions for significant reform.

The regulatory burden on schools and residency programs is great, and the standards of one agency are not always consistent with those of others. Among the possibilities for better integrating and coordinating standards for accreditation, certification, and licensing is establishing a single oversight body for medical education. At the same time, funding of academic medicine needs to be made more transparent and fair; this will entail aligning finances with missions in both medical schools and teaching hospitals.

The reforms we propose would bring important changes to the external forces of regulation and financing that so powerfully affect medical education, coordinating them with forces internal to medical education that are already exerting pressure for much-needed reforms to promote educational excellence, curricular innovation, and reform of pedagogy. Individuals and groups within programs and institutions are trying to counterbalance the effects of the pace and commercial nature of health care. In the next chapter, we look at how strong central leadership and innovative organizational structures are fostering attention to excellence and supporting standardization and individualization, integration, habits of inquiry and improvement, and identity formation at all levels of medical education.

6

LEADERSHIP FOR ORGANIZATIONAL CHANGE

JUST AS EXTERNAL FORCES create pressures on medical education, so do internal forces. An important internal force is the vision and energy of highly effective leaders, from deans to individual faculty members, who over recent decades have been transforming medical education from within, course by course, program by program. Whether by overhauling courses or clerkships and residency programs or implementing broad institutional curricular initiatives, many educational leaders have been changing the culture of their school. Although bringing about fundamental change in institutional culture might seem daunting, or even insurmountable, in the course of our study we found a number of examples of inspiring leaders whose efforts have radically changed educational programs to improve teaching and learning for their students and residents.

In this chapter, after an overview of the internal organization of medical education, we describe how leaders at every level are accomplishing institutional change. In our examples, we draw on real cases derived from our site visits and review of the literature on leadership and organizational change. To keep the focus on the dynamics of leadership and the change process, we do not identify either the institutions or the people involved.

Organization

Although their organizational structures vary considerably, medical schools share many similarities. They are large organizations that employ on average one thousand full-time faculty members with a range from one hundred to nearly eight thousand, and three times that number of support staff; they enroll 164–1,381 medical students and three times that many residents and fellows (Association of American Medical Colleges, 2008). As suggested by the discussion of financing in Chapter Five, teaching hospitals are multimillion- or billion-dollar businesses. It should be noted that the size of the faculty is determined by the needs of the clinical and research enterprises as well as the number of faculty needed to educate students and residents; thus faculty size is not necessarily related to medical student class size.

In 2007, for example, total enrollment of medical students per school averaged 553 students (138 per class), but enrollment at individual schools varied considerably, from 164 total students (41 students per class) at the Mayo Clinic College of Medicine to 1,381 (345 students per class) at the University of Illinois (Association of American Medical Colleges, 2008). Of late, with the intention of increasing medical student enrollment nationally by 30 percent, existing medical schools are expanding class size and new medical schools are being created across the country.

Locus of Responsibility

UME is the responsibility of the dean of the medical school, although this function is typically delegated to the vice or associate dean for medical education. In some schools, assistant or associate deans deal with admissions, student affairs, curricular affairs, and an office of medical education. GME is much more decentralized than UME, with the institution and the specialty sharing responsibility. Although the office of graduate medical education typically houses the "designated institutional official" (usually with the title of associate dean for graduate medical education) who is responsible for overseeing all residency and fellowship programs at that institution and serves as the liaison to the ACGME, each residency program has its own program director who coordinates the program within that specialty.

For UME, this central, integrative function requires strong leadership on the part of the dean and associate deans as well as an active and engaged curriculum committee and subcommittees. The impetus to innovate in medical education can come from a variety of sources, among them the dean, associate dean for curriculum, national reports, accreditation reports, faculty members, or students. However, it is the responsibility of the school's curriculum committee to oversee the design, conduct, evaluation, and revision of the curriculum. Curriculum committees ensure faculty oversight and involvement even though the administrative responsibility for the curriculum rests with the dean.

Supporting Innovation

Although every medical school has a curriculum committee, some exert visionary leadership, inspiring innovation, and some perform essential management functions, establishing educational guidelines and monitoring performance. Others do very little. Where there is strong leadership, central resources to support medical education, and an inspiring vision, innovative educational programs abound; this is the subject of our discussion in this chapter.

To encourage creativity and innovation, some schools award educational innovation grants to improve teaching and learning. These funds are often allocated for use in projects associated with curriculum reform, pedagogical improvement, strengthened assessment, or educational research. A few medical schools we visited are intentionally blurring the boundary between UME and GME as innovations in one domain cross over to the other. For instance, electronic performance evaluation systems and teacher rating systems are used in both UME and GME, as are electronic portfolios. Some schools are developing common curriculum organized around shared competencies that could be used in UME, GME, and continuing medical education. We strongly support these synergistic changes.

Indeed, in the course of our study we noted many ingredients of successful change, but often they were particular to local settings. Among those that can be generalized across settings, five appear to be necessary for transforming medical education:

1. Effective leaders and productive teams
2. An institutional culture of creativity, inquiry, and continuous improvement
3. Organizational structures that promote action, discipline, and innovation
4. Educational resources and support services to fuel innovation and excellence
5. Academic communities that advance the scholarship of teaching and learning

These key ingredients for successful innovation and reform are the primary focus of this chapter.

Effective Leaders and Productive Teams

Medical education programs thrive when there are effective leaders, productive work teams, and collaborative relationships among administrators, faculty members, staff members, and learners. Indeed, we found excellent educational leaders and vigorous leadership teams at all of the medical schools we visited. Their excitement, shared vision, collegiality, educational innovation, and commitment to excellence were clearly evident. Although it is impossible to disentangle entirely the role of leadership from the organizational culture and resources, we found leaders and guiding coalitions that have helped their school make the creative leap into new programs.

We observed leadership in action at various levels. For example, at some schools deans have played a pivotal role in initiating and guiding curriculum reform; at others, vice and associate deans have been instrumental in effecting educational transformation. At the departmental level, chairs, clerkship directors, and residency program directors have dramatically improved education. What was consistent, however, is that in every instance these leaders have worked collaboratively to improve the quality of medical education and in the process achieved remarkable results. Consider this case:

○

When a new dean was recruited to a medical school in a rural state, he found a small, state-sponsored, community-based medical school with a mission to educate primary care physicians for the state. He was attracted to the strong educational focus of the school, even though the curriculum and facilities were dated. On arrival, this enthusiastic and affable dean began to articulate a new and exciting vision for an innovative educational program that would make the university a leader in medical education. He spoke passionately and enthusiastically about the importance of medical student education and worked persistently on behalf of the educational mission. He assembled a new leadership team and inspired its members to reform the curriculum from a traditional discipline-based approach to a problem-based, integrated structure for the first two years of study. He then appointed a curriculum planning task force, selecting faculty members who were open to reform, and instructed the members to learn about educational innovations occurring nationally and visit other medical schools that had already made significant changes. From their review of curriculum reform nationally and a "wipe-the-slate-clean" approach, together they designed and later implemented a new curriculum. Accomplishing this goal took persistence, hard work, and leadership at every level of the organization.

The dean supported the process by providing additional resources and political guidance and by making public speeches that articulated the vision and importance of educational reform. Recognizing that clinical skills are an important but underemphasized component of the curriculum, he established and built a clinical skills center to be used by both medical students and residents. Oversight of the curriculum was centralized in the dean's office, and medical educators were recruited to support the endeavor. With the full approval of the medical students to underwrite enhancements, additional technology was made available and tuition was increased for three consecutive years.

A major reason for the continuing success of the new curriculum has been the dean's unwavering commitment to medical student education, a guiding coalition of faculty leaders, and investment of additional resources in the educational endeavor.

○

The approach of the dean in this case is congruent with the literature on the essential behaviors or practices of successful leaders: they articulate vision and generate excitement for change, attract and empower others, build a creative culture, establish organizational structures that ensure disciplined action, act with integrity and humility, demonstrate unwavering resolve to do what it takes, and garner and use resources effectively (Kouzes & Posner, 1995; Kotter, 1996; Collins, 2001, 2005).

Successful leaders also continuously learn and scan the environment for new ideas. They do this by listening attentively, reading widely, digging deeper into problems, spotting opportunities, challenging prevailing practices, and promoting organizational learning. Creative leaders see possibilities where others might see impediments to further progress and they break down barriers to achieve successful action (Bereiter & Scardamalia, 1993). Leaders are able to articulate an emerging vision and inspire others to achieve common goals and work in a self-motivated manner (Collins, 2005). They are also able to communicate a sense of urgency and take disciplined action, developing plans, organizational cultures, and structures.

In every school and residency program we visited, we observed examples of strong educational leadership teams. These teams include not only the dean and vice or associate deans for education but also committee chairs, faculty leaders, staff members, and, in some cases, the medical center CEO. Schools and programs organize their change initiatives differently, but they have in common an impressive level of enthusiasm and dedication of the team members working together in pursuit of a mutual goal of promoting exceptional educational experiences for students and residents and an outstanding product: competent and compassionate physicians.

Some leadership teams are assembled to design and implement an innovation in a particular area of the curriculum, such as clerkship education, as this example illustrates:

---
o

After reforming the curriculum for the first two years of UME, the medical school's central leaders turned to the task of revising clinical clerkships. The vice dean had expressed concern about the discontinuities students experienced as part of their clinical clerkship experiences and the failure of the current clinical environment to meet the educational needs of third-year clerks. In response to his call for change, several clerkship site directors at one community hospital planned a full-scale restructuring of the entire third-year clerkship experience with the purpose of dramatically improving the educational experience for students. Aided by support from the dean's office and the hospital CEO, these enthusiastic and creative clerkship site directors set about generating a new vision for clinical education, one so sweeping that it might also change the culture of the institution.

The initial planning team comprised a variety of stakeholders, approached the work collaboratively, and celebrated creativity. Leaders facilitated open dialogue and identified guiding principles and evidence in the literature to support the incipient program concepts. The leaders clearly and repeatedly expressed commitment to a broad and inspiring vision of clinical education. They organized their work so they could address problems as they arose. They developed functional leadership structures that could compel change through communal work in naming and addressing barriers to success. The result: they developed an ambulatory-oriented, integrated, patient-centered, yearlong, longitudinal clerkship experience.

---
o

Assembling the right people and empowering them to excel is the primary task of institutional leaders—in this case, the vice dean, who understood that the leadership team in the community hospital would be crucial to the success of the innovation. As the literature suggests, the first task of institutional leaders is selecting members of the team—"getting the right people on the bus," to use Collins's phrase (2001, 2005).

Change is fundamentally a team sport (Kouzes & Posner, 1995; Kotter, 1996; Wright et al., 2000; Gardner, 2007; Loeser, O'Sullivan, & Irby, 2007).

We also observed that committed and persistent leadership is essential to achieving major curricular change, especially when changing circumstances necessitate adapting to new procedures and relationships, as another case suggests:

○

During his long tenure, an enthusiastic associate dean worked on a variety of important education initiatives. Early on, he established an energetic team of educational leaders who over the ensuing decades developed numerous educational innovations, from curriculum reform to clinical performance exams, a society of teaching scholars, and mission-based management. The enthusiasm generated by this group is palpable, and the team of administrators, faculty members, and staff members genuinely enjoy contributing to the formation of future physicians. Moreover, the team has consistently sought input from learners, making them important and valuable partners in the academic improvement process.

One of the associate dean's initiatives was mission-based budgeting, a means of linking funds intended for education with their allocation. Although it took several years to refine data-collection criteria and processes and to help the teaching faculty fully understand that their time teaching was not "voluntary," mission-based budgeting has become critical to valuing the educational mission and appreciating faculty members as teachers.

Another success at this school was development of a community of teachers, not just through budgeting but by honoring them. The Society of Teaching Scholars supports faculty members in continuing to learn about teaching, and it recognizes, celebrates, and rewards them for their contributions to teaching and learning. The Office for Program Evaluation and Faculty Development establishes a foundation for continuous quality improvement through regular feedback about students' progress, faculty members' effectiveness in teaching, courses and clerkships, and the overall education program. This evaluation program monitors progress and constitutes a basis for continuous curriculum renewal.

The associate dean was persistent in his pursuit of these innovations and helped focus the faculty on the benefits that would accrue from them. This persistence was especially important in the formative period, when problems emerged and frustration flared up.

Yet perseverance and openness to input allowed the programs to go forward and ultimately improve the educational programs at this university.

---

o

Research on leadership also suggests that no one set of attributes is universally appropriate across contexts, times, and organizations (Fiedler, 1967; Vroom & Yetton, 1973). Each situation demands its own type of leader. This situational or contingency theory of leadership asserts that there is an interaction between the qualities of the leader and the needs and culture of the organization (Bolman & Deal, 2003). For example, a school or program might need a visionary and inspirational leader to initiate change but a very tough negotiator in fiscally lean times in order to cut budgets and shrink programs. The real key to effective leadership, according to this theory, is the appropriate match of the individual leader to the organization and its environment.

If innovation involves major curricular change, then a substantial political process ensues. Successful leaders build coalitions to support change, and they foster advocacy for reform (Kotter, 1996; Bolman & Deal, 2003; Loeser et al., 2007). The institutional leader must empower faculty leaders who can champion the reform and successfully guide it through to approval and implementation (Loeser et al., 2007). In addition, persistence in pursuit of change (or, said differently, the professional will of the leader) is essential to surviving the short-term problems that inevitably arise as a result of major change (Collins, 2005). Change is inherently disruptive, unsettling, and anxiety-provoking. New approaches and new procedures must be invented, and the twin processes of inventing and implementing it are challenging. In the life cycle of innovation and change, there is a predictable course of events, often referred to as the J curve (Jellison, 2006). For example, organizations that are underperforming may initiate a change process and discover that performance initially dips until the new routines are invented and new competencies are well established. It is impossible to anticipate all of the problems that arise in this early phase, often from unexpected places. As competence in managing the new programs grows, the performance of the organization typically exceeds that prior to the intervention. Therefore complaints about innovation are most strident during the initial period, and unless the leadership can keep the faculty focused on the new model and allay fears and frustrations innovations will flounder and fail—not because the innovation was ill conceived but because the leadership was unable to persist in the face of resistance and anxiety during the initial implementation.

A Culture of Creativity, Innovation, and Continuous Improvement

Although effective leadership is essential to managing change, the culture of the institution is equally important and can make or break attempts at educational reform. Institutional culture is the collective beliefs, values, language, symbols, rituals, norms, practices, assumptions, and accumulated wisdom of the group—"who we are and how we do things here." The institutional culture drives, and is reflected in, performance: "The essence of high performance is spirit . . . not just finding the right people and designing an appropriate structure" (Bolman & Deal, 2003, p. 262). However, institutional culture not only defines what its participants do but can also empower them to continuously improve: "A profession is defined by what it does, not just what it knows, and by doing what it does better all the time, not just doing it well" (Batalden & Davidoff, 2007, p. 1059).

Institutional culture varies from school to school, hospital to hospital, and department to department. Some medical schools highly value their educational mission while others begrudgingly acknowledge it. Some schools are hothouses for educational innovation while others are trapped in the past. Innovative medical schools share the norms of collaborative problem solving and idea generation, value and support innovations, and pursue continuous quality improvement; in short, they are a community of inquiry. A number of the schools and programs we visited exemplified such a culture of innovation, as this case illustrates:

○

At a small medical school that has a particularly strong and unifying culture of seeking to provide the best care to every patient, every time, continuous improvement in patient care is also connected to continuous improvement in education. The dean, working collaboratively with the associate dean for faculty affairs, developed a program to support faculty who teach and take on educational leadership roles. Together, they developed a system of financial support connected with faculty development. Any faculty member who wishes to teach must complete a series of faculty development workshops. The offerings are rich: there are dozens of workshops related to teaching and learning, instructional methods, assessment, educational technology, academic skills, and leadership. After the faculty members have taken a certain number of workshops, the productivity standards for their patient care are reduced for teaching sessions as they step into the teaching role. Teaching faculty members who take on a greater leadership role in education, such as being a course or clerkship director, must enroll in additional workshops to appropriately prepare for those responsibilities. A clinician-educator award program funds time and resources for educational projects judged meritorious through a faculty peer-reviewed mentoring process. This close connection between assignment of faculty responsibilities, a career development pathway, advancement opportunities for teachers, and faculty development is exemplary; it creates a culture focused on doing what is right for the patient, the learner, and the faculty member.

○

Medical schools, like the universities of which they are a part, are knowledge-building organizations. As such, they intently focus on advancing knowledge by creating a culture where growth is an ongoing expectation. Once faculty members master routine problems, they then focus their energies on new challenges and engage in progressive problem solving, addressing problems at progressively higher levels. These norms involve use of inquiry, discovery of promising alternative solutions to problems, articulation of explanations, and discussion of alternatives. Such pursuit of knowledge flourishes best in a culture that encourages collaborative work, interdisciplinary engagement, openness to innovation, free dialogue across boundaries and among people with differing frames of reference, and optimism in seeing opportunities for improvement and growth. Everyone works at the highest edge of competence, which means that each person keeps growing and learning (Bereiter & Scardamalia, 1993).

The culture must also be consonant with the core values of the profession. Consequently, any organizational change needs to be connected to the values of professionalism in medicine, as is illustrated in this case:

○

The president of an academic medical center was concerned about the culture of professionalism at his institution. Working with faculty members from all schools and staff from the medical center, he created a comprehensive program designed to change the culture and reclaim the soul of the healing professions. The program, which involves faculty members, staff members, health care professionals, residents, and students, is rooted in a professionalism charter, and every member of the university community is required to pledge: "On my honor, as a member of this university community, I pledge to act with integrity, compassion and respect in all my academic and professional endeavors."

Every policy and program is viewed through the lens of profession-alism. For example, mission-based budgeting was a failure because there was nothing altruistic or inspiring about it. In other words, it did not fit the culture of professionalism and thus was abandoned. The program also deals with violations of professionalism, monitor-ing patient and learner satisfaction surveys, furnishing an anonymous reporting site on the Web, and addressing any problems directly with the individuals involved and through a student honor council for medical students. On the staff level, this has reduced turnover from 33 percent to 14 percent and has made the medical center one of the best places to work in its metropolitan area. Because institutional culture changes slowly, the transformation had to be championed and led with consistency and persistence, across several fronts, and over the long run.

○

Creating a culture of professionalism and innovation takes time and effort: time to establish new behaviors and procedures and effort to maintain them, often in the face of resistance. As we discuss in the sections that follow, strategies to encourage creativity and innovation include educational innovation funds, collaborative research by medical faculty members and educational researchers, and pilot-testing promising new ideas.

Organizational Structures That Promote Action, Discipline, and Innovation

As our discussion of financing and regulation in Chapter Five indicated, U.S. academic medical centers are among the largest and most complex organizations in the world. The locus of power is often spread across several areas, and the relationships among them may be such that no one person, not even the dean or medical center CEO, has all the power needed to effect change. However, some medical schools have created outcome-oriented governance structures that are able to take action and promote innovation, even though many academic organizations are prone to bouts of extended deliberation that stymie action. As we noted earlier in this chapter, many of the schools we visited have strong central leadership in the dean's office and activist committees who were driving innovation. In schools and GME programs where this is not the norm, we found that innovation happens in pockets, without overall support or direction. Such orphan innovations are not likely to flourish or make a significant contribution to changing the culture unless they are connected to organizational structures that permit oversight and manage educational programs, ensure that change occurs, maintain discipline, and promote innovation.

Organizational structure defines the pattern of relationships, expectations, responsibilities, and accountability of participants inside and outside the institution. Like the framework of a building, the structure both enhances and constrains what the organization can accomplish (Bolman & Deal, 2003). Through specialization and division of labor, an organization can enhance efficiency. However, to increase effectiveness it must also create appropriate forms of coordination and control so that organizational goals are achieved across units.

When the dean's office is the central locus of leadership, it serves the important structural role of integrating and directing resources to educational programs. Departments, divisions, research centers, and clinical services cluster faculty members with specialized knowledge and skill into smaller organizational units. But to integrate resources for teaching purposes, this differentiation must be managed through effective networking and collaboration. Excessive autonomy of faculty members, organizational units, and services impedes interdependent work. Therefore many medical schools are creating new, integrative structures to connect what have traditionally been organizationally separate units.

In the schools of medicine we visited, we noted collaborative working relationships among educational administrators (typically vice or associate deans for education, curriculum, and graduate medical education), faculty members, staff members, and learners. These teams, like innovative companies, constantly search for promising ideas from inside and outside the school, share information across the organization, and test promising ideas (Hargadon & Sutton, 2000). Still, many schools have long had dysfunctional organizational structures, and as another case illustrates the first task of new a leader is often to redesign them:

<hr>

○

An energetic and creative faculty member was recruited to be vice dean for education and charged by the dean with transforming the entire medical school curriculum to better prepare students to be physicians for the twenty-first century. She began by appointing a new steering committee of senior faculty to oversee the process. They approved her guiding principles and plan to start with a blank slate in designing a curriculum based on core competencies. The hallmark of this curricular plan was an integrated, multidisciplinary curriculum that emphasized small-group instruction, self-directed learning, and flexibility. It took nine months of intensive committee work to develop a vision and achieve consensus on the broad outline of the plan, which was then presented to and approved by the medical faculty. Accordingly, the dean announced a commitment of $3 million to facilitate planning and implementation and to support development of the infrastructure necessary to oversee and evaluate the new curriculum. The following year, the vice dean appointed six interdisciplinary course module teams to design specific content for the revised curriculum. Development of a four-year curricular blueprint was approved by the medical faculty senate, and the six module leaders, each responsible for a specific module or section of the curriculum, reported to the vice dean and to the curriculum committee.

To achieve this transformation, the vice dean also had to create a new organizational structure to implement and manage the curriculum. The curriculum committee is appointed by and reports to the vice dean for education and gives annual reports to the faculty senate. The committee meets every other month, but its real work is carried out by the executive committee: six faculty members who are responsible for directing the six core modules of the curriculum and are paid 20 percent time for this leadership. They meet twice monthly with the vice dean to monitor the ongoing curriculum and oversee quality improvement efforts. The ongoing dialogue with this faculty leadership team is invaluable and enhances faculty ownership of the curriculum.

The companion organizational change was establishing central support services to ensure that faculty members succeed. The academic programs office comprises four offices responsible for managing the curriculum: a curriculum office, evaluation and assessment office, information technology, and standardized patients program. The new structure combines central administrative oversight and support with faculty engagement with the curriculum as expressed through the curriculum committee.

○

Central administration serves the important structural role of integrating resources for the educational programs, and many schools we visited had created new structures to connect historically separate units. However, as another case illustrates, sometimes oversight for innovation and policy need to be separate functions:

○

The vice and associate deans for medical education observed that the faculty committees charged with operational management of the curriculum (for example, course and clerkship committees) were not able to envision new possibilities or hold their colleagues accountable because they were too overwhelmed with running existing courses and fearful of challenging their peers. Thus the associate dean for curriculum established oversight committees for preclerkship and clerkship education to engage in visioning, policy setting, and discipline. The committees were formed with faculty members who were familiar with the issues in their arena but were not responsible for operations and thus had a broader perspective on education and the needs of the institution. This new organizational structure promoted innovation at the policy level and creativity in implementation at the operational level. Committee chairs were carefully chosen for their ability to be conceptual thinkers and action-oriented leaders.

○

In our site visits, we discovered that some schools and residency programs pilot-tested educational innovations to gain experience with the strategy and obtain approval to enact change. This strategy is often less risky and more likely to be approved than immediate full-scale implementation. Some schools employ rapid prototyping for these pilots, a process adapted from high-technology companies. Teams are encouraged to develop prototypes of promising products and get them out to users as quickly as possible. Because 80 percent of the time involved in creating a new product is spent on the last 20 percent of development, new products are sent out for testing once they are 80 percent ready and users are asked to test the product, identify problems, and make suggestions for improvement. This collaborative process between manufacturers and end users is much more time-efficient than trying to complete the whole process internally. Translated into medical education, this means a new educational program or curriculum does not have to be 100 percent perfect before it is put into action, as the faculty might wish. Giving the faculty permission to work at 80 percent success on the initial launch is good enough, provided that learners are encouraged and empowered to work collaboratively with the faculty to improve the educational program and the faculty are not punished for initial failures.

As these examples illustrate, effective organizational structures ensure discipline by setting high standards, monitoring performance, and taking action if benchmarks are not met. This requires clarity of objectives, rigorous evaluation, strategically aimed educational research, creative action planning, ongoing monitoring, and disciplined leadership.

Educational Resources and Support Services to Fuel Innovation and Excellence

Quality educational programs for medical students and residents require adequate resources and strong support services. For example, in the schools that we visited funding for educational programs in UME and GME increased under effective leaders and during periods of curriculum reform. This has often included expanded funding for teachers; curriculum, course, clerkship, and residency program directors; educational technology; clinical skills and simulation centers; new classroom buildings; academies of medical educators and faculty development programs; evaluation and assessment programs; student advising and mentoring services; and expanded offices of medical education. All of these add expense to the bottom line of the medical school budget, but they also add significant value to the educational mission of the school.

Offices of medical education and skilled medical educators, both Ph.D. and M.D., are critical assets in promoting the innovation and excellence in medical education. Over the past fifty years medical education has come of age, and the majority of medical schools have offices of medical education dedicated to collaborating with educational researchers to optimize the outcomes of curricular, pedagogical, and assessment practices. This large and strategic investment is unique in higher education.

More particularly, and unique among the professions, medicine has a long-standing commitment to incorporating researchers into medical schools and residency programs as a means of guiding and improving educational practice. In medicine, it is common practice to seek consultation from a subspecialty expert; therefore seeking consultation from a specialist in education is a logical approach to dealing with problems of curriculum, instruction, and evaluation (Miller, 1980). What began with a handful of educational researchers working in medical schools in the 1950s is now commonplace. In 2007, the Society of Directors of Research in Medical Education, the professional society for offices of medical education, listed sixty-four member offices in North America. This trend continues internationally as well (Davis, Karunathilake, & Harden, 2005).

A number of the schools and residency programs we visited have hired educators who have a doctorate in education to consult with faculty members on curriculum development, instructional design, faculty development, assessment and program evaluation, and educational technology. At the school level, these educators work in either the dean's office or a separate office of medical education; thus, generally a centralized model prevails. This vignette is thus typical:

○

As part of curriculum reform, the dean hired a medical educator to work as a generalist, offering faculty assistance with testing, program evaluation, and faculty development. However, as the challenges of curriculum reform grew, more specialized educators were hired to lend assistance with instructional technology, research design and measurement, curriculum development, and performance assessment. Now there are four Ph.D. educators working collaboratively with faculty members to take a scholarly approach to teaching and academic programs.

○

Faculty development to improve pedagogical practices is a key responsibility for these educators, because until recently medical school faculty members rarely had any preparation for teaching before taking on these responsibilities (Steinert, Cruess, Cruess, & Snell, 2005; Steinert et al., 2006; Wilkerson & Irby, 1998). The schools and programs we visited have faculty development programs, usually workshops on such topics as leading small-group discussion, creating and using educational technology, writing test items, giving feedback, teaching in clinical settings, teaching procedural skills, and developing curriculum. In many schools, this episodic approach to faculty development is being augmented by yearlong teaching scholars programs that offer more in-depth exposure to learning theory, curriculum development, educational technology, educational research, leadership, and organizational change. These programs typically last one or two years, meet weekly to monthly, and include an educational project such as creating a new course or conducting educational research. The intent of these programs is to create a cadre of educational leaders who are equipped to take a major leadership role in medical education at their institution (Searle, Hatem, Perkowski, & Wilkerson, 2006; Searle, Thompson, & Perkowski, 2006). A number of master's and doctoral programs in medical and health sciences education are serving those faculty members who wish to continue developing their educational knowledge and research abilities, and an increasing number of physicians are choosing to pursue these programs. Another trend is for teaching improvement programs to go beyond faculty members and include residents and medical students. In some schools, students enroll in elective courses in medical education, participate in teaching assignments, develop medical school curriculum, and complete a teaching-focused project. At the GME level, many programs, offered within and across departments, prepare residents to teach (Wamsley, Julian, & Wipf, 2004).

As we have noted, the centralized model of medical education research is predominant; however, there are alternative models at the department level. For example, individual departments may employ educators to strengthen their performance in medical student and resident education—a more decentralized improvement strategy. Several schools that we visited employed this decentralized, departmental model, sometimes in addition to the centralized model. Departments of family medicine and internal medicine have long hired educators because they historically received grant support from the federal government to promote primary-care education. More recently, departments of surgery and obstetrics and gynecology have followed suit, as illustrated in two cases:

---

o

A department of surgery hired an enthusiastic and energetic educator to improve student and resident education. As an educational researcher, she worked with the surgery faculty on nontraditional curriculum and assessment systems in the clerkship and residency programs, formal skills laboratory instruction for students and residents, faculty development, and educational research. Over time, her collaboration with the faculty has transformed teaching and learning in the department. Working closely with her department chair, she created a think-tank retreat to envision new educational models for resident education. Among the outcomes of the retreat, new structures for resident rotations were implemented. Leadership at the local level has also led to leadership for surgical education nationally.

---

o

At another university, a medical educator works within a department of surgery, providing support for curriculum development, technology development, program evaluation, and educational research. Working closely with the chairman, he has formed and coordinates the Surgical Education and Performance Group, which comprises nurse educators, the skills coordinator, and a skills coach as well as those surgeons who are particularly interested in educational innovation, educational research, practice behavior research, and outcomes research. The research and innovation conducted by members of this group is designed to understand and resolve problems affecting the surgery training programs, and to improve their quality through systematic innovations. He supports the group's

efforts by conducting his own program of research and by supporting
the research of others through data collection, data analysis, research
conceptualization, data interpretation, and manuscript writing.

○

As these two examples suggest, important educational innovation
and research can be generated at the department level as well as at
the school level. In each case, having formally trained medical educators working collaboratively with other faculty members was critical to
success. To afford such a resource, the Institute of Medicine (Committee on the Health Professions Education Summit, 2003) recommended
that Congress set up a competitive grant program to support medical
education innovation, and others have called for an NIH section on
research in health professions education (Wartman, 2004). This would
facilitate broadening the culture of creativity and innovation in medical
education.

Academic Communities That Advance the Scholarship of Teaching and Learning

The scholarship of teaching and learning arises out of close examination
of instructional processes: design and delivery of curriculum and instruction, interactions with learners, evaluation, reflection, and redesign. The
work of planning and delivering such instruction occurs primarily within
the minds, classrooms, and clinical settings of individual faculty members and thus tends to be invisible to others. The challenge is to create
a community of scholars who care passionately about teaching and give
them opportunities to come together in forums that focus on issues of
teaching and learning. These forums are "teaching commons," a real or
virtual space in which faculty members can engage in discourse about
teaching and learning (Huber & Hutchings, 2005). These intellectual
spaces, or communities of interest, are created locally through educational workshops, seminars, work-in-progress conferences, education
retreats, teaching scholars programs, offices of medical education, and
academies of medical educators; globally, they occur through professional
conferences and Web-based collaborative working environments.

Although medical schools, as with higher education in general, have
focused on teaching excellence, the new approach is intended to ensure
that teaching is more scholarly—that is, it builds on the work of others,
makes its own successes and failures public so that others can learn, and
thus advances the field. The Carnegie Foundation for the Advancement
of Teaching has been in the forefront of efforts to expand the concept

of scholarship to include scholarly teaching (Boyer, 1990) and create communities of scholars that address issues of teaching and learning (Glassick, Huber, & Maeroff, 1997) by continuously studying "the quality of their work, its fidelity to their missions, and its impact on students intellectually, practically, and morally" (Shulman, 2005a, p. vi).

To encourage this type of careful reflection on teaching, Glassick, Huber, and Maeroff (1997, p. 36, Exhibit 2.1) identify six assessment standards, each presented with a guiding question:

1. Clear goals: Are the purposes and objectives clear and appropriate?

2. Adequate preparation: Does the scholar understand the scholarship in the field and have the skills needed to do the work?

3. Appropriate methods: Does the scholar create an appropriate learning environment and use appropriate instructional methods?

4. Significant results: Are the goals achieved and do they add consequentially to the field?

5. Effective presentation: Does the scholar use a suitable style and effective organization to present his or her work with clarity and integrity?

6. Reflective critique: Does the scholar critically evaluate and improve his or her own work?

The teaching programs we visited both UME and GME, used a variety of mechanisms to encourage this type of scholarship and create a community of teachers. The most common approach is to use curriculum committees and curriculum reform work to promote quality improvement. Many schools have assigned a faculty member, usually one of the school's medical educators, to scan the education literature to help inform debate about various curricular and instructional methods, and then lead discussion of educational research and theory.

Another mechanism for creating a teaching commons is a relatively new organizational structure called an academy or a society of medical educators. The academy movement is flourishing nationally and internationally (Searle et al., 2010). Three essential structural characteristics of academies distinguish them from faculty development programs: (1) a formal schoolwide organizational structure that is separate from the dean's office or department, with leadership by members of the organization; (2) designated resources to fund mission-related initiatives; and (3) membership of qualified faculty educators identified through a rigorous peer-review selection process that values teaching, educational leadership, and educational scholarship.

The oldest academy appears to be the one at the Medical College of Wisconsin, founded in 1990 (Simpson et al., 2000); there are now more than thirty academies in medical schools around the country and more are being created every year (Dewey, Friedland, Richards, Lamki, & Kirkland, 2005). All share some components of the mission to advance and support teachers, carry out faculty development, promote curriculum improvement, and advocate for the educational mission of the university. Here is a description of the origins of one such academy:

○

For decades, a research-intensive medical school had treated the educational mission with benign neglect. Faculty members taught in isolation from one another and did so without any expectation that the mission would be a valued contribution to the university or to their own academic career. Faculty members recognized that research is what brought advancement, and so the common adage was "teach at your own peril." Today, the culture has changed dramatically, in part because of strong leadership in education, curriculum reform, an office of medical education, and the Academy of Medical Educators. These last two have fueled educational innovation and scholarship through innovation funding, Academy Day events, educational scholarship programs, faculty development, and educational advocacy. Through the academy application process, the educator's portfolio has become a standard way of presenting evidence regarding educational contributions to the university. This, along with admission to the academy, has led to accelerated advancements and promotions for academy members. The academy offers an opportunity to publicly honor the very best teachers, and create an intellectual commons for sharing creative ideas in education as well as an organizational structure to serve all teachers. The academy has become a symbol of the school's commitment to teaching and to educational innovation and scholarship. Palpable excitement about education reflects this cultural change on the campus.

○

To further extend the local dialogue about teaching and learning, new forums are being created to encourage students and faculty members to work together to improve the curriculum. Students share their perceptions of courses, curricula, materials, exercises, and pedagogy, and they work with faculty members on course improvements. Some schools hire students to partner with faculty members to improve the curriculum and work on course syllabi, self-instructional materials, quizzes, examinations, evaluation of a course, and any other task that improves learning. This has helped speed up innovation and curricular improvement.

Scholarly teaching involves building on the work and best practices of others, and the scholarship of teaching requires making one's work public, submitting it to peer review, and disseminating it. This is now happening at the national level with MedEdPortal at an AAMC website (http://www.aamc.org/mededportal). This peer-reviewed repository of educational materials and programs in medical education offers medical educators a place to share their best work, have it peer reviewed, and make it available for others to adopt or adapt; it offers other educators curricular products that can be used "as is." Another national repository for sharing educational objects, the Health Education Assets Library (http://healcentral.org), is a database that focuses on individual objects or assets, such as images, animations, video clips, or illustrations, that can be incorporated by educators into new educational products. These peer-reviewed repositories offer an important mechanism for dissemination and scholarship of educational products.

Professional organizations also advance this form of scholarship. As an example, the AAMC and the American Educational Research Association both offer venues for sharing research and best practices in medical education. Medical specialty organizations have created education-related organizational structures and national meetings as well; one can point to the Society of Surgical Educators, the Society of Teachers of Family Medicine, the Clerkship Directors in Pediatrics, and the Association of Directors of Medical Student Education in Psychiatry, to name just a few. These professional organizations serve as a scholarly community that offers opportunities for those with a passion for teaching to discuss key challenges facing medical education and share their research.

The scholarship of teaching and learning in medical education is advanced by a number of journals, among them *Academic Medicine*, *Advances in Health Sciences Education*, *Medical Education*, *Medical Teacher*, *Teaching and Learning in Medicine*, and *Evaluation in the Health Professions*. In addition, medical specialty journals publish theme issues and educational supplements.

Perhaps most important, faculty members who lead educational programs now have guidelines to help them document their teaching contributions for academic promotion purposes (Simpson et al., 2007). Every dimension of educational work can be done in a scholarly manner and promote the scholarship of teaching and learning: teaching, curriculum development, advising and mentoring, educational leadership and administration, and learner assessment (Simpson et al., 2007).

This scholarly approach to professional education, as represented by academies of medical educators, offices of medical education, professional conferences and organizations, and scholarly journals, is unique in higher education generally and in education for the professions specifically, and it constitutes an important resource for reform efforts.

Leading Change: The Work Ahead

In spite of the resource constraints and complexities that medical education faces, as outlined in Chapter Five, we found that change is afoot in the medical schools and residency programs we visited. Effective and energetic leaders working with productive leadership teams are changing the curricula, creating cultures of inquiry and improvement, and redesigning organizational structures to promote action and discipline. Companion investments in educational resources and support services are fueling innovation and advancing the scholarship of teaching and learning. As the examples in this chapter illustrate, significant change in medical education is possible, offering tangible proof that the reform called for in the next chapters is attainable. However, the work ahead is considerable, and successful reform depends on both programmatic and policy actions that support individuals, institutions, and indeed the system of medical education. It also depends on leadership at every level, from individual programs through national organizations. In the two closing chapters, we offer recommendations for such actions.

PART FOUR

MEETING TOMORROW'S CHALLENGES: A VISION OF THE POSSIBLE

7

REALIZING THE VISION

TRANSFORMING MEDICAL EDUCATION

AT THE UNDERGRADUATE AND GRADUATE LEVELS, U.S. medical education has both shortcomings and strengths. We believe that by building on innovation and creativity, as well as the commitment to excellence that we observed in our fieldwork, U.S. medical schools and residency programs can make critically needed reforms in the education of medical students and residents. Doing so, however, will entail meaningful programmatic and policy changes, and in Chapter Eight we discuss the policy reforms that would support excellence and facilitate transformation. In the Introduction to this book and in Chapter One, we described in detail a set of goals that we believe medical education should strive for. In this chapter, we describe how, through new programmatic approaches, medical education might attain these goals of standardizing learning outcomes and individualizing the learning process; integrating knowledge and clinical experiences, roles, and responsibilities; developing habits of inquiry and improvement; and explicitly addressing professional formation. We begin by presenting the principles behind these goals and strategies for enacting them. Then, to make these ideas concrete, we present examples that illustrate how implementing promising educational approaches, from medical school through residency, would advance the four goals.

Essential Educational Goals

Our observation of the strengths and weaknesses of U.S. medical education, as well as our synthesis of the contributions of the learning sciences, yield a set of principles about curriculum, pedagogy, and assessment that are broadly applicable; they can—and should—be widely employed, regardless of specific teaching objective or level of learner:

o With respect to curricular content, educators must distinguish more clearly between core material and everything else (diFrancesco et al., 2005; Core Committee, 2002). Given that the medical knowledge base and the skills required to practice effectively are constantly evolving, it is crucial that curricular material with a five- or ten-year date stamp be minimized.

o Learners at all levels should not be obliged to spend time unproductively repeating clinical activities once they have already mastered the competencies appropriate to their level. Medical education must make much more use of readiness assessments and design curricula that are sufficiently flexible to allow individual learners to engage at various levels of difficulty. Eliminating noncore activities will free up time for medical students and residents to develop additional depth in areas of individual interest and to explore the nonclinical roles of the physician.

o At every level, the approaches to teaching must emphasize that *competence* means *minimal standard*; it is the level of performance that all aspiring physicians must attain with respect to the core (see, for example, Brooks, 2009). It is essential that the aspirational nature of the quest for excellence be communicated to and inculcated in learners. For this reason, we believe that medical schools and residency programs must encourage students to form a lifelong commitment to pursuing excellence, instilling in students and residents the understanding that learning continues beyond the formal four-to-six-year training period, and preparing them to continuously incorporate the advancing knowledge base and procedural innovations of contemporary medicine.

o The fundamental pedagogy of medical education aims to have learners develop the motivation and skill required to teach themselves, stimulated by their clinical experiences, information about the effectiveness of their care, and interactions with others in the clinical environment (Hoff, Pohl, & Bartfield, 2004). This "learning spiral" connecting prior knowledge, clinical experience, identification of next questions, and formal study should be presented to medical students and residents as the basis for metacognitive monitoring of their own approaches to learning (ten Cate, Snell, Mann, & Vermunt, 2004). To the greatest extent possible, learners should approach curricular material, including the sciences foundational to medicine, through questions arising out of clinical work; this is as important for residents as it is for early medical students.

o Throughout their medical education, students and residents require strong, engaged relationships with faculty members that provide challenge, support, and strong role modeling, as well as the opportunity for individual guidance (Haidet & Stein, 2006; Kendrick et al., 1993).

o At both the UME and GME levels, medical education must ensure, through assessment, that learners achieve predetermined standards of competence with respect to knowledge and performance in core domains. Assessment should use a common set of competency domains over the entire learning continuum, with actual benchmarks specified by learner level; there are successful examples of this kind of assessment over a developmental spectrum from which medical education should learn (Wilson & Scalise, 2006). Such benchmarking, shared nationally, would allow medical schools, residencies, and learners to understand how programs compare in terms of the capabilities of their entering learners, and what the education they supply adds as measured by the performance of their graduates.

o Assessment must go beyond what students and residents know and can do to address learner ability to identify gaps and next steps for learning, because it is appreciation of those gaps that should drive lifelong learning (Miflin, Campbell, & Price, 2000; Teunissen & Dornan, 2008). To discourage learners' segmentation of knowledge and skills, and to reinforce development of well-networked understanding of medical phenomena, assessment across the competencies should be integrated and cumulative.

o Commitment to excellence is a hallmark—some would maintain *the* hallmark—of professionalism in medicine (Leach, 2002), and accordingly expertise is likewise a commitment, not an attribute. This concept is fundamental to our view of medical education and knits together the goals of standardization and individualization, integration, innovation and improvement, and identity formation. Assurance of quality accomplished through standardization; an educational process of individualization that treats learners humanely, respects their interests, abilities, and experiences and that encourages high achievement; the expectation that physicians play a broad role in society, even during training; and insistence that all physicians participate in field building are all goals referring to a dimension of the professional identity of physicians. Although, for the purposes of highlighting each of these goals, we have talked about designs that emphasize individualization, integration, inquiry, and formation, every choice in education has implications for professional formation of students and residents. Programs must be deliberate about learners' experiences and vigilant about the implicit and explicit messages conveyed by the curriculum, pedagogy, and assessment; otherwise, the professional development outcomes desired by the program may be distorted or subverted.

How might these principles be enacted? Our vision for medical education, grounded in research on both medical education and learning sciences and stimulated by educational innovations that we observed, is intended to inspire and foster excellence in education and ultimately patient care. Accordingly, we offer these recommendations for programmatic reform of medical education:

1. Standardize learning outcomes and individualize learning processes

   - Set clear, progressive expectations for learning outcomes, and assess competencies over time

   - Establish common competency domains across the UME-GME-CME continuum, with appropriate developmental benchmarks for learners

   - Individualize learning within and across levels, allowing flexibility in approach to learning and offering opportunities to pursue areas of interest beyond core learning outcomes

2. Integrate knowledge and clinical experience, roles, and responsibilities

   - Closely connect formal knowledge and clinical experience, including provision of early clinical immersion and later revisiting of the sciences

   - Examine diseases and clinical situations from multiple perspectives

   - Give learners access to different roles and responsibilities of physicians

   - Promote learners' ability to work collaboratively with other health professionals to effectively deliver patient care in complex systems

3. Develop habits of inquiry and improvement

   - Focus on development of both routine and adaptive expertise

   - Engage learners in challenging problems and knowledge-building endeavors

4. Address professional identity formation explicitly

   - Offer formal ethics instruction, feedback, and reflective opportunities related to professional development

   - Support learner and teacher relationships that advance the highest values of the profession

- Encourage exploration of the roles of the physician-citizen
- Create collaborative learning and practice environments committed to excellence and continuous improvement

Programmatic Approaches: Eleven Possibilities

What would these ideas look like in operation? To stimulate the creative thinking of those who lead medical education, we offer in Table 7.1 eleven programmatic approaches: four at the early medical school level, two for later students, two for early residents, and three for advanced

Table 7.1. Eleven Programmatic Approaches

| Approach | Goals | | | |
	Standardization and Individualization	Integration	Innovation and Improvement	Professional Identity
Early medical school				
Core and depth	✓			
Clinically driven cumulative learning		✓		
Curiosity and field building			✓	
Joining a moral community				✓
Late medical school				
Advancing professional commitments	✓		✓	
Settings and perspectives		✓		
Early residency				
Problem reformulation	✓			
Uncertainty, confidence, and responsibility				✓
Advanced residency				
Impact of physicians		✓		
Everyday innovation and big improvement			✓	
Taking responsibility for excellence				✓

residents. Although, in developing these approaches, we recognized that a school or residency program might by virtue of its history, mission, or current circumstances begin its improvement effort by addressing one or two of the four goals, we regard all of them as equally critical. Our sole purpose in isolating and focusing on, in most cases, one goal for each approach is to bring into high relief how curriculum, pedagogy, and assessment must together support the goal.

The thumbnail sketches and hypothetical learner stories we present to illustrate these approaches are intended as examples, as schools and programs consider how they might address the goals not only in individual courses, clerkships, and residencies but more broadly across their institution. The examples are not intended to be prescriptive; rather, we hope to stimulate others to generate more approaches.

It may be challenging to implement some of the approaches in the clinical settings currently used for medical education. However, without new thinking to push them, systems will sustain the same inertia that has resulted in a remarkable lack of evolution in clinical education over the past century, despite sweeping changes in medical science and health care and revolutionary advances in our understanding of how people learn (Christakis, 1995). It is our hope that these examples of what medical education can look like will be galvanizing, a catalyst that starts medical educators moving toward needed change.

Early Medical School

○

Anna Sheffield is a first-year medical student at her state's public medical school. A thirty-two-year-old anthropology major, Anna was a Peace Corps volunteer when she first thought of becoming a physician. However, she married shortly after returning from Guinea Bissau and quickly found herself pregnant with her first child. She had her second baby while completing postbaccalaureate premedical requirements. She was delighted to discover that, though not as inexpensive as she might have hoped, the school of medicine at her public university offered a number of features she regarded as critical. Most important, it respects the diversity of backgrounds and interests of its students. The first three months of the curriculum are devoted to "evening out" the preparation of students before they begin a highly integrated common core. This relatively individualized introductory program, the Art and Science of Medicine, gives science majors required and elective offerings in the social and behavioral sciences and medical humanities. Anna, with her strong background and experience in the social sciences, took biochemistry and a seminar in which students discussed research papers describing key scientific advances relevant to medicine. When the common core course Foundations of Health, Disease, and Health Care began in January of the first year, Anna felt well prepared to handle material based in the natural sciences, such as pharmacology. At the beginning of winter quarter, the first-year students read a set of medical oaths and explored the dimension of professional responsibility in preparation for creation of a collective statement titled Our Ideals as Physicians. Anna is sure that exploration of science for her, and the social sciences and patient narratives for many of her classmates, made this collaborative exercise easier and its product broader.

Because Anna has significant family responsibilities and wants neither to deprive her children nor to miss out on the joys and tribulations of motherhood, the flexible schedule offered by her school was a real draw. Students in good standing can complete school in as little as three years or as much as five years, for the standard four years of tuition. While interviewing, Anna met students taking advantage of this flexibility for a host of reasons. All reported that the school facilitated arrangements that best met their needs and that residents and faculty were supportive of their nonclinical activities.

Finally, Anna was pleased to discover as an applicant that her school had an extensive program in global health. She had assumed that as a clinician and mother she would have to set aside her interests in international health. However, while taking "The Art and Science of Medicine," she was able to attend a program at which medical students, residents, and faculty members presented their work in global health. She met two residents, both young parents, who had worked abroad during residency; they also assured her that she could continue to deepen her commitment to global health and that the school would assist her. Encouraged, Anna joined the global health interest group and has signed up for a spring quarter elective on health care in developing countries. She is looking forward to opportunities afforded later in medical school to work as part of a team on an overseas project; seeing near-peers who are successfully contributing to global health has made Anna optimistic that she can sustain this interest while in medical school and residency.

o

The first phase of medical school should establish the patterns that physicians will use throughout their lives to link their clinical work to continuing learning. Specifically, it must introduce students to the dialectical relationships that establish the "spiral learning helix," in which clinical experience is framed by prior knowledge stimulating further study and formal learning and leading to conceptual and procedural advances, with the cycle then repeating at a higher level (Hewson, 1991). In addition, the early phase of medical school invites students into the community of physicians and builds skills in social learning and collaborative performance (Palincsar, 1998). It should facilitate establishment of a foundational knowledge base that students can build on cumulatively; likewise, students should acquire introductory clinical skills to allow their work in clinical settings to be educationally productive and, to the extent possible, clinically authentic (Lave & Wenger, 1991). Finally, the early years of medical school lay the groundwork for establishment of the professional identity of the physician, building on the desire for service and other commendable dispositions that students bring to their medical studies (Forsythe, 2005).

CORE AND DEPTH.   The early years of medical school do not have to be one-size-fits-all. To illustrate how a school honoring the principles of individualization and standardization might work, we describe a "core and depth" program for the first phase of medical school. This approach recognizes that medical students begin their studies with diverse intellectual backgrounds, to a much greater degree than characterizes doctoral students in the sciences or the humanities. Medical students with a humanities or social science background often fear the "hard science" component of medical education, specifically biochemistry, molecular biology, and to some extent pharmacology, while students with a strong natural sciences background may not appreciate what the humanities and fields such as anthropology contribute to the work of the physician. A variously prepared class of students can promote diversity of perspective, but a common and unfortunate consequence is teaching to the lowest common denominator, resulting in presentation of scientific material at a level that is not challenging for the students with a strong science background. Likewise, material in the behavioral and social sciences may be watered down and oversimplified to make it accessible to students who are unfamiliar with those domains. The humanities and narrative medicine are often not taught at all or are offered only as electives.

To address these challenges, we imagine a program in which students are required to demonstrate a level of mastery across the domains of natural science, the social and behavioral sciences, and the humanities before beginning the shared or common coursework of medical school (standardization of outcome). To accomplish this, our design has medical school beginning with an omnibus course, like Anna's Art and Science of Medicine. This course consists of four elements: (1) advances in molecular biology and genetics, (2) foundational social sciences for medicine (anthropology, psychology, and sociology), (3) biostatistics and introduction to epidemiology, and (4) medical humanities. Students are expected to take the two elements in which they did the least course work as undergraduates or in which they showed the least proficiency on placement testing. In the first quarter of medical school, students spend the bulk of their time in the Art and Science of Medicine in conjunction with early clinical work.

Early patient contact allows students to work together in groupings other than their Art and Science of Medicine section. Introductory contact with patients is linked to formal didactic content across the four content areas. In the second quarter of medical school, students begin Foundations of Health, Disease, and Health Care, consisting of shared or common coursework, while continuing for a second quarter with one of the elements of Art and Science of Medicine. In this manner, students who bring to medical school a strong background in the sciences engage with literature as it pertains to such topics as the role of the physician or the nature of suffering. The kinds of experiences that have been explored by a number of medical schools, in which students are asked to hone their skills of observation by considering works of art, could also be offered within this program. Meanwhile, a student with an undergraduate degree in art history and postbaccalaureate completion of the premedical requirements would take the advanced molecular biology and biostatistics components. With this kind of individualized leveling out, topics in all four domains will be tackled more ambitiously when they appear in the shared course Health and Disease.

The teaching approaches most suitable for content within the Art and Science of Medicine would vary from domain to domain, but the predominant teaching approach is small-group discussion. In addition, online individual and group learning would allow students to tackle modules supporting self-paced exploration of unfamiliar topics and fields. Students (perhaps classmates or students in the class ahead) serve as near-peer or peer teachers; for example, a student with an art history degree might serve as a group leader or docent for the museum course "Art" of Observation, while a classmate who did honors work in biology as an undergraduate would be a facilitator or cofacilitator for students with a humanities background in their seminar Advanced Topics in the Life Sciences.

A school adopting "core and depth" will use assessment to support the program in multiple ways. For example, placement tests give credit for prior experience to students who mastered material in one of the four domains at an advanced level. The same placement tests would be used to identify students for the components of the Art and Science of Medicine. These uses of assessment support individualization. Assessment would also be used to demonstrate that all students were prepared to begin the shared Health and Disease coursework and, at completion, that they have mastered its content, as mandated by the commitment to standardization of outcomes.

To support both standardization of outcome and individualization of process, a medical school program will also allow flexible pacing to accommodate family responsibilities or in-depth pursuit of nonclinical interests. As Anna's story illustrates, a powerful way to express this support is to allow students in good academic standing to take a variable amount of time to proceed to medical school graduation, perhaps three years to five years, all at the same tuition.

CLINICALLY DRIVEN CUMULATIVE LEARNING. All of the senses in which we use the term *integration* can and should be powerfully represented in the early years of medical school. The "clinically driven cumulative learning" approach features careful integration of formal knowledge and clinical experience (Teunissen et al., 2007). From the earliest days of medical school, the students' clinical experience is organized to support a series of intentionally planned and sequenced learning objectives. Student learning develops out of these sequenced experiences. The primary objective is to inculcate the habit of using clinical experiences to drive learning across all the domains that underlie effective medical practice: the foundational or basic sciences, the social and behavioral sciences, clinical knowledge and procedures, and policy and the health care system. Some formal didactics would be offered, but the content would always be linked to clinical conditions that the students have seen. Thus students would spend time in the office of a community clinician, learning how outpatient medicine works and practicing their physical examination skills; but they also have sessions in the pulmonary practice as they learn about pulmonary diseases and visit the ICU to observe ventilated patients as they learn about pulmonary physiology. The array of conditions that cause abdominal pain would be considered in a variety of clinical settings: ob-gyn clinic, pediatrics clinic, the operating room, and the emergency department. The impracticality of having every student encounter every setting is converted to a virtue as students share their experiences in small-group collaborative learning sessions.

In a clinically driven cumulative learning approach, instruction begins with an attempt to make students aware of their own learning. Students are introduced early to the concepts of "spiral learning" and the metacognitive skills required for optimal learning (Croskerry, 2003; Kuiper & Pesut, 2004). A shortcoming of workplace learning can be that learners become adept at workplace procedures without developing deeper conceptual understanding of the rationale for the practices they are learning. To avoid this, instructors will emphasize the importance of using experiences in clinical settings to identify opportunities to advance conceptual understanding in addition to practical skills (Billett, 1996; Prawat, 1993). As appropriate, simulation and other approaches that allow decomposition of clinical experiences concentrate the students' attention on skills or concepts that are deemed particularly important (Grossman et al., 2009). For example, the practice of using simulations to teach critical concepts in the pathophysiology of shock, as many schools are beginning to do, is entirely consistent with attention to integration in this approach.

To advance the goal of integration, assessment avoids partitioning material and assessing by discipline or skill. For example, an OSCE station presents a patient with a palpable spleen; the exercise allows direct observation of a student's ability to establish rapport with an anxious patient and perform a systematic and focused abdominal exam. The most proficient students might discern that the patient's spleen is enlarged, but detection of the splenomegaly is not the primary point. All students are told that the abdominal exam reveals splenomegaly and that laboratory findings include anemia, marked leukocytosis, and moderate thrombocytosis; they are asked to generate a differential diagnosis and discuss the molecular genetics of the most likely diagnosis. In this manner, a single OSCE station is used and in an integrated manner to assess interpersonal skills, physical examination techniques, fundamentals of problem formulation, and basic science understanding. Similarly, in an approach based on clinically driven cumulative learning students are held accountable for previously covered material. Thus, in a block devoted to cancer, its molecular mechanisms, and presentation, the case of a patient presenting with superior vena cava syndrome could be used to assess students' understanding of vascular anatomy as well as their appreciation of the epidemiology of lung cancer. In this way, the curriculum and assessment of students' growing proficiency are truly integrated and cumulative.

There are other, equally important forms of integration that beginning medical students should experience. Perhaps none is more important in our health care system than sophisticated understanding of how health care professionals work together to accomplish desired outcomes for patients (Baker, Salas, King, Battles, & Barach, 2005). Medical education has failed to adequately prepare learners to function together effectively as members of an integrated health care team, with well-developed appreciation of the roles and responsibilities of every member of the team. Curricula must regularly place medical students together with future colleagues—other early health profession learners, nursing students, pharmacists, physical therapists, and so on—to complete team-based work together on problems over time, with a single team grade awarded.

CURIOSITY AND FIELD BUILDING. A challenge for early education in medicine is representing the dynamic nature of medical knowledge and the provisional nature of medical "truth." Students come to medical studies with a great respect for the accumulated mass of medical learning and often an unwarranted confidence that what they are being taught is truth for the ages (Mylopoulos & Regehr, 2009). Even if they recognize that current understanding is imperfect, they think of medical knowledge as improving by successive and linear steps, with every year bringing closer approximations of the truth. This contrasts with the perspective of graduate students in the natural sciences, who begin their doctoral work committed to building their field, disproving unhelpful models, and introducing more helpful ones, either through an incremental process or, even better, by contributing a paradigm-shifting insight (Bereiter & Scardamalia, 1993). Medicine should cultivate a similar spirit in its students.

A curriculum committed to engaging even early medical learners in inquiry and improvement explicitly represents physician work to first-year students as developing new understandings and approaches. It is important that this field building not be identified solely with classical bioscientific research, as important as this work is. Students need to understand that opportunities to make things better for patients and improve the health of the public are diverse; all efforts to improve our understanding and effectiveness are valuable. A second feature of the "curiosity and field building" curriculum is its open structure. Rather than a closely scheduled curriculum with the majority of time committed to didactic instruction, the students' week presents them with problems and allows them to individually and collectively explore and discover solutions (Martin, Rayne, Kemp, Hart, & Diller, 2005). Faculty members (and some students) may resist this design as inefficient, but this claim has merit only if the sole goal is unidirectional transfer of today's knowledge. A substantial body of empirical work at multiple educational levels supports the idea that, to inculcate understanding of so dynamic a field and to engage students as field builders, learners need the opportunity to participate in this work, even if they are rediscovering established knowledge and concepts (Norman & Schmidt, 1992). As students' skills progress, the curriculum shifts from preselected problems, designed, as in a problem-based learning curriculum, to guarantee that students encounter key domains and concepts, to a more naturalistic method in which students frame problems and questions out of their own clinical experience.

The curiosity-and-field-building educational design demands an appropriate pedagogy. Teachers should encourage inquisitiveness and skepticism about received truths, even when they emanate from the teacher's own mouth (Schwartz & Martin, 2004). Approaches to teaching support simultaneous development of routine and adaptive expertise. By routine expertise, we mean fluent, accurate, and effective handling of familiar situations; these situations may be common or relatively uncommon, high-stakes or low-stakes, but they have characteristic features and can be counted on to respond predictably to medical intervention.

Adaptive expertise, by contrast, involves something out of the ordinary (Barnettt & Koslowski, 2002; Baroody, 2003; Hatano & Oura, 2003). Adaptive expertise requires, first of all, the ability to recognize that something is different and that routine procedures are inappropriate; and second, the capacity to fall back on fundamental understandings, rather than automatic responses, to invent an approach more likely to be appropriate to the situation. It can be tempting to think that routine expertise should be acquired before moving on to adaptive expertise, but this linear sequencing may foster overreliance on routine expertise (Feltovich et al., 1997).

Again, doctoral level work in the natural sciences offers some insight into how teaching might support development of adaptive expertise among early learners in a curiosity-and-field-building medical school. In the natural sciences, a graduate student joins a lab and becomes a member of a research group. At the same time that students are being taught the procedures integral to the investigations that the lab conducts and are familiarizing themselves with the relevant scientific literature, they are confronted with and included in discussion of the questions the lab is exploring. Indeed, the more rapidly they can orient to their domain, its established understandings, and open questions, and the more quickly they become facile with the procedures of their laboratory (developing routine expertise), the more authentically and completely they can engage in its real work of inventing and testing new understandings. The teacher's stance is an important element of the pedagogy for curiosity and field building; key features are a strongly collegial relationship, provision of an appropriate level of challenge, and supportive mentoring.

Assessment in a program that stresses curiosity and field building would attend to domains beyond mastery of facts and attainment of routine expertise, as important as these achievements are. Students' commitment to contributing new knowledge, their ability to identify situations where "good enough" really is not and to define productive and important questions from their clinical experience, and their creativity and resilience in the face of difficult problems are also important attributes. These dimensions can be documented through global assessment of collaborators and mentors and, perhaps most important, through methods that capture the process of engaging with problems itself. A component of a portfolio having some of the features of the lab notebook that wet lab researchers use serves this purpose well (Carraccio & Englander, 2004).

JOINING A MORAL COMMUNITY.   As we have emphasized, a critical dimension of medical education (perhaps the most critical) is transformation of identity; this is what we refer to as becoming a physician. At one level, everything we do in medical education, and every goal that we address in these illustrations of programmatic approaches, carries its own messages about the fundamental purposes and values of medicine. Much of this messaging is, however, implicit. Schools are becoming more overt in calling out values and in emphasizing to students that, although it may be three or four years before they can write "M.D." after their name, they have already entered the community of physicians and begun to share its privileges and responsibilities. We offer an approach to first-year medical education that is focused on this dimension of medical education.

A key curricular activity in the "joining a moral community" approach is negotiation of a statement of personal commitment, perhaps modeled on the "This I Believe" radio series pioneered by Edward R. Murrow and revived in 2004 by Norman Gediman. As Anna Sheffield has experienced, this program begins with the student writing a brief essay capturing his or her beliefs about the calling of medicine. These essays are discussed in a small group; their common features and points of difference are explored. This beginning collective negotiation of an understanding of professional values sets the context for investigation of the history of medical ethics, the various oaths taken by physicians, contemporary professionalism compacts, and the challenges posed as a diverse physician workforce cares for an even more diverse patient population. In joining a moral community, students are asked to periodically consider how their experiences with patients affect their statement of Our Ideals as Physicians and note examples of physicians who exemplify key values described in their statement. Importantly, in the approach of joining a moral community, faculty members in both the clinical departments and the foundational sciences are engaged. The program expects them to write their own Ideals as Physicians statement; there is explicit attention to characteristics such as promptness, preparation, and respectful engagement with divergent viewpoints as professional attributes; both students and faculty are expected to uphold high standards across the board, whether patients are present or not.

Storytelling, rituals, and role models are important elements in students' formation as physicians. Faculty members recognize the importance of their relationships with students as a pedagogical element (Haidet et al., 2008; Kenny et al., 2003). Because students see patients early in a program focusing on joining a moral community, it is appropriate to have the "white coat ceremony" at the beginning of medical school, as most schools currently do (Huber, 2003). However, because students are assaulted throughout medical school by challenges to their professional identity, the "joining a moral community" program would periodically hold professional development sessions in which students can share their inspirations and disappointments. Small groups established in the first year would reconvene for these discussions; in addition to trusted faculty facilitators, students one and two years ahead would be invited to participate. In these forums, students would give each other formative feedback. For example, they might be asked to identify attributes among their small-group mates that they particularly admire; reciprocally, they select something they are working on as learners and enlist one of their group members to collaborate with them. The focus of these collaborative projects need not be earthshaking (for example, a student may simply decide that he wants to participate more regularly in small-group discussion; another may focus on preparing more thoroughly); the point is that the students serve as coaches to one another in these self-selected areas. In this way, interdependence and mutual accountability are encouraged.

Because the highest values of medicine do not reside only in the "doctoring" course but are owned across the curriculum (Goldstein et al., 2006), all faculty members would participate in assessing professionalism. Although there are mechanisms for identifying and counseling students with significant deficits, because this is a relatively uncommon problem more emphasis is placed on helping all students with the aspirational dimensions of professionalism: accountability, humanism, excellence, and altruism (Arnold & Stern, 2006). Central to the assessment process would be student narrative self-assessment; students would also write comments for their partners in the collaborative self-improvement project just described.

Late Medical School

○

Harris Roberts is a third-year student who has always wanted to be a scientist. Initially, he thought he would be a chemist, but in high school he became interested in human disease and decided he could better meet his goals by obtaining an M.D. In high school, he worked in a lab as a summer volunteer, and he coauthored a paper and presented at a national meeting while still an undergraduate. He knows that the life of a physician-investigator is not easy and wants to be sure he gets sound training, but he has been reluctant to take the extra time to get a Ph.D. as well as his M.D.

Because he already had a good relationship with the principal investigator (PI) in the lab where he worked as an undergrad, Harris was happy to learn that the medical school at his university has a strong commitment to fostering innovation and discovery; so he remained there for medical school. At the orientation, school leaders talked to the arriving class about medicine as a "field-building discipline," with all its practitioners expected to question current practice, innovate, and improve. Being quite lab-focused, he was surprised by the breadth of inquiry that was included under the umbrella of the school's support. Harris grew to enjoy the sense of common cause he felt during the first two years with classmates who were looking forward to improving the health care delivery system or to writing about the patient-physician relationship.

By the time he began his third year, Harris had been working in his area of systems biology for more than six years. The prospect of suspending this portion of his professional life for the last two years of medical school and three to five years of residency and fellowship training was unappealing. Fortunately, his school had recently developed a longitudinal ambulatory structure in the third year. Although the primary purpose of the redesign was to involve each third- or fourth-year student with a panel of outpatients for whom the student would care in a team-based model over two years, the new curriculum proved to have a number of secondary benefits. The third- and fourth-year classes are organized into four-person teams of mixed levels. During any month, three of the students are involved in the care of their panel and other clinical activities, while one student is engaged in nonclinical work. This has allowed Harris to have three months of full-time research during his third year as well as one or two half-days per week during most of the months when he is doing clinical work. This has required some juggling, but he has seen his PI balance different aspects of his professional life in the same manner. For his fourth year, Harris considered proceeding directly to internship. The internal medicine residency program at his school reserves some internship slots for aspiring physician-scientists, providing special mentoring, research opportunities during residency, and preferred consideration for fellowship positions. However, having spent eight years at the same institution, he feels ready for a change and is confident he can find residency programs that will support his interest in bench science.

Meanwhile, having performed well in clinical work as a third-year student, he plans to commit minimal time to clinical work in his fourth year; he feels confident his residency will further those skills. By scheduling only three clinical months—a subinternship in medicine, an intensive care rotation, and a clinical elective—Harris will have eight months in the fourth year to devote to his research. This predominance of nonclinical activities would not be permitted had he not consistently performed very well in the clinical domain since the beginning of medical school, and most importantly, in the third year.

o

The later phase of medical school serves to advance students' ability to participate in caring for inpatients and outpatients and to appreciate the course of illness and recovery for a number of important disease processes. Although the third year has been conventionally organized around the specialties of medicine, in our view the point is really not the factual content of the various rotations. Rather, more advanced students should be deepening their understanding of patient care, enriching their appreciation of the patient's experience, learning how physicians collaborate across disciplines to provide effective care for complex problems, and gaining enough appreciation of the various specialties to prepare themselves for internship (Hauer, O'Brien, & Poncelet, 2009; Hirsh et al., 2007). At the same time, they should not have to give up major commitments they have made to global health, bench science, the medical humanities, or improving health care delivery.

The programmatic approaches we describe here illustrate how the goals of individualization and standardization, integration, inquiry and improvement, and formation of professional identity can be addressed in the third and fourth years of medical school.

ADVANCING PROFESSIONAL COMMITMENTS. By the third year, the disparities of students' prior preparation that were the focus of the core-and-depth approach become less relevant. An approach that focuses on advancing professional commitments creates the opportunity for individualized learning, primarily nonclinical, in the midst of a very intense period of clinical learning. This approach addresses the goals of standardization of outcomes and individualization of process; the individualized element houses students' work in inquiry and improvement.

In this program, as Harris experienced it, the clinical component of the third year occurs in a longitudinal integrated format. Organized in groups of four, students care as a team for a panel of patients. One student is always off, doing individualized inquiry and improvement work. Therefore the students spend on average 75 percent of the third year on clinical work and 25 percent on nonclinical work, with the clinical component moderately adjustable according to attainment of competencies. If the year is initially structured so that students have twenty-five half-day sessions of internal medicine outpatient practice, fifteen sessions of obstetrics and gynecology, and twelve sessions of psychiatry practice, and if for example a particular student meets the internal medicine competencies more promptly than he does the psychiatry competencies, the session numbers can be adjusted midyear to support additional focus on psychiatry. In addition to allowing emphasis on more slowly acquired competencies, scheduling flexibility facilitates earlier advanced clinical work or increased time for individual inquiry and improvement. The fourth year offers substantial time (as Harris enjoyed) for students to deepen their expertise in an area of nonclinical interest. It is possible for selected students to short-track from the end of the third year directly into the PG1 year of specialty training. Because students are sharing a panel of patients and moving in and out of the clinical environment, a de facto element of the curriculum of a program focused on deepening professional commitments is collaborative team care, hand-offs, and clinical communication.

A distinctive pedagogical feature of a program focused on deepening professional commitments is participation over time in communities of interest that involve students, residents, and faculty members together. Anna Sheffield glimpsed such a community when, at the beginning of medical school, she met with residents who had worked in Africa. Harris is a long-standing member of a systems biology lab. Access to advanced opportunities is facilitated through longitudinal relationships with faculty mentors with whom the student shares a substantial professional interest. Because these relationships are abiding, they can tolerate the coming and going that the focus on clinical learning requires in the third year. Recognizing that students set their own goals, they create an individual learning plan (ILP) in collaboration with a mentor for their inquiry and improvement work. The clinical and nonclinical components of the approach both explicitly feature carefully designed experiences (often called "deliberate practice" in the expertise literature) through which students advance their knowledge and skills in domains where they might otherwise lag (Moulaert, Verwijnen, Rikers, & Scherpbier, 2004).

Assessment in the clinical component of such an approach would be strongly competency-oriented (Ringsted et al., 2006), allowing identification of areas where the student needs further experience and learning as well as areas where she has reached level-appropriate competencies. Work products in the nonclinical domain would be captured through portfolio assessment; project mentors provide formative feedback and global assessment. The clinical teams are held accountable for the quality of patient care and clinical outcomes (Haan et al., 2008); in the individualized inquiry and improvement component, the primary focus of evaluation is the work product itself.

SETTINGS AND PERSPECTIVES. The structure of the typical third year, with its sequential disciplinary blocks, does not promote integrated learning. The focus is on the knowledge and skills associated with the specialty in which the student is currently engaged, and by and large the differences and discontinuities between specialties and settings of care are featured more than their similarities and interrelations are. As we mentioned in Chapter Three, some schools are beginning to experiment with alternative models intended to give students a more integrated perspective on the care of patients by structuring the third year as a longitudinal, primarily outpatient-focused endeavor (Ogur & Hirsh, 2009). A variety of frames can be applied to these longitudinal clinical structures; we offer an approach we call "settings and perspectives."

In a program focused on this approach, the curricular emphasis is on the general knowledge and skills needed to take good care of patients in the hospital, in outpatient settings, at home, and in the community; this contrasts with the priority currently accorded to specialty-specific knowledge in traditional clerkships. Students would observe patients moving from one setting to another and gain appreciation for how the approach to a condition is influenced by the context in which it is being treated. Rather than a snapshot or a still frame of a moment in an illness, students can see the movie of the illness unfolding, from diagnosis to determination and implementation of the treatment plan implemented, as well as response to treatment. Instead of the "binge and purge" that, as we noted in Chapter Three, is a hallmark of the preclerkship learning process and the sequential block-style clerkship year, students would recognize that the skills they are acquiring are cumulative and generally applicable across disciplinary domains. Thus, for example, a student would perceive that techniques and approaches learned in the psychiatry preceptorship are relevant in managing an anxious surgical patient.

A key goal of the settings-and-perspectives approach is to give students a broader understanding of the variety of health professionals and informal caregivers involved in the care of patients with complex illnesses, an appreciation of the varying perspectives of these members of the health care team, and a sense of how physicians collaborate with one another to the benefit of the patient (Hall & Weaver, 2001). This is in contrast to students' almost complete focus on the residents in the sequential disciplinary clerkship. Longitudinal outpatient-based programs instead build strong relationships between learners and their patients; students must deal with differences between the physician's viewpoint and the preferences of patients and their families. Furthermore, they see, from the patient's perspective, the discontinuities and contradictions of the health care delivery system, the implications for an ill and frightened patient of a management disagreement between the primary care clinician and a key subspecialist, and the consequences of discharge planning poorly coordinated between the inpatient and home-care teams.

Pedagogy would support the integration that a settings-and-perspectives approach encourages across disciplines. As students manage their learning goals and choose issues to pursue prompted by their clinical encounters, faculty would encourage students to consider how a topic might be encountered in a discipline other than the one it has arisen in. How, for example, does acute renal failure present in internal medicine, pediatrics, and surgery? What are the similarities and differences in the approaches of physicians in these disciplines? Integrative pedagogies encourage students to monitor their own learning to ensure that clinical experiences are being used to stimulate learning about the underlying science, psychosocial issues, and the system in which care is being delivered as well as the core clinical content and practical how-to issues (Dornan et al., 2005). In this way, students develop a sophisticated "concept map" that integrates the knowledge and understanding of different and distinctive cognitive domains (West et al., 2002).

Assessment to promote integration would focus on the students' ability to understand and apply skills acquired in one context to another and to collaborate. In a portfolio exercise, students might be asked to include notes (with patient identifiers removed) on patients with the same or similar conditions seen in at least two settings (for example, an inpatient service, an ambulatory care practice, a skilled nursing facility, or at home). The portfolio entry would include a brief reflection on continuities and discontinuities, similarities and dissimilarities. Similar exercises would focus on perspective. Students could be asked to consider a complex patient they had come to know well and discuss a clinical episode from three among the perspectives of the patient, a close family member or friend, the principal clinician, and a subspecialty consultant. In more knowledge-focused assessments, students would be expected to manifest cumulative growth across all disciplines and be able to discuss a condition from the perspective of a number of specialties. Assessment at an OSCE station would require students, for example, to counsel a family medicine patient with prostate cancer who is asking about treatment options, relative effectiveness, and long-term complications. They would be expected to display basic understanding of the therapeutic options and some skill in helping the patient negotiate an area of considerable uncertainty and controversy. After the counseling exercise, the student might do a writing exercise describing which elements of the discussion he would leave to the treating surgeon and why. Feedback from these multiple sources would be used both as an assessment modality and as formative information for students as they learn about differing perspectives on patient care and teamwork.

Early Residency

○

Shalini Prasad, twenty-four, is completing her PG1 year in family medicine. She graduated from medical college in New Delhi with an MBBS degree and scored very well on USMLE Step 1 and Step 2. She chose to do her residency training in the United States because she was interested in the challenge and in broadening her perspective. However, unlike some of her friends who are pursuing residency training in this country, she does not plan to emigrate; she intends to return to India, where she hopes to combine direct patient care and work at the health-systems level.

Shalini found she was a competitive applicant in family medicine and chose a program in a plains state, rather than one of the urban programs she considered, because it offered her the full breadth of family medicine, including deliveries and experience with simple surgical procedures, thus approximating the scope of her future practice in India. Her residency program is based at a community hospital in a town of thirty thousand; it is the only GME program the medical center sponsors. Nevertheless, in the community there are two general internists, a cardiologist, a pediatrician, and a general surgeon, in addition to six family physicians. Other subspecialists can be found at the state capital, ninety minutes away.

Once the excitement of her successful match subsided, Shalini approached her residency with some trepidation. All of her family is in India, and although she visited the United States during high school her group then toured only the big cities. So, in addition to the anxieties that all new interns feel, Shalini was worried about adapting to the rural Midwest and being accepted by the patients there. These concerns were familiar to her program director; typically about half the intern class consists of international medical graduates. The family medicine program has developed a set of programs to ease new interns into the culture of the region and facilitate their acceptance in the community. The internship itself begins in the third week of June, but interns are encouraged to arrive at least two weeks earlier for a series of orientation and assessment activities. The program conducts a six-station OSCE focused on the new interns' command of a new patient history and physical exams, as well as their ability to generate a differential diagnosis and identify an acute or unstable situation in which help is required. The OSCE also assesses English-language skills and the interns' approach to challenging interpersonal negotiations, as in working with a substance-abusing patient and discussing end-of-life issues. There are enrichment opportunities for those whom the OSCE identifies as needing additional work in one or more areas.

When Shalini was considering residencies, she was especially attracted to the "community partners" program, a curricular element of the residency she chose. Families who have had a member hospitalized within the past two years are offered the opportunity to host a new intern. The responsibilities of the host family include attending a preinternship welcome party, having their intern to brunch or dinner once a month, and including the resident in routine community activities such as church and special celebrations such as the Fourth of July. The goal is to create a home base for residents who are far from home, help each intern develop an appreciation for the history and culture of the community, and give the intern some insight into how the townspeople perceive the hospital and the care it provides. Although the community partners initiative got off to a slow start, it has become very popular; parents of high school students in particular appreciate the chance to have their children meet a young doctor from another culture. Several exchanges have taken place, with the parents of a resident hosting a visitor from the community partners' family in their country.

Shalini also very much appreciated her experience with her family medicine preceptor. Each intern has a primary placement with one of the town's six family physicians, with whom he or she works one or two half-days every week. This placement functioned as Shalini's clinical home base. As intended, her preceptor took a strong interest in both her clinical progress and her personal life and future plans. She was quickly integrated into the practice, and although all of her preceptor's patients recognized that she was a trainee, a number of them saw her as their main physician.

All of this support notwithstanding, Shalini's internship year had its ups and downs. She had a one-month inpatient rotation with a third-year resident whose expectations she could never fully discern, much less live up to. During this rotation, in a dreary January that threatened to go on forever, a fourteen-year-old boy admitted with influenza and shortness of breath died; in the M and M conference, the resident suggested that Shalini's decisions about ventilator management contributed to his death. She was profoundly shaken by this episode and did not begin to come to terms with it until the next quarterly intern retreat in February. Her program director uses the retreats to have the interns write about high points, low moments, and team and patient conflicts. They are then shared and discussed.

By contrast, a high point of the year was the month during which Shalini focused on organization and delivery of pediatric service in the region. She had been scheduled to do a second month of outpatient pediatrics in the office of the community's pediatrician in March, but she had met the competencies expected at the intern level by the end of her first month. Accordingly, another intern in her class who was still working on intern-level competencies picked up her month and Shalini was able to undertake a project with the faculty pediatrician and the state department of public health. This was her first real taste of the type of health-system work she hopes to do in India, and she found it very exciting.

○

The early stage of residency serves a purpose similar to the third year of medical school. PG1s, and in the case of the longer residency programs PG2s, are familiarizing themselves with the broad knowledge base and fundamental procedures of their chosen specialty. Third- and fourth-year students' exposure to the specialties of medicine occurs through their care of inpatients and outpatients and by observing how the physicians in the specialty interact with one another and with other members of the health care team. The eight to fourteen weeks that a student going into internal medicine or surgery works in that specialty during the latter phase of medical school affords only an overview. Thus medical school graduates arrive at residency training in need of systematic exposure to the conditions under which physicians in their chosen specialty provide care; an opportunity to build a flexible and rich knowledge base through a careful mix of clinical, didactics, and experience; and developmentally sequenced exposure to the procedures of the specialty sufficient to allow development of proficiency while ensuring that patients are well and safely cared for.

As we explained in Chapter Four, because the curriculum is determined by the early resident's assignment and duties (Jagannathan et al., 2009; Ringsted et al., 2006; Sheehan et al., 2005), the key educational decisions about PG1s and PG2s concern deployment of the house staff. Too often, these decisions begin with assessment of the volume of patients seen on various inpatient services; most early residents are assigned to the busiest services. Early residents live right in the middle of the system of layered supervision we described in Chapter Four; they observe their senior residents negotiating diagnostic formulations with the attending physicians (Rogoff et al., 2003); serve as the implementers and effectors of treatment plans that, at the outset, they may have contributed to only minimally; and, in academically based residencies connected with medical schools, supervise the third-year students in refining their skills in physical diagnosis, learning and practicing basic procedures, and building skills in clinical communication. Although early residents attend didactic sessions such as grand rounds and clinical conference, the significant majority of their learning occurs through interaction with near peers. Assessment tends to emphasize the PG1's effectiveness in the implementer role; thus such attributes as organization, time management, efficiency, cooperativeness, and ability to get along with others lead to positive evaluations.

We believe, however, that assignment of residents to clinical services should begin with consideration of what residents at that level need to learn and which clinical settings and activities support this learning. If learning needs are identified that cannot be met through assignment of early residents to existing inpatient services, programs should hold themselves responsible for developing new placements that can. Accordingly, we offer a number of approaches.

PROBLEM REFORMULATION.   Because residents are integral to the work of hospitals, the challenge of creating the flexibility to support individualization and also to ensure standardization of outcomes is significant. It is much simpler to assign residents to months of service, trusting that all of them will find every assignment well matched to their developmental educational needs and relevant given their ever-more-specific career focus. However, common sense argues that some residents are likely to need five months of a particular experience to achieve the competence that a peer can attain in two, and that the same rotation may not be appropriate at all for a resident heading in a different professional direction. Nonetheless, sick patients require care, and residents need to see an adequate number of patients on each rotation to support their learning. Thus it is not feasible, from either an educational or a clinical standpoint, to have services be uncertain from month to month as to how many residents will be participating in patient care. How might a training program reconcile its commitment to individualization of experience and standardization of outcomes for residents given the realities of administering a complex patient care enterprise?

First, every clinical rotation for residents must be of demonstrable educational value and should contribute distinctively to the aggregate of the residents' learning (Maddaus et al., 2008). A residency program designed in this manner would begin from first principles: What are the clinical experiences that a newly minted physician in this specialty should have encountered under supervision? How many instances should she have seen? What level of proficiency or sophistication should she have attained?

The second step is to identify clinical opportunities that can predictably offer residents the desired experiences under good educational conditions—meaning at an appropriate pace, with adequate time for reading and reflection, and supported by a thoughtful, challenging, and supportive faculty. Because no residency program can have just the right mix of clinical opportunities, this design process involves setting aside potential clinical rotations that, despite their many positive features, are simply the third, fourth, or fifth example of opportunities already well represented in the program. Such careful planning will reveal that there are experiences that residents require but that are lacking and must be developed. The most obvious example of such a gap is the full array of functional outpatient rotations for residents in all specialties. A program committed to the principles of individualization of experience and standardization with respect to competence across the core domains of the specialty would ensure that residents have a chance to become proficient in caring for patients in a variety of outpatient settings. For example, in her PG2 year Shalini will pick up a small panel of nursing-home and home-bound patients for whom she will provide care where they live.

Offering an appropriate array of productive clinical experiences for residents is necessary in meeting core competencies, but it does not address the challenging problem of supporting individualization while ensuring that the various rotations are adequately staffed. A solution is to have residents engage in the work of a rotation at different levels, depending on their capabilities at the time they arrive. In Shalini's case, a colleague was conveniently available to pick up her second month of outpatient pediatrics. Had this not occurred, the faculty pediatrician would simply not have had a resident with him that month. The situation is a bit more complicated, though not insoluble, for inpatient services. For example, two internal medicine residents are scheduled to do a cardiac care unit rotation in February of their PG2 year. One resident is still acquiring the knowledge, procedural skills, and experience to deliver solid competent care to patients with acute and unstable cardiac conditions; the second resident, whether by virtue of previous experiences, aptitude, or motivation, has already mastered the fundamentals expected of a PG2. Both residents would take turns admitting patients overnight, supervising the PG1s. But they would spend the bulk of their days differently. The first resident would remain on the unit, under the supervision of faculty members and fellows, refining his skills in the clinical care of patients in the cardiac care unit. The second resident would make work rounds with the team but would then be free to tackle more advanced problems in cardiac disease, perhaps continuing work initiated by a prior resident in community outreach, or working on a problem in patient flow or care delivery. In this way residents assigned to the same service can tackle the problems seen there at a level appropriate to their own professional development.

Clearly, supporting the learning of interns and residents in a system such as this requires considerable ability on the part of individual faculty members to benchmark the attainment of residents and deliver teaching that meets their needs, and on the part of residency programs to link teachers to residents as the need arises. Because procedures are observable, residency programs in surgery are more able to teach residents at the growing edge of their competence, at least in the dimension of technical competence, than are the cognitive specialties; faculty development focusing on "entrustable professional activities" may help teachers in the nonprocedural specialties become more aware of the level of competence of their resident (ten Cate & Scheele, 2007).

Across specialties, a structural factor that facilitates discerning assessment of resident capabilities is adequate duration of the pairing of a faculty member with a resident. An abiding relationship facilitates development of detailed understanding of resident capabilities and allows attendings to construct learning opportunities for residents that are focused on the next thing the resident needs to tackle. This is particularly obvious in surgery, where faculty members faced with an unfamiliar resident will adopt the conservative position that the resident requires assistance. Assisting residents to do things they can accomplish unassisted diminishes the educational value of the experience for the resident. More durable faculty-resident pairings permit more accurate assessment of resident capabilities, performance by residents of more advanced elements of care, and consequently better preparation for independent practice. For this problem-reformulation approach to work properly, reliable competency-based assessment is necessary to identify the resident who needs additional clinical experience and the one who, although at the same level of training, is ready to focus on, for example, redesign of processes of care.

UNCERTAINTY, CONFIDENCE, AND RESPONSIBILITY. The internship year is famously stressful and demanding, and in many ways it serves as a forge of professional formation. Helping newly minted doctors cope with the burdens of medical practice, uncertainty, the death of patients, team conflict, and their own negative emotional responses is the core of a curriculum for early residency focused on professional formation. Just the workload, even with the duty-hour reduction, is oppressive and discouraging. As a new resident describes it, "The low point was returning to rounds at 5:00 p.m., then having my resident give me another 100 things to do on top of the 100 things she/he gave me to do before clinic, then realizing that she/he probably could have done 50 or 75 of those things while I was at clinic but did nothing" (Ackerman, Graham, Schmidt, Stern, & Miller, 2009, p. 30).

Unfortunately, many residency programs neglect this dimension of intern experience or deal with it inadequately (Levine et al., 2006). Though not attempting a formal didactic curriculum, Shalini's residency has created several forums for discussion of these issues. In addition to the intern retreat, Shalini found her family medicine preceptor to be a useful confidant, moral support, and advisor. Additionally, because the culture of her residency program is open and trusting, a number of other residents came up to her after the M and M conference and indicated they felt she was treated poorly.

The pedagogy in a program that helps residents move from uncertainty to confidence and responsibility locates the teaching within several key relationships, particularly with the program director and the faculty preceptors. For example, in Shalini's program several of the family medicine preceptors are graduates of the program and thus have a strong sense of generational continuity and commitment. Before beginning as preceptors, they have a formal faculty development session with the program director in which the importance of this dimension of their role is emphasized and they are given specific instruction in empathic listening. The preceptors meet several times a year, usually following the intern retreats, so that the program director can advise them if any of the interns need particular assistance. A key issue that preceptors are encouraged to explore with their interns is the tension between requesting assistance when required and maintaining and promoting their professional credibility (Kennedy, Regehr, Baker, & Lingard, 2009). Because family medicine is a specialty in which knowing when to consult is a critical attribute of competence, preceptors are encouraged to tell stories from their work as physicians and share their own struggles with this issue.

Assessment to support the growth of residents from uncertainty to confidence and responsibility is explicit, but largely formative. The key evaluators would be the supervising residents and the family medicine preceptor. The assessment might focus on the resident's initiative, engagement with the inpatient team and preceptor's practice, calling for help, and functioning as principal physician.

Advanced Residency

---------------------------------------o---------------------------------------

Dr. Dan Chen is looking forward to his upcoming interview for a faculty position in which he will spend a third of his time assisting the director of the simulation center and two-thirds as a vascular surgeon. He developed an interest in medical education toward the end of medical school and is eager to continue some of the research he started in residency, on use of simulation to improve the postoperative care provided by interprofessional surgical teams.

Dr. Chen knew he wanted to be a doctor as early as junior high and worked hard to prepare for medical school. He performed well on the MCAT but was devastated to find that he had difficulty with the interview process and was not accepted at any medical school.

He spent the next year shadowing several physicians, volunteering in two clinics, and learning how better to communicate with patients and health professionals. When he reapplied to medical school, he was much more comfortable talking to people and received two acceptances.

During the first two years of medical school, he continued to work hard on communication and interpersonal skills. By the middle of his third year, he felt comfortable applying his knowledge, using his skills in clinical settings, and interacting with patients and colleagues in the role of a novice professional. Dr. Chen especially enjoyed his experiences in surgery, where the intensity and the tangible sense of accomplishment along with the teamwork and collaboration in the OR excited him. He also had some exceptional role models and mentors in surgery. He was paired with a vascular surgeon, Dr. Card, during the third year and worked with this surgeon for most of a four-week block. During that time he followed three patients closely from pre-op visits, through their surgery, to their recovery and post-op care. Dr. Card fully involved Dr. Chen in the care of these patients, treating him more like a junior partner than a student. Dr. Card also suggested how Dr. Chen could focus his learning in other specialties to benefit and enrich the surgical perspective he would develop in the future.

After experiencing the power of the simulation center for learning basic procedural skills, Dr. Chen decided to enroll in an elective course on medical education and joined a project studying use of simulation to improve intra-operative team communication. This stimulated his interest in completing a formal elective program that involved more courses in medical education and a guided research project on operating room communication. He chose to use the fourth year of medical school to focus on this research.

Dr. Chen entered a surgical residency program at another university with a strong simulation center program. Although he was not able to spend much time during residency in the center, he did find that his research was applicable to several studies currently under way at that center. He was able to work with the surgery faculty members involved in the research, building on medical school experience. As a result of his work on operating room communication, he was invited to participate in a hospital quality improvement committee that sought to improve team functioning in the OR.

One reason he selected this surgery program is that it was an opportunity to fast-track into a surgical fellowship. So, after three years of general surgical training, meeting all his competencies, Dr. Chen

entered the vascular surgery fellowship. This program offered him not
only the opportunity to progress in his competencies but also research
and development work in training future vascular surgeons in how to
use task trainers in the simulation center.

○

Advanced residency serves a distinctly different purpose from the
internship year. At this point in training, residents are preparing for
independent and unsupervised practice. Rather than implementing the
plan of a more senior physician from an understanding of the clinical
situation that may be largely received, advanced residents are expected
to tackle "raw" clinical problems, rapidly distinguish important features
from distracting ones in the patient's presentation, deploy an extensive
knowledge base, perform complex procedures proficiently, and demonstrate both routine and adaptive expertise. Furthermore, although the
faculty supervisor is legally responsible for the conduct of patient care,
advanced residents have extensive responsibility for workflow on their
services, serve as the moment-to-moment leader of their clinical team,
supervise their immediate juniors, and are responsible for much of the
teaching that all members of the team receive. In the three-year residency
specialties, the leadership function begins early in the second year; in
surgery (a five-year residency), it occurs intermittently in the third year
but characterizes the fourth and fifth years.

An educational program designed to nurture this set of advanced
capabilities will necessarily look quite different from one intended to
develop intern level skills. As we explained in Chapter Four, both the
procedurally oriented residencies such as surgery and the nonprocedural
specialties such as family medicine and neurology achieve this developmental progression by having more advanced residents do more advanced
clinical work. This can be accomplished by having the residents take on
more challenging roles in the care of patients with common and familiar
problems, or by assigning them to patients whose condition or treatment
is more challenging. Although the first of these two strategies is more
typical of the nonprocedural specialties and the second characterizes
the procedural disciplines, the fundamental educational challenge is the
same: to create an experience that allows the resident, in a graduated
way, to encounter increasing clinical challenge and decreasing supervisory
intervention while maintaining sufficient oversight to ensure the safety
of patients and permit accurate characterization of the advanced resident's capabilities. Residents at this point should be largely self-sufficient
and self-directed learners; however, teachers can assist their residents in

developing nuanced approaches and a broadened repertory of responses by sharing their experience.

IMPACT OF PHYSICIANS.   Physicians play a number of roles in society; residency programs must offer opportunities for trainees to experience the impact of physicians working in nonclinical capacities. Dr. Chen's participation in both simulation and communication research and his committee work on quality improvement exemplify this kind of opportunity. Other residents may choose to become involved with the community in which their GME program is located, and still others may elect to engage with their specialty professional organization. These physician-citizen roles allow residents to see medicine in a broader context and appreciate the perspective of payers, employers, government, and policy makers. Preparing residents for their role as physician-citizen is part of the broad responsibility of residency training programs (Gruen et al., 2004). The kinds of experiences that are now available for medical students under names such as "scholarly concentration," "pathways to discovery," and "areas of concentration" must be developed for residents as well. As at the UME level, it is important that these programs be broadly conceived; we do not envision this simply as a bioscience research opportunity. Rather, residents should have the opportunity to work in a public health department, serve on a national committee of their specialty's professional organization, and do an externship with the health committee of their state legislature.

Assessment addressing these types of activities will focus on such resident characteristics as initiative, self-direction, ability to collaborate, and leadership. Of course, the effectiveness of the work undertaken as part of the "impact of the physician" work is relevant as well. The perspectives of the resident himself, colleagues, and mentors are obtained and used for formative feedback as well as for summative assessment.

EVERYDAY INNOVATION AND BIG IMPROVEMENT.   In a residency program that is organized around everyday innovation and big improvement, residents collaborate with other health professionals to maximize the efficiency of care processes. Residents have a detailed, ground-level experience of how systems of care in the hospital are working, or not. Too often, however, this knowledge is not captured and converted to the benefit of patients. In addition to the missed opportunity to improve our systems of health care, this contributes to a sense of diminished agency on the part of the house staff and deprives them of opportunities to learn important skills in change management, organizational development, and program evaluation. Residents continue to care for patients at the level of sophistication and independence appropriate to their skills, but because they are not being called on to perform myriad clerical and other nonclinical tasks or to provide care that is not contributing to their education, most residents have time available to undertake projects that improve the systems of care in which they work. These projects may be individual or group, ambitious or quite discrete, sustained or short in duration; "everyday innovation" is Mylopoulos and Scardamalia's term (2008) to describe the ordinary adjustments that physicians, at least some physicians, make in response to unsatisfactory processes of care. The projects should arise out of residents' interests and recognition of opportunities to make care better and should create an opportunity for the resident or residents to work with the larger community of those charged with improving safety and patient outcomes. Advanced residents who are interested should serve on all committees and task forces concerned with delivery of care and its quality. Other residents may be more interested in improving the health of the community from which their patients come.

Teaching that supports everyday innovation and big improvement would encourage residents to consider not only what they know about a patient's situation but also how the system in which they work supports or interferes with delivery of effective care to their patient. A program focused on everyday innovation and big improvement would be constructed broadly and could work as well in a community-based residencies program as in an academic one. Engaged faculty members would connect with residents and assist them in understanding how to be effective in improving patient care in the environment in which they work. Communities of interest formed around improving care outcomes would allow residents and faculty members to collaborate on projects. Residents would be encouraged to suggest projects, participate in improvement work, and disseminate what they learn.

Assessment would of course focus on the residents' projects. Outcome measures consider the success of the resident's project in producing the change it intended and the importance of the issue addressed, and this could be documented in a portfolio (Carraccio & Englander, 2004). In addition, team members would assess their collaborators' initiative, collegiality, and productivity (Farmer, Beard, Dauphinee, LaDuca, & Mann, 2002).

TAKING RESPONSIBILITY FOR EXCELLENCE. A residency program organized around taking responsibility for excellence would build into its professional formation an insistence on excellence. Investing effort to achieve the best possible outcomes for a patient or patients collectively is a critical professional attribute that is both distributed and individually held. A program focused on this goal would take advantage of the powerful positive formative influence of learning in an environment that is consistently focused on improving patient outcomes. In such a program, residents (and students) would be incorporated into microsystems dedicated to improvement in quality (Nelson, Godfrey, Batalden et al., 2008). The key curricular element would be the work of improvement itself, but particularly for all levels of learners there would be explicit discussion of the habits of mind, problem reformulation, and effortful reinvestment that is professional practice, as we discussed in Chapter Two. More fundamentally, attention would be drawn to excellence as an aspirational dimension of physicians' professional identity. Residents and medical students would be encouraged to observe the work of near-peers and faculty members as they go beyond simple disease-oriented knowledge to improving patient care.

The primary pedagogy for work of this nature is coaching. Residents benefit from and grow in response to collegial relationships with peers and supervisors in an environment in which commitment to excellence is a shared value (Viggiano et al., 2007). When these learning environments are working well, self-assessment and mutual accountability are regarded as fundamental processes for improving quality and patient outcomes; student see their teachers modeling approaches (such as the debrief) as a way to explore how better care might be achieved. The importance of the various perspectives represented by an interprofessional team is recognized; residents and students learn to seek feedback from their nonphysician colleagues, not because of an ideological commitment to interprofessional work but because it produces better outcomes for patients (Eva & Regehr, 2005).

The environment itself and the people in it reinforce the aspirational quality of striving for excellence.

Accordingly, assessment strategies would focus on the learner's self-assessment. Although the nature of this work requires that motivation for action be internalized, the work is also highly interdependent and collaborative. Thus project teams might, for example, collectively assess the success of their work and the effectiveness of their collaborative processes, as well as routinely give one another feedback. Portfolio assessment would also be particularly well suited to assessment of residents' growth in taking responsibility for excellence.

Taking Action for Change

Medical school and residency program curriculum committees need to actively engage in the process of thinking creatively about how to implement—and improve on—these recommendations within their individual programs. Each program will have to examine its unique circumstances and adapt the designs to meet local needs. To support programs in learning about and implementing reform, the profession must communicate about and collaborate on improvement efforts just as it does in issues of patient care. However, the effect of these programmatic efforts will be limited without accompanying changes in the regulation and financing of medical education. In Chapter Eight, we consider the policy changes that would facilitate and support the excellence in medical education we envision.

8

SUPPORTING
EXCELLENCE THROUGH
EFFECTIVE POLICY

MEDICINE AS A PROFESSION has thrived in the United States in part because medical education's considerable array of stakeholders has continued to insist on high standards for education and practice. Among these stakeholders are medical school deans; faculty and faculty leaders; CEOs of teaching hospitals; medical directors; residency program directors and deans of graduate medical education; leaders of accrediting, certifying, and licensing organizations; leaders of medical professional organizations; federal and state government officials; foundation leaders; payers; and patients. In various ways, they all influence the design, implementation, and funding of medical education. Therefore, even though curriculum deans, residency program directors, and course and clerkship directors have immediate responsibility for design and delivery of educational programs, they respond to the demands of and work within constraints imposed by external entities. The programmatic recommendations we presented in Chapter Seven must be facilitated by changes at the state and national levels in financing and regulating U.S. medical education. Indeed, for medical schools and residency programs to successfully innovate, the funders, regulators, and professional organizations that control and influence medical education must be actively engaged in this reform effort. Moreover, this engagement must be collaborative and coordinated among all the stakeholder groups; individually and collectively, each stakeholder has a role in facilitating a new vision of medical education.

We propose that medical education's key stakeholders take seven major steps to advance U.S. medical education and, ultimately, the health of the public:

1. AAMC and medical schools work together to revise premedical course requirements and admission processes.

2. Accrediting, certifying, and licensing bodies together develop a coherent framework for the continuum of medical education and establish effective mechanisms to coordinate standards and resolve jurisdictional conflicts.

3. CEOs of teaching hospitals and directors of residency programs collaborate to improve both patient care and clinical education and develop educational programs that are consistent with practice requirements.

4. Deans of medical schools and CEOs of teaching hospitals support the teaching mission by providing financial support, mentoring, faculty development, recognition, and academic advancement.

5. Deans of medical schools and CEOs of teaching hospitals collaboratively make funding for medical education transparent, fair, and aligned with the missions of medical schools and teaching hospitals.

6. AAMC, AMA, ACGME, medical specialty societies, and medical schools advocate for sustained private, federal, and state funding commitments to support infrastructure, innovation, and research in medical education.

7. AAMC, AMA, ACGME, medical specialty societies, and medical schools collaborate on developing a medical workforce policy for the United States. A variety of interventions are required to address the cost of medical education, length of training, and practice viability to ensure that the country has the mix of specialty and subspecialty physicians to meet the needs of the population.

1. Revising Course Requirements and Admission Processes

More than a hundred years ago, Flexner and others developed a list of prerequisite courses for medical school. The list is still in use. Yet much has changed since then; entirely new fields are now regarded as foundational to medicine, among them genetics, molecular science, statistics and population sciences, psychology, sociology, and the learning sciences. Working together, AAMC and medical schools must develop a broader, more current, and more forward-looking set of prerequisites that accurately reflect the integrated nature of the basic, clinical, and social sciences and broadly represent the core competencies expected of a physician (Emanuel, 2006).

AAMC and Howard Hughes Medical Institute's *Scientific Foundations for Future Physicians* (2009) addresses both premedical and medical school scientific competencies. The report also recognizes the importance of communicating to colleges and universities recommendations about science courses, to admissions committees about admissions processes, to AAMC regarding MCAT test construction, to medical school curriculum committees about incorporating foundational science competencies, and to the NBME to test for these competencies. Enacting these recommendations will entail concerted effort and coordination among these entities.

It is critical that the medical profession and thus medical school classes be diverse; this requires a well-qualified and diverse pipeline. Diversity enhances the quality of education for all students and results in more culturally competent physicians who are better prepared to serve varied patient populations. In addition, physicians underrepresented in medicine are more likely to practice in underserved communities and speak languages other than English, thus addressing linguistic and cultural barriers that contribute to health disparities (Coleman et al., 2008). More pipeline programs are needed to prepare students from populations now underrepresented in medicine for admission to medical school.

The admissions process itself has to be redesigned to select applicants with the potential to achieve competencies expected of all physicians. Unfortunately, the selection process in most medical schools focuses on basic science knowledge and fails to adequately assess the breadth of attributes required for medical practice. Furthermore, current admissions practices compromise the diversity of entering classes; applicants are typically screened on the basis of grade point average and MCAT scores, and this initial screen, mechanically applied, may disadvantage underrepresented minority applicants. The standard interview worsens the problem because interviewers tend to favor applicants who look much like themselves (Kreiter et al., 2004). Innovative practices, such as the multiple mini-interview (MMI), can more realistically assess noncognitive factors in the selection process and should be widely adopted (Eva, Reiter, Rosenfeld, and Norman, 2004a, 2004b; Eva, Rosenfeld, et al., 2004; Lemay, Lockyer, Collin, & Brownell, 2007; Reiter & Eva, 2005; Reiter, Salvatori, Rosenfeld, Trinh, & Eva, 2006; Rosenfeld, Reiter, Trinh, & Eva, 2008). The AAMC needs to promote best practices in the admissions process and help medical schools adopt these processes at the local level.

2. Framework for Continuum of Medical Education and Effective Mechanisms

Organizations charged with ensuring the safety of the public—that is, accrediting, certifying, and licensing agencies—must more tightly coordinate expectations and define appropriate areas of jurisdiction. As we explained in Chapter Five, there is no single agency responsible for regulating and financing medical education; multiple agencies participate in this process and often hold conflicting expectations of programs and learners. Working together, however, the LCME, the ACGME and its multiple residency review committees, and the Accrediting Council for Continuing Medical Education could establish common competency domains, from UME, through GME and CME, with performance standards appropriate for each level. Doing so would increase the coherence of medical education, improve the quality of every level of training, give faculty and learners consistent language, and reduce the burden on schools and training programs (Committee on the Health Professions Education Summit, 2003).

Licensing and certification should similarly be updated and aligned. As we explained in Chapter Five, physicians in the United States must demonstrate the knowledge base required for the practice of medicine by passing the three-step USMLE and then applying for a license in the state in which they wish to practice. The USMLE's steps, offered at the end of the foundational science curriculum (second year), toward the close of clerkship education (fourth year), and at the end of internship, reflect the three stages of medical education that were in place by 1920; but they are poorly timed with respect to contemporary medical education and retard the integration and flexibility we advocate. Indeed, as earlier clinical immersion becomes the norm in the first two years of the curriculum, USMLE Step 1, which focuses solely on basic science knowledge, has become archaic. Likewise, USMLE Step 3 is an anachronism from the era when preparation for general practice included only an M.D. degree and one year of internship. The current situation persists because the examining entities (the NBME, the FSMB, and the ABMS) have distinct and dissimilar interests.

The FSMB argues that a national examination prior to licensure is a necessity so that states have a uniform metric for assessing candidates for licensure. We do not disagree. However, licensure for independent practice is premature at the end of the PG1 year, and the content of USMLE Step 3 is inappropriate for all but the small number of medical school graduates who do transitional internships.

Instead, we recommend a single USMLE examination at the end of the third year or early in the fourth year to permit integrated assessment of foundational science, clinical knowledge, and clinical skills. USMLE Step 3, currently taken during internship, should be dropped in favor of a requirement that all physicians be certified by their specialty's board in order to practice independently. This would establish a rational two-step national examination series: an integrated USMLE examination toward the end of medical school for supervised practice, and the specialty board examination on completion of residency training that all states could use for licensing for independent practice.

The competing interests of these various agencies serve neither medical education nor patient care well. The public deserves assurance that residents completing training are ready for independent practice and that clinicians are continuing to advance their knowledge and skills over their lifetime in practice. If the jurisdictional disputes cannot be adjudicated, a national oversight body must be created to coordinate all accrediting, certifying, and licensing agencies associated with medical education. Similarly, to create a more vigorous and credible educational system in the postresidency period that can support physicians in maintaining competence over a lifetime of professional practice, the expectations and goals of specialty certification, medical licensure, and CME accreditation bodies must be rationalized and their efforts coordinated.

3. Aligning Patient Care and Clinical Education with Practice Requirements

Physicians in training learn in the context of providing patient care and working within systems that promote or inhibit excellence. High-quality patient care is the best "learning laboratory" for establishing the habits of practice we expect of future professionals. Clinical practices used for learning, regardless of setting, must support continuous redesign of health care delivery that is directly linked to quality patient outcomes in a patient-centered way. Students, residents, and fellows can help drive such patient safety and quality-improvement initiatives (Spear, 2006).

However, not just the trainees are responsible for quality. Hospital and clinical administrators and faculty physicians must ensure that students and residents are working in an environment where the patient comes first. Teaching hospitals should be a beacon of excellence showing the way to better health care delivery and should demonstrate how to improve the health of populations and communities as well as individual patients (Committee on the Roles of Academic Health Centers in the 21st Century, 2003).

An element of effective patient care is good teamwork. Physicians in training, both students and residents, need the opportunity to work and learn in well-functioning teams together with other health professions trainees. Again, the culture of the clinical environment strongly influences how physicians, nurses, and other health professionals work together and the models that trainees see (Gittell, 2009).

Residency programs must offer training that is tightly coupled with the performance expectations for professional practice. Specifically, clinical education needs to move away from a predominantly inpatient and service-driven training model to include other settings such as outpatient clinics that better reflect actual future practice for the majority of physicians. To accomplish this, the ACGME must focus on the outcomes of patients cared for by residents. The ability of residency programs to characterize the outcomes of patients cared for by individual residents and to assist residents in improving those outcomes should be part of the assessment of residency programs. Finally, the funds flowing to support residency education should go to the educators, rather than to medical center CEOs.

4. Financial Support, Mentoring, Faculty Development, Recognition, and Academic Advancement

Achieving the innovation and reform that U.S. medical education needs is not possible without faculty members who are invested in, and prepared and honored for, their role as teacher. With increasing pressure for clinical productivity, time to teach is compromised. These circumstances are unacceptable; teaching must be supported. In addition, as curriculum reform transforms the structure of medical education, faculty will have new roles and responsibilities. These new teaching responsibilities require faculty development and mentoring from skilled and experienced senior faculty.

Faculty development has traditionally been the mechanism for extending pedagogical training to faculty members, generally in the form of workshops to develop instructional skills (Steinert et al., 2006). In addition to these episodic efforts, broader programs, like the Teaching Scholars Programs described in Chapter Six, are needed to equip teaching faculty with the knowledge, skills, and values needed to succeed in their roles as educators (Gruppen, Frohna, Anderson, & Lowe, 2003).

Teachers also require a community of fellow teachers and scholars, sometimes referred to as "a teaching commons" (Huber & Hutchings, 2005)—a place where issues of teaching and learning can be dealt with in a scholarly manner. In Chapter Six, we discussed academies; these academies advance and support teachers, offer faculty development, promote curriculum improvement, and advocate for the teaching mission of the school and the university.

In addition, faculty members who invest heavily in education should be able to offer documentation of their teaching contributions for academic promotion purposes (Simpson et al., 2007). To reward and advance faculty members with major teaching responsibilities, university promotion committees must incorporate these forms of scholarship into their advancement criteria and documentation of teaching requirements. In addition, dean's offices, offices of medical education, and academies can promote educational innovation and the scholarship of teaching and learning through funding support for these activities and infrastructure support for educational evaluation and research.

5. Making Funding Transparent, Fair, and Aligned with the Mission

The funding sources that support medical schools and teaching hospitals include patient care services, faculty practice, research grants, philanthropy, patent royalties, tuition, student fees, and payers (prominently Medicare and Medicaid). As we noted in Chapter Five, resources generated for one purpose often pay for another. Indeed, private insurance companies do not cover their fair share of medical education expenses, which then must be covered by other sources. Faculty practice revenue is generally taxed to support education and sometimes research programs. This cost shifting or cross-subsidization strategy has worked reasonably well in the past, but it is being challenged by the lack of excess revenues in one mission to cover the expenses of another and regulations prohibiting such cost transfers.

Many medical schools and teaching hospitals are moving toward mission-based management as a way of apportioning mission-related revenue to mission-related expenses while still protecting funding for education as a strategic priority. Faculty and department contributions to the educational, research, patient care, and community service missions of the institution are thus accounted for, and revenues are apportioned on the basis of those contributions and aligned with strategic priorities. We recommend that medical schools adopt transparent mechanisms that are administratively simple, predictable, fair, and accountable (Detmer & Steen, 2005).

6. Sustained Funding Commitments to Support Infrastructure, Innovation, and Research

Medical education is, fundamentally, learning in action: a process of learning a practice and learning to continuously revise and improve that practice. However, this view of medical education as learning in action does not diminish the fact that it requires an infrastructure, faculty resources and capabilities, and a research base of its own, distinct from that of the clinical enterprise. Medical education is not simply a byproduct of clinical work. Funding agencies such as governments and foundations can advance change with innovation grants, much as Flexner did after publication of his report in 1910. As secretary of the General Education Board supported by John D. Rockefeller's foundation, Flexner channeled millions of dollars to medical schools to improve their educational programs, an effort that may have been as important as his critique in improving the quality of medical education in North America (Ludmerer, 1999).

A similar infusion of innovation funding today would help guide and fuel educational reform as well. Best practices identified through such an initiative could be broadcast. The AAMC, AMA, ACGME, medical specialty boards, and foundations can facilitate the educational reform process by jointly convening national forums for sharing innovative ideas and stimulating local action, and by publicizing these recommendations to its members.

To guide educational program decisions with empirical research and maximize educational innovation, a significant and sustainable mechanism for funding research on medical education must be developed. Without such resources, educational research will continue to be a marginal contributor to the educational policy debate. Multi-institutional research that employs powerful research methods requires funding not currently available for medical education. However, only with such funding will the field know if changes being made in education and financing actually improve medical education and make a difference in patient care outcomes and costs.

7. Medical Workforce Policy for the United States

Medical education is a public good that must be supported by society. State governments have traditionally funded much of undergraduate medical education; the federal government has funded graduate medical education through Medicare and Medicaid. However, both mechanisms are being reduced as a proportion of the total cost of educating physicians in training. This erosion must be reversed.

In most developed countries, specifically in many European Union countries that achieve better health outcomes than does the United States, medical students pay little or no tuition (Ginsburg et al., 2008). In the United States, with dwindling state support for medical education, the cost of tuition continues to rise at both public and private universities, along with student debt. Soon only the wealthy will be able to afford a medical education, and it will become impossible for young physicians to repay their debts and make a reasonable living in all but a few specialties of medicine, further compounding the problem of maldistribution of specialties. A variety of initiatives would help address this problem: improved and sustained government support of medical schools and residency programs; scholarships, low- or no-interest loans; and debt forgiveness programs, such as the National Health Service Corps, that are designed to attract physicians to practice in underserved areas and specialties.

Funding of GME is particularly problematic in at least two respects. First, as an unintended consequence of the recognition that care at teaching hospitals has some training-related expenses, the Centers for Medicare and Medicaid Services (CMS) have become responsible for training residents. In addition to inappropriately binding residents to inpatient settings, CMS caps the total number of residents supported by Medicare, in order to control costs. The rising complexity of health care in inpatient and outpatient settings, limitations on resident duty hours, and the greater size of medical school graduating classes all militate for expanding the number of funded residency positions. Facilitating the flexibility and innovation that GME redesign demands requires a more broad-based, less politicized flow of funds. Medicare has made a number of programmatic changes recently to recognize that medical care is entirely different from what it was forty-five years ago, when the program was enacted. Initiatives such as Part D funding for outpatient medication are a response to the fact that much medical care occurs, and expenses are incurred, outside the hospital. Whether federal funding for medical education continues to flow through CMS or is otherwise organized, it must be structured in a way that supports the participation of residents from all specialties in outpatient care.

Second, the recipient of the IME and DME funding intended to support the expenses associated with the education of residents is not necessarily the entity responsible for this education. In other words, medical centers receive medical education funding associated with resident education, but academic departments, which are responsible for the salaries of residency program directors, associate program directors, and a host of other cost centers related to resident education, often do not receive that funding. Funds arriving at a medical center for resident education should be managed by those responsible for designing and conducting residency educational programs.

A Concerted Effort

The imperative for change is clear. The U.S. system of medical education cannot continue to look back to the innovations of a century past. Profound changes in society, in the nature and delivery of health care, and in technology and communication alone argue for new conceptions of medical education. Insights from the learning sciences and extensive empirical work on medical student and resident learning further suggest that transformative change in medical education is overdue.

Strong advocacy is required on the part of the medical community to ensure accomplishment of these recommendations for policy action. Although mobilization of the key stakeholders in medical education will be challenging, powerful and visionary leadership can make this happen. Action can be promoted at every level, from course and program innovation within a school or residency program to local and national policy changes, to advocacy for funding reforms. Taken together, our recommendations offer a blueprint for the future of medical education at every level—and an agenda for action.

By acting on these recommendations for policy reform and supporting the programmatic goals we offered in Chapter Seven, decision makers who believe in improving the education of physicians will benefit the health of the public. Implementation of these recommendations will drive medical education to new heights of excellence, establishing it as the model for professional education worldwide. Most important, preparing physicians who have a firm professional identity, who continuously seek excellence through inquiry, and who are engaged as members of a moral community will ensure the highest-quality care for patients.

REFERENCES

Aagaard, E., Teherani, A., & Irby, D. (2004). Effectiveness of the one-minute preceptor model for diagnosing the patient and the learner: Proof of concept. *Academic Medicine, 79*(1), 42–49.

Accreditation Council for Graduate Medical Education. (2001). ACGME highlights its standards on resident duty hours—May 2001. Retrieved from http://www.acgme.org/acWebsite/resInfo/ri_OSHAresp.asp

Accreditation Council for Graduate Medical Education. (2007). Common program requirements: General competencies. Retrieved from http://www.acgme.org/outcome/comp/GeneralCompetenciesStandards21307.pdf

Accreditation Council for Graduate Medical Education. (2009). Retrieved from http: www.acgme.org/acWebsite/newsResleases/newsRel_11_05_08.pdf

Ackerman, A., Graham, M., Schmidt, H., Stern, D., & Miller, S. (2009). Critical events in the lives of interns. *Journal of General Internal Medicine, 24*(1), 27–32.

Albanese, M. (2000). Problem-based learning: Why curricula are likely to show little effect on knowledge and clinical skills. *Medical Education, 34*(9), 729–738.

Alexander, P. (2003). The development of expertise: The journey from acclimation to proficiency. *Educational Researcher, 32*(8), 10–14.

Alguire, P. (1998). A review of journal clubs in postgraduate medical education. *Journal of General Internal Medicine, 13*(5), 347–353.

Allison, J., Kiefe, C., Weissman, N., Person, S., Rousculp, M., Canto, J., et al. (2000). Relationship of hospital teaching status with quality of care and mortality for Medicare patients with acute MI. *Journal of the American Medical Association, 284*(10), 1256–1262.

Anderson, G., Greenberg, G., & Wynn, B. (2001). Graduate medical education: The policy debate. *Annual Review of Public Health, 22*, 35–47.

Anderson, J. (1980). *Cognitive psychology and its implications.* San Francisco: W. H. Freeman.

Arnold, L., Shue, C., Kalishman, S., Prislin, M., Pohl, C., Pohl, H., et al. (2007). Can there be a single system for peer assessment of professionalism among medical students? A multi-institutional study. *Academic Medicine, 82*(6), 578–586.

Arnold, L., & Stern, D. (2006). What is medical professionalism? In D. Stern (Ed.), *Measuring medical professionalism* (pp. 15–38). New York: Oxford University Press.

Arora, V., Guardiano, S., Donaldson, D., Storch, I., & Hemstreet, P. (2005). Closing the gap between internal medicine training and practice: Recommendations from recent graduates. *American Journal of Medicine, 118*(680–685).

Association of Academic Health Centers (2009). Criteria for membership. Retrieved from http://www.aahcdc.org/about/members.php

Association of American Medical Colleges. (2008). *AAMC data book: Medical schools and teaching hospitals by the numbers 2008.* Washington, DC: Association of American Medical Colleges.

Association of American Medical Colleges, Ad Hoc Council of Deans. (2004). *Educating doctors to provide high quality medical care: A vision for medical education in the United States.* Washington, DC: Association of American Medical Colleges.

Association of American Medical Colleges & Howard Hughes Medical Institute. (2009). *Scientific foundations for future physicians.* Washington, DC: Association of America Medical Colleges.

Ayanian, J., & Weissman, J. (2002). Teaching hospitals and quality of care: A review of the literature. *Milbank Quarterly, 80*(3), 569–593.

Babbott, S., Beasley, B., Hinchey, K., Blotzer, J., & Holmboe, E. (2007). The predictive validity of the internal medicine in-training examination. *American Journal of Medicine, 120*(8), 735–740.

Baker, D., Salas, E., King, H., Battles, J., & Barach, P. (2005). The role of teamwork in the professional education of physicians: Current status and assessment recommendations. *Journal on Quality and Patient Safety, 31*(4), 185–202.

Barnes, L. (1994). *Teaching and the case method: Text, cases and readings.* Boston: Harvard Business School Press.

Barnett, S., & Koslowski, B. (2002). Adaptive expertise: Effects of type of experience and the level of theoretical understanding it generates. *Thinking and Reasoning, 8*(4), 237–267.

Baroody, A. (2003). The development of adaptive expertise and flexibility: The integration of conceptual and procedural knowledge. In A. Baroody & A. Dowker (Eds.), *Development of arithmetic concepts and skills: Constructing adaptive expertise* (pp. 1–34). Mahwah, NJ: Erlbaum.

Barzansky, B., & Etzel, S. (2004). Educational programs in U.S. medical schools, 2003–04. *Journal of the American Medical Association, 292*(9), 1025–1031.

Batalden, P., & Davidoff, F. (2007). Teaching quality improvement: The devil is in the details. *Journal of the American Medical Association, 298*(9), 1059–1061.

Batalden, P., Leach, D., Swing, S., Dreyfus, H., & Dreyfus, S. (2002). General competencies and accreditation in graduate medical education. *Health Affairs, 21*(5), 103–111.

Bates, D., Shore, M., Gibson, R., & Bosk, C. (2003). Patient safety forum: Examining the evidence: Do we know if psychiatric inpatients are being harmed by errors? What level of confidence should we have in data on the absence or presence of unintended harm? *Psychiatric Services, 54*(12), 1599–1603.

Bell, D., Fonarrow, G., Hays, R., & Mangione, C. (2000). Self-study from web-based and printed guideline materials. A randomized, controlled trial among resident physicians. *Annals of Internal Medicine, 132*(12), 938–946.

Bell, S., Krupat, E., Fazio, S., Roberts, D., & Schwartzstein, R. (2008). Longitudinal pedagogy: A successful response to the fragmentation of the third-year medical student clerkship experience. *Academic Medicine, 83*(5), 467–475.

Benner, P. (1984). *From novice to expert: Excellence and power in clinical nursing practice.* Menlo Park, CA: Addison-Wesley.

Benner, P., Sutphen, M., Leonard, V., & Day, L. (2009). *Educating nurses: A call for radical transformation.* San Francisco: Jossey-Bass.

Benner, P., Tanner, C., & Chesla, C. (1996). *Expertise in nursing practice: Caring, clinical judgment, and ethics.* New York: Springer.

Bereiter, C., & Scardamalia, M. (1993). *Surpassing ourselves: An inquiry into the nature and implications of expertise.* Chicago: Open Court.

Berry, P. (2008). Achieving independence: A decision-making framework for doctors in training. *Clinical Medicine, 8*(5), 512–514.

Bhandari, M., Montori, V., Devereaux, P., Dosanjh, S., Sprague, S., & Guyatt, G. (2003). Challenges to the practice of evidence-based medicine during residents' surgical training: A qualitative study using grounded theory. *Academic Medicine, 78*(11), 1183–1190.

Bilimoria, K., Kmiecik, T., DaRosa, D., Halverson, A., Eskandari, M., Bell, R., et al. (2009). Development of an online morbidity, mortality, and near-miss reporting system to identify patterns of adverse events in surgical patients. *Archives of Surgery, 144*(4), 305–311.

Billett, S. (1996). Situated learning: Bridging sociocultural and cognitive theorising. *Learning and Instruction, 6*(3), 263–280.

Billett, S. (2001). *Learning in the workplace: Strategies for effective practice.* Crows Nest, Australia: Allen & Unwin.

Billett, S. (2002). Workplace pedagogic practices: Co-participation and learning. *British Journal of Educational Studies, 50*(4), 457–481.

Billett, S. (2006). Constituting the workplace curriculum. *Journal of Curriculum Studies, 38*(1), 31–48.

Bleakley, A., & Bligh, J. (2008). Students learning from patients: Let's get real in medical education. *Advances in Health Sciences Education Theory and Practice, 13*(1), 89–107.

Bodenheimer, T., Berenson, R., & Rudolf, P. (2007). The primary care-specialty income gap: Why it matters. *Annals of Internal Medicine, 146*(4), 301–306.

Boex, J., Boll, A., Franzini, L., Hogan, A., Irby, D., Meservey, P., et al. (2000). Measuring the costs of primary care education in the ambulatory setting. *Academic Medicine, 75*(5), 419–425.

Boex, J., & Leahy, P. (2003). Understanding residents' work: Moving beyond counting hours to assessing educational value. *Academic Medicine, 78*(9), 939–944.

Bolman, L., & Deal, T. (2003). *Reframing organizations: Artistry, choice, and leadership.* San Francisco: Jossey-Bass.

Bordage, G. (1994). Elaborated knowledge: A key to successful diagnostic thinking. *Academic Medicine, 69*(11), 883–885.

Bordage, G., & Lemieux, M. (1991). Semantic structures and diagnostic thinking of experts and novices. *Academic Medicine, 66*(9S), S70–S72.

Boshuizen, H., & Schmidt, H. (1992). On the role of biomedical knowledge in clinical reasoning by experts, intermediates, and novices. *Cognitive Science, 16*(2), 153–184.

Boud, D., Cohen, R., & Sampson, J. (Eds.). (2001). *Peer learning in higher education: Learning from and with each other.* Sterling, VA: Stylus.

Boyer, E. (1990). *Scholarship reconsidered: Priorities of the professoriate.* Princeton: Carnegie Foundation for the Advancement of Teaching.

Bragard, I., Razavi, D., Marchal, S., Merckaert, I., Delvaux, N., Libert, Y., et al. (2006). Teaching communication and stress management skills to junior physicians dealing with cancer patients: A Belgian interuniversity curriculum. *Support Care Cancer, 14*(5), 454–461.

Brancati, F. (1989). The art of pimping. *Journal of the American Medical Association, 262*(1), 89–90.

Branch, W., Jr. (2000). Supporting the moral development of medical students. *Journal of General Internal Medicine, 15*(7), 503–508.

Branch, W., Jr., Hafler, J., & Pels, R. (1998). Medical students' development of empathic understanding of their patients. *Academic Medicine, 73*(4), 361–362.

Branch, W., Jr., & Paranjape, A. (2002). Feedback and reflection: Teaching methods for clinical settings. *Academic Medicine, 77*(12 Pt 1), 1185–1188.

Branch, W., Jr., Pels, R., Lawrence, R., & Arky, R. (1993). Becoming a doctor: Critical-incident reports from third-year medical students. *New England Journal of Medicine, 329*(15), 1130–1132.

Bransford, J., Brown, A., & Cocking, R. (1999). *How people learn: Brain, mind, experience and school.* Washington, DC: National Academies Press.

Brooks, M. (2009). Medical education and the tyranny of competency. *Perspectives in Biology and Medicine, 52*(1), 90–102.

Busari, J., & Scherpbier, A. (2004). Why residents should teach: A literature review. *Journal of Postgraduate Medicine, 50*(3), 205–210.

Buyx, A., Maxwell, B., & Schone-Seifert, B. (2008). Challenges of educating for medical professionalism: Who should step up to the line? *Medical Education, 42*(8), 758–764.

Carraccio, C., Benson, B., Nixon, L., & Derstine, P. (2008). From the educational bench to the clinical bedside: Translating the Dreyfus developmental model to the learning of clinical skills. *Academic Medicine, 83*(8), 761–767.

Carraccio, C., & Englander, R. (2004). Evaluating competence using a portfolio: A literature review and web-based application to the ACGME competencies. *Teaching and Learning in Medicine, 16*(4), 381–387.

Cave, M., & Clandinin, D. (2007). Revisiting the journal club. *Medical Teacher, 29*(4), 365–370.

Christakis, N. (1995). The similarity and frequency of proposals to reform U.S. medical education: Constant concerns. *Journal of the American Medical Association, 274*(9), 706–711.

Chumley-Jones, H., Dobbie, A., & Alford, C. (2002). Web-based learning: Sound educational method or hype? A review of the evaluation literature. *Academic Medicine, 77*(10S), S86–S93.

Clark, J., & Simpson, A. (2008). Integrating basic science into clinical teaching initiative (IBS-CTI): Preliminary report. *Journal of Pediatrics, 153*(5), 589–590e2.

Cohen, P., (2009). Training for expertise: The Harvard Medical School Cambridge Integrated Clerkship tutorial. *The Clinical Teacher, 6*(3), 28–33.

Coates, W., Crooks, K., Slavin, S., Guiton, G., & Wilkerson, L. (2008). Medical school curricular reform: Fourth-year colleges improve access to career mentoring and overall satisfaction. *Academic Medicine, 83*(8), 754–760.

Coleman, A., Palmer, S., & Winnick, S. (2008). *Roadmap to diversity: Key legal and educational policy foundations for medical schools.* Washington, DC: Association of American Medical Colleges.

Collins, J. (2001). *Good to great: Why some companies make the leap and others don't.* New York: HarperCollins.

Collins, J. (2005). *Good to great and the social sectors.* Boulder, CO: Jim Collins.

Colliver, J. (2000). Effectiveness of problem-based learning curricula: Theory and practice. *Academic Medicine, 75*(3), 59–76.

Colthart, I., Bagnall, G., Evans, A., Allbutt, H., Haig, A., Illing, J., et al. (2008). The effectiveness of self-assessment on the identification of learner needs, learner activity, and impact on clinical practice: BEME Guide no. 10. *Medical Teacher, 30*(2), 124–145.

Committee on the Health Professions Education Summit, Institute of Medicine. (2003). *Health professions education: A bridge to quality.* Washington, DC: National Academies Press.

Committee on Quality of Health Care in America, Institute of Medicine. (2000). *To err is human: Building a safer health system.* Washington, DC: National Academies Press.

Committee on Quality of Health Care in America, Institute of Medicine. (2001). *Crossing the quality chasm: A new health system for the 21st century.* Washington, DC: National Academies Press.

Committee on the Roles of Academic Health Centers in the 21st Century, Institute of Medicine. (2003). *Academic health centers: Leading change in the 21st century.* Washington, DC: National Academies Press.

Commonwealth Fund. (2003). *Envisioning the future of academic health centers. Final report of the Commonwealth Fund Task Force on Academic Health Centers.* New York: Commonwealth Fund.

Cook, D. (2006). Where are we with web-based learning in medical education? *Medical Teacher, 28*(7), 594–598.

Cooke, M., Irby, D., & Debas, H. (2003). The UCSF Academy of Medical Educators. *Academic Medicine, 78*(7), 666–672.

Core Committee, Institute for International Medical Education. (2002). Global minimum essential requirements in medical education. *Medical Teacher, 24*(2), 130–135.

Coverdill, J., Adrales, G., Finlay, W., Mellinger, J., Anderson, K., Bonnell, B., et al. (2006). How surgical faculty and residents assess the first year of the Accreditation Council for Graduate Medical Education duty-hour restrictions: Results of a multi-institutional study. *American Journal of Surgery, 191*(1), 11–16.

Cox, K. (2001). Stories as case knowledge: Case knowledge as stories. *Medical Education, 35*(9), 862–866.

Croskerry, P. (2003). The importance of cognitive errors in diagnosis and strategies to minimize them. *Academic Medicine, 78*(8), 775–780.

Croskerry, P. (2005). The theory and practice of clinical decision-making. *Canadian Journal of Anesthesiology, 52*(6), R1–R8.

Cruess, R., & Cruess, S. (2006). Teaching professionalism: General principles. *Medical Teacher, 28*(3), 205–208.

Custers, E. (2008). Long-term retention of basic science knowledge: A review study. *Advances in Health Sciences Education: Theory and Practice.* Retrieved from http://www.springerlink.com/content/e77v5w36j07n7576/

DaRosa, D., Bell, R., Jr., & Dunnington, G. (2003). Residency program models, implications, and evaluation: Results of a think tank consortium on resident work hours. *Surgery, 133*(1), 13–23.

Davis, D. (2005). Knowledge translation: The next big thing. *Canadian Journal of Continuing Medical Education, 17*(4), 102–106.

Davis, D., O'Brien, M., Freemantle, N., Wolf, F., Mazmanian, P., & Taylor-Vaisey, A. (1999). Impact of formal continuing medical education: Do conferences, workshops, rounds, and other traditional continuing education activities change physician behavior or health care outcomes? *Journal of the American Medical Association, 282*(9), 867–874.

Davis, D., & Ringsted, C. (2006). Accreditation of undergraduate and graduate medical education: How do the standards contribute to quality? *Advances in Health Sciences Education: Theory and Practice, 11*(3), 305–313.

Davis, M., Karunathilake, I., & Harden, R. (2005). AMEE education guide no. 28: The development and role of departments of medical education. *Medical Teacher, 27*(8), 665–675.

de Virgilio, C., Chan, T., Kaji, A., & Miller, K. (2008). Weekly assigned reading and examinations during residency, ABSITE performance, and improved pass rates on the American Board of Surgery examinations. *Journal of Surgical Education, 65*(6), 499–503.

Department of Veterans Affairs. (2004). *VERA educational funds guidelines.* Washington, DC: Department of Veterans Affairs.

Detmer, D., & Steen, E. (2005). *The academic health center: Leadership and performance.* New York: Cambridge University Press.

Detsky, A. (2009). The art of pimping. *Journal of the American Medical Association, 301*(13), 1379–1381.

Dewey, C., Friedland, J., Richards, B., Lamki, N., & Kirland, R. (2005). The emergence of academies of educational excellence: A survey of U.S. medical schools. *Academic Medicine, 80*(4), 358–365.

Dienstag, J. (2008). Relevance and rigor in premedical education. *New England Journal of Medicine, 359*(3), 221–224.

diFrancesco, L., Pistoria, M., Auerbach, A., Nardino, R., & Holmboe, E. (2005). Internal medicine training in the inpatient setting: A review of published educational interventions. *Journal of General Internal Medicine, 20*(12), 1173–1180.

Dornan, T., Boshuizen, H., King, N., & Scherpbier, A. (2007). Experience-based learning: A model linking the processes and outcomes of medical students' workplace learning. *Medical Education, 41*(1), 84–91.

Dornan, T., Hadfield, J., Brown, M., Boshuizen, H., & Scherpbier, A. (2005). How can medical students learn in a self-directed way in the clinical environment? Design-based research. *Medical Education, 39*(4), 356–364.

Downing, S. (2002). Assessment of knowledge with written test forms. In G. Norman, D. Newble, & C. van der Vleuten (Eds.), *International handbook of research in medical education* (pp. 647–672). Dordrecht, Netherlands: Kluwer.

Dreyfus, H., & Dreyfus, S. (1986). *Mind over machine: The power of human intuition and expertise in the era of the computer.* New York: Free Press.

Driessen, E. (2009). Portfolio critics: Do they have a point? *Medical Teacher, 31*(4), 279–281.

Driessen, E., van Tartwijk, J., van der Vleuten, C., & Wass, V. (2007). Portfolios in medical education: Why do they meet with mixed success? A systematic review. *Medical Education, 41*(12), 1224–1233.

Dweck, C. (2000). *Self-theories: Their role in motivation, personality and development.* Philadelphia: Psychology Press.

Elger, W. (2006). Managing resources in a better way: A new financial management approach for the University of Michigan Medical School. *Academic Medicine, 81*(4), 301–305.

Emanuel, E. (2006). How to redefine a medical education. *Chronicle of Higher Education, 53*, B12–B15.

Epstein, R. (1999). Mindful practice. *Journal of the American Medical Association, 282*(9), 833–839.

Epstein, R. (2007). Assessment in medical education. *New England Journal of Medicine, 356*(4), 387–396.

Epstein, R., & Hundert, E. (2002). Defining and assessing professional competence. *Journal of the American Medical Association, 287*(2), 226–235.

Ericsson, K. (2002). Attaining excellence through deliberate practice: Insights from the study of expert performance. In M. Ferrari (Ed.), *The pursuit of excellence through education* (pp. 21–55). Mahwah, NJ: Erlbaum.

Ericsson, K. (2004). Deliberate practice and the acquisition and maintenance of expert performance in medicine and related domains. *Academic Medicine, 79*(10S), S70–S81.

Ericsson, K. (2007). An expert-performance perspective of research on medical expertise: The study of clinical performance. *Medical Education, 41*(12), 1124–1130.

Eva, K. (2005). What every teacher needs to know about clinical reasoning. *Medical Education, 39*(1), 98–106.

Eva, K., & Cunnington, J. (2006). The difficulty with experience: Does practice increase susceptibility to premature closure? *Journal of Continuing Education in the Health Professions, 26*(3), 192–198.

Eva, K., Cunnington, J., Reiter, H., Keane, D., & Norman, G. (2004). How can I know what I don't know? Poor self-assessment in a well-defined domain. *Advances in Health Sciences Education, 9*(3), 211–224.

Eva, K., & Regehr, G. (2005). Self-assessment in the health professions: A reformulation and research agenda. *Academic Medicine, 80*(10S), S46–S54.

Eva, K., Reiter, H., Rosenfeld, J., & Norman, G. (2004a). The ability of the multiple mini-interview to predict pre-clerkship performance in medical school. *Academic Medicine, 79*(10S), S40–S42.

Eva, K., Reiter, H., Rosenfeld, J., & Norman, G. (2004b). The relationship between interviewer characteristics and ratings assigned during a multiple mini-interview. *Academic Medicine, 79*(6), 602–609.

Eva, K., Rosenfeld, J., Reiter, H., & Norman, G. (2004). An admissions OSCE: The multiple mini interview. *Medical Education, 38*(3), 314–326.

Farmer, E., Beard, J., Dauphinee, W., LaDuca, T., & Mann, K. (2002). Assessing the performance of doctors in teams and systems. *Medical Education, 36*(10), 942–948.

Feltovich, P., Spiro, R., & Coulson, R. (1997). Issues of expert flexibility in contexts characterized by complexity and change. In P. Feltovich, K. Ford, & R. Hoffman (Eds.), *Expertise in context: Human and machine* (pp. 125–146). Menlo Park, CA: AAAI/MIT Press.

Feudtner, C., Christakis, D., & Christakis, N. (1994). Do clinical clerks suffer ethical erosion? Students' perceptions of their ethical environment and personal development. *Academic Medicine, 69*(8), 670–679.

Fiedler, F. (1967). *A theory of leadership effectiveness.* New York: McGraw-Hill.

Flexner, A. (1910). *Medical education in the United States and Canada.* New York: Carnegie Foundation for the Advancement of Teaching.

Flexner, A. (1925). *Medical education: A comparative study.* New York: Macmillan.

Flexner, A. (1940). *I remember: The autobiography of Abraham Flexner.* New York: Simon and Schuster.

Flexner, A. (1943). *Henry S. Pritchett: A Biography.* New York: Columbia University Press.

Forsythe, G. (2005). Identity development in professional education. *Academic Medicine, 80*(10S), S112–S117.

Foster, C., Dahill, L., Golemon, L., & Tolentino, B. (2005). *Educating clergy: Teaching practices and pastoral imagination.* San Francisco: Jossey-Bass.

Gardner, H. (2007). *Responsibility at work: How leading professionals act (or don't act) responsibly.* San Francisco: Wiley.

Garg, M., Boero, J., Christiansen, R., & Booher, C. (1991). Primary care teaching physicians' losses of productivity and revenue at three ambulatory-care centers. *Academic Medicine, 66*(6), 348–353.

Gbadebo, A., & Reinhardt, U. (2001). Economists on academic medicine: Elephants in a porcelain shop? *Health Affairs, 20*(2), 148–152.

Ginsburg, J., Doherty, R., Ralston, J. Jr, Senkeeto, N., Cooke, M., Cutler, C., et al. (2008). Achieving a high-performance health care system with universal access: What the United States can learn from other countries. *Annals of Internal Medicine, 148*(1), 55–75.

Gittell, J. (2009). *High performance healthcare: Using the power of relationships to achieve quality, efficiency and resilience.* New York: McGraw Hill.

Glassick, C., Huber, M., & Maeroff, G. (1997). *Scholarship assessed: Evaluation of the professoriate.* San Francisco: Jossey-Bass.

Goldman, L., Caldera, D., Southwick, F., Nussbaum, S., Murray, B., O'Malley, T., et al. (1978). Cardiac risk factors and complications in non-cardiac surgery. *Medicine, 57*(4), 357–370.

Goldstein, E., Maestas, R., Fryer-Edwards, K., Wenrich, M., Oelschlager, A., Baernstein, A., & Kimball, H. (2006). Professionalism in medical education: An institutional challenge. *Academic Medicine, 81*(10), 871–876.

Golub, J., Weiss, P., Ramesh, A., Ossoff, R., & Johns, M., III. (2007). Burnout in residents of otolaryngology—head and neck surgery: A national inquiry into the health of residency training. *Academic Medicine, 82*(6), 596–601.

Gore, D. (2006). National survey of surgical morbidity and mortality conferences. *American Journal of Surgery, 191*(5), 708–714.

Grady, M., Batjer, H., & Dacey, R. (2009). Resident duty hour regulation and patient safety: Establishing a balance between concerns about resident fatigue and adequate training in neurosurgery. *Journal of Neurosurgery, 110*(5), 828–836.

Grant, H., & Dweck, C. (2003). Clarifying achievement goals and their impact. *Journal of Personality and Social Psychology, 85*(3), 541–553.

Grantcharov, T., Bardram, L., Funch-Jensen, P., & Rosenberg, J. (2003). Learning curves and impact of previous operative experience on performance on a virtual reality simulator to test laparoscopic surgical skills. *American Journal of Surgery, 185*(2), 146–149.

Greenhalgh, T. (2001). Storytelling should be targeted where it is known to have greatest added value. *Medical Education, 35*(9), 818–819.

Greeno, J. (2006). Learning in activity. In K. Sawyer (Ed.), *The Cambridge handbook of the learning sciences* (pp. 79–96). New York: Cambridge University Press.

Gross, C., Donnelly, G., Reisman, A., Sepkowitz, K., & Callahan, M. (1999). Resident expectations of morning report: A multi-institutional study. *Archives of Internal Medicine, 159*(16), 1910–1914.

Grossman, P., Compton, C., Igra, D., Ronfeldt, M., Shahan, E., & Wiliamson, P. (2009). Teaching practice: A cross-professional perspective. *Teachers College Record, 111*(9), 2055–2100. Retrieved from http://www.tcrecord.org

Gruen, R., Pearson, S., & Brennan, T. (2004). Physician-citizens: Public roles and professional obligations. *Journal of the American Medical Association, 291*(1), 94–98.

Gruppen, L., & Frohna, A. (2002). Clinical reasoning. In G. Norman, D. Newble, & C. van der Vleuten (Eds.), *International handbook of research in medical education* (pp. 205–230). Dordrecht, Netherlands: Kluwer.

Gruppen, L., Frohna, A., Anderson, R., & Lowe, K. (2003). Faculty development for educational leadership and scholarship. *Academic Medicine, 78*(2), 137–141.

Guest, C., Regehr, G., & Tiberius, R. (2001). The lifelong challenge of expertise. *Medical Education, 35*(1), 78–81.

Haan, C., Edwards, F., Poole, B., Godley, M., Genuardi, F., & Zenni, E. (2008). A model to begin to use clinical outcomes in medical education. *Academic Medicine, 83*(6), 574–580.

Hafferty, F. (1998). Beyond curriculum reform: Confronting medicine's hidden curriculum. *Academic Medicine, 73*(4), 403–407.

Hafferty, F. (2006). Professionalism: The next wave. *New England Journal of Medicine, 355*(20), 2151–2152.

Hafferty, F., & Franks, R. (1994). The hidden curriculum, ethics teaching, and the structure of medical education. *Academic Medicine, 69*(11), 861–871.

Haidet, P., Hatem, D., Fecile, M., Stein, H., Haley, H., Kimmel, B., et al. (2008). The role of relationships in the professional formation of physicians: Case report and illustration of an elicitation technique. *Patient Education and Counseling, 72*(3), 382–387.

Haidet, P., Kelly, P., Bentley, S., Blatt, B., Chou, C., Fortin, A., et al. (2006). Not the same everywhere: Patient-centered learning environments at nine medical schools. *Journal of General Internal Medicine, 21*(5), 405–409.

Haidet, P., Kelly, P., Chou, C., & Communication, Curriculum, and Culture Study Group (2005). Characterizing the patient-centeredness of hidden curricula in medical schools: Development and validation of a new measure. *Academic Medicine, 80*(1), 44–50.

Haidet, P., & Stein, H. (2006). The role of the student-teacher relationship in the formation of physicians. The hidden curriculum as process. *Journal of General Internal Medicine, 21*(1S), S16–S20.

Hall, P., & Weaver, L. (2001). Interdisciplinary education and teamwork: A long and winding road. *Medical Education, 35*(9), 867–875.

Hamdy, H., Prasad, K., Anderson, M., Scherpbier, A., Williams, R., Zwierstra, R., et al. (2006). BEME systematic review: Predictive values of measurements obtained in medical schools and future performance in medical practice. *Medical Teacher, 28*(2), 103–116.

Hammond, I., Taylor, J., Obermair, A., & McMenamin, P. (2004). The anatomy of complications workshop: An educational strategy to improve the training and performance of fellows in gynecologic oncology. *Gynecologic Oncology, 94*(3), 769–773.

Hamstra, S., Dubrowski, A., & Backstein, D. (2006). Teaching technical skills to surgical residents: A survey of empirical research. *Clinical Orthopedics and Related Research, 449*, 108–115.

Hansen, L., Brandt, S., Christopherson, C., Gilmore, H., Halverson, K., Hinkley, L., et al. (1992). The Yankton Model Program. *South Dakota Journal of Medicine, 45*(4), 103–107.

Hargadon, A., & Sutton, R. (2000). Building an innovation factory. *Harvard Business Review, 78*(3), 157–166.

Hart, L., Skillman, S., Fordyce, M., Thompson, M., Hagopian, A., & Konrad, T. (2007). International medical graduate physicians in the United States: Changes since 1981. *Health Affairs, 26*(4), 1159–1169.

Hatala, R., Brooks, L., & Norman, G. (2003). Practice makes perfect: The critical role of mixed practice in the acquisition of ECG interpretation skills. *Advances in Health Sciences Education, 8*(1), 17–26.

Hatano, G., & Oura, Y. (2003). Commentary: Reconceptualizing school learning using insight from expertise research. *Educational Researcher, 32*(8), 26–29.

Hauer, K., O'Brien, B., & Poncelet, A. (2009). Longitudinal, integrated clerkship education: Better for learners and patients. *Academic Medicine, 84*(7), 821.

Hebert, R., & Wright, S. (2003). Re-examining the value of medical grand rounds. *Academic Medicine, 78*(12), 1248–1252.

Hemmer, P., Hawkins, R., Jackson, J., & Pangaro, L. (2000). Assessing how well three evaluation methods detect deficiencies in medical students' professionalism in two settings of an internal medicine clerkship. *Academic Medicine, 75*(2), 167–173.

Hewson, M. (1991). Reflection in clinical teaching: An analysis of reflection-on-action and its implications for staffing residents. *Medical Teacher, 13*(3), 227–231.

Hirsh, D., Gutterson, W., Batalden, M., Beck, S., Bernstein, C., Callahan, J., et al. (2006). The Harvard Medical School-Cambridge Integrated Clerkship. *Journal of General Internal Medicine, 21*(S4), 186.

Hirsh, D., Ogur, B., Thibault, G., & Cox, M. (2007). "Continuity" as an organizing principle for clinical education reform. *New England Journal of Medicine, 356*(8), 858–866.

Hitchcock, M. (2002). Introducing professional educators into academic medicine: Stories of exemplars. *Advances in Health Science Education, 7*(3), 211–221.

Hoff, T., Pohl, H., & Bartfield, J. (2004). Creating a learning environment to produce competent residents: The roles of culture and context. *Academic Medicine Special Themes: Educating for Competencies, 79*(6), 532–540.

Hoffman, K., & Donaldson, J. (2004). Contextual tensions of the clinical environment and their influence on teaching and learning. *Medical Education, 38*(4), 448–454.

Hogan, A., Franzini, L., & Boex, J. (2000). Estimating the cost of primary care training in ambulatory settings. *Health Economics, 9*(8), 15–26.

Holmboe, E. (2004). Faculty and the observation of trainees' clinical skills: Problems and opportunities. *Academic Medicine, 79*(1), 16–22.

Holmboe, E., Lipner, R., & Greiner, A. (2008). Assessing quality of care: Knowledge matters. *Journal of the American Medical Association, 299*(3), 338–340.

Horwitz, I., Horwitz, S., Daram, P., Brandt, M., Brunicardi, F., & Awad, S. (2008). Transformational, transactional, and passive-avoidant leadership characteristics of a surgical resident cohort: Analysis using the multifactor leadership questionnaire and implications for improving surgical education curriculums. *Journal of Surgical Research, 148*(1), 49–59.

Howe, A. (2002). Professional development in undergraduate medical curricula: The key to the door of a new culture? *Medical Education, 36*(4), 353–359.

Huber, M., & Hutchings, P. (2005). *The advancement of learning: Building the teaching commons.* San Francisco: Jossey-Bass.

Huber, S. (2003). The white coat ceremony: A contemporary medical ritual. *Journal of Medical Ethics, 29*(6), 364–366.

Humphrey, H., Smith, K., Reddy, S., Scott, D., Madara, J., & Arora, V. (2007). Promoting an environment of professionalism: The University of Chicago "Roadmap." *Academic Medicine, 82*(11), 1098–1107.

Hundert, E., Hafferty, F., & Christakis, D. (1996). Characteristics of the informal curriculum and trainees' ethical choices. *Academic Medicine, 71*(6), 624–642.

Hutchins, E. (1995). *Cognition in the wild.* Cambridge, MA: MIT Press.

Iglehart, J. (1999). Support for academic medical centers: Revisiting the 1997 Balanced Budget Act. *New England Journal of Medicine, 341*(4), 299–304.

Iglehart, J. (2008). Medicare, graduate medical education, and new policy directions. *New England Journal of Medicine, 359*(6), 643–650.

Irby, D. (2007). Educational continuity in clinical clerkships. *New England Journal of Medicine, 356*(8), 856–857.

Irby, D., Cooke, M., Lowenstein, D., & Richards, B. (2004). The academy movement: A structural approach to reinvigorating the educational mission. *Academic Medicine, 79*(8), 729–736.

Irby, D., & Wilkerson, L. (2003). Educational innovations in academic medicine and environmental trends. *Journal of General Internal Medicine, 18*(5), 370–376.

Issenberg, S., McGaghie, W., Petrusa, E., Gordon, D., & Scalese, R. (2005). Features and uses of high-fidelity medical simulations that lead to effective learning: A BEME systematic review. *Medical Teacher, 27*(1), 10–28.

Jacobsohn, V., DeArman, M., Moran, P., Cross, J., Dietz, D., Allen, R., et al. (2008). Changing hospital policy from the wards: An introduction to health policy education. *Academic Medicine, 83*(4), 352–356.

Jagannathan, J., Vates, G., Pouratian, N., Sheehan, J., Patrie, J., Grady, M., et al. (2009). Impact of the Accreditation Council for Graduate Medical Education work-hour regulations on neurosurgical resident education and productivity. *Journal of Neurosurgery, 110*(5), 820–827.

Jarrell, B., Mallot, D., Peartree, L., & Calia, F. (2002). Looking at the forest instead of counting the trees: An alternative method for measuring faculty's clinical education efforts. *Academic Medicine, 77*(12), 1255–1261.

Jeffe, D., Andriole, D., Sabharwal, R., Paolo, A., Ephgrave, K., Hageman, H., et al. (2006). Which U.S. medical graduates plan to become specialty-board certified? Analysis of the 1997–2004 National Association of American Medical Colleges Graduation Questionnaire database. *Academic Medicine, 81*(10S), S98–S102.

Jellison, J. (2006). *Managing the dynamics of change: The fastest path to creating an engaged and productive workforce.* New York: McGraw-Hill.

Johnson, S., & Finucane, P. (2000). The emergence of problem-based learning in medical education. *Journal of Evaluation in Clinical Practice, 6*(3), 281–291.

Jones, R., & Korn, D. (1997). On the cost of educating a medical student. *Academic Medicine, 72*(3), 200–210.

Kane, R., Bershadsky, B., Weinert, C., Huntington, S., Riley, W., Bershadsky, J., et al. (2005). Estimating the patient care costs of teaching in a teaching hospital. *American Journal of Medicine, 118*(7), 767–772.

Kanna, B., Deng, C., Erickson, S., Valerio, J., Dimitrov, V., & Soni, A. (2006). The research rotation: Competency-based structured and novel approach to research training of internal medicine residents. *BMC Medical Education, 6*(52). Retrieved from http://www.biomedcentral.com/1472–6920/6/52

Kendrick, S., Simmons, J., Richards, B., & Roberge, L. (1993). Residents' perceptions of their teachers: Facilitative behaviour and the learning value of rotations. *Medical Education, 27*(1), 55–61.

Kennedy, T., Lingard, L., Baker, G., Kitchen, L., & Regehr, G. (2007). Clinical oversight: Conceptualizing the relationship between supervision and safety. *Journal of General Internal Medicine, 22*(8), 1080–1085.

Kennedy, T., Regehr, G., Baker, G., & Lingard, L. (2005). Progressive independence in clinical training: A tradition worth defending? *Academic Medicine, 80*(10SS), S1–S6.

Kennedy, T., Regehr, G., Baker, G., & Lingard, L. (2009). Preserving professional credibility: Grounded theory study of medical trainees' requests for clinical support. *BMJ, 338*(b128). Retrieved from http://www.bmj.com/

Kenny, N., Mann, K., & MacLeod, H. (2003). Role modeling in physicians' professional formation: Reconsidering an essential but untapped educational strategy. *Academic Medicine, 78*(12), 1203–1210.

Knapp, R. (2002). Complexity and uncertainty in financing graduate medical education. *Academic Medicine, 77*(11), 1076–1083.

Kneebone, R. (2005). Evaluating clinical simulations for learning procedural skills: A theory-based approach. *Academic Medicine, 80*(6), 549–553.

Koh, G., Khoo, H., Wong, M., & Koh, D. (2008). The effects of problem-based learning during medical school on physician competency: A systematic review. *Canadian Medical Association Journal, 178*(1), 34–41.

Kotter, J. (1996). *Leading change.* Boston: Harvard Business School Press.

Kouzes, J., & Posner, B. (1995). *The leadership challenge: How to keep getting extraordinary things done in organizations.* San Francisco: Jossey-Bass.

Krajewski, K., Siewert, B., Yam, S., Kressel, H., & Kruskal, J. (2007). A quality assurance elective for radiology residents. *Academic Radiology, 14*(2), 239–245.

Kravet, S., Howell, E., & Wright, S. (2006). Morbidity and mortality conference, grand rounds, and the ACGME's core competencies. *Journal of General Internal Medicine, 21*(11), 1192–1194.

Kreiter, C., Yin, P., Solow, C., & Brennan, R. (2004). Investigating the reliability of the medical school admissions interview. *Advances in Health Sciences Education: Theory and Practice, 9*(2), 147–159.

Kuiper, R., & Pesut, D. (2004). Promoting cognitive and metacognitive reflective reasoning skills in nursing practice: Self-regulated learning theory. *Journal of Advanced Nursing, 45*(4), 381–391.

Kuo, A., Irby, D., & Loeser, H. (2005). Does direct observation improve medical students' clerkship experiences? *Medical Education, 39*(5), 518–555.

Lai, C., Aagaard, E., Brandenburg, S., Nadkarni, M., Wei, H., & Baron, R. (2006). Brief report: Multiprogram evaluation of reading habits of primary care internal medicine residents on ambulatory rotations. *Journal of General Internal Medicine, 21*(5), 486–489.

Lave, J., & Wenger, E. (1991). *Situated learning: Legitimate peripheral participation.* Cambridge, England: Cambridge University Press.

Leach, D. (2002). Competence is a habit. *Journal of the American Medical Association, 287*(2), 243–244.

Lemay, J., Lockyer, J., Collin, V., & Brownell, A. (2007). Assessment of noncognitive traits through the admissions multiple mini-interview. *Medical Education, 41*(6), 573–579.

Levine, R., Haidet, P., Kern, D., Beasley, B., Bensinger, L., Brady, D., et al. (2006). Personal growth during internship: A qualitative analysis of interns' responses to key questions. *Journal of General Internal Medicine, 21*(6), 564–569.

Levine, R., O'Boyle, M., Haidet, P., Lynn, D., Stone, M., Wolf, D., et al. (2004). Transforming a clinical clerkship with team learning. *Teaching and Learning in Medicine, 16*(3), 270–275.

Liaison Committee on Medical Education (2008). Functions and structure of a medical school: Standards for accreditation of medical education programs leading to the M.D. degree. Retrieved from http://www.lcme.org/functions2008jun.pdf

Lingard, L., Schryer, C., Garwood, K., & Spafford, M. (2003). "Talking the talk": School and workplace genre tension in clerkship case presentations. *Medical Education, 37*(7), 612–620.

Linn, M. (2007). Creating lifelong science learners: What models form a firm foundation? *Educational Researcher, 25*(5), 18–24.

Littlefield, J., DaRosa, D., Paukert, J., Williams, R., Klamen, D., & Schoolfield, J. (2005). Improving resident performance assessment data: Numeric precision and narrative specificity. *Academic Medicine, 80*(5), 489–495.

Loeser, H., O'Sullivan, P., & Irby, D. (2007). Leadership lessons from curricular change at the University of California, San Francisco, School of Medicine. *Academic Medicine, 82*(4), 324–330.

Long, D. (2000). Competency-based residency training: The next advance in graduate medical education. *Academic Medicine, 75*(12), 1178–1183.

Ludmerer, K. (1985). *Learning to heal: The development of American medical education.* New York: Basic Books.

Ludmerer, K. (1999). *Time to heal: American medical education from the turn of the century to the era of managed care.* Oxford, England: Oxford University Press.

Ludmerer, K. (2000). Time and medical education. *Annals of Internal Medicine, 132*(1), 25–28.

Lyon, H., Healy, J., Bell, J., O'Donnell, J., Shultz, E., Moore-West, M., et al. (1992). PlanAlyzer, an interactive computer-assisted program to teach clinical problem solving in diagnosing anemia and coronary artery disease. *Academic Medicine, 67*(12), 821–828.

Maddaus, M., Chipman, J., Whitson, B., Groth, S., & Schmitz, C. (2008). Rotation as a course: Lessons learned from developing a hybrid online/on-ground approach to general surgical resident education. *Journal of Surgical Education, 65*(2), 112–116.

Madsen, P., Desai, V., Roberts, K., & Wong, D. (2006). Mitigating hazards through continuing design: The birth and evolution of a pediatric intensive care unit. *Organization Science, 17*(2), 239.

Mallon, W. (2009). Introduction: The history and legacy of mission-based management. *Academic Medicine, Management Series: Mission-Based Management.* Retrieved from http://journals.lww.com/academicmedicine/Documents/00001888–200604001–00001.pdf

Mandin, H., Harasym, P., Eagle, C., & Watanabe, M. (1995). Developing a "clinical presentation" curriculum at the University of Calgary. *Academic Medicine, 70*(3), 186–193.

Mandin, H., Jones, A., Woloschuk, W., & Harasym, P. (1997). Helping students learn to think like experts when solving clinical problems. *Academic Medicine, 72*(3), 173–179.

Martin, T., Rayne, K., Kemp, N., Hart, J., & Diller, K. (2005). Teaching for adaptive expertise in biomedical engineering ethics. *Science and Engineering Ethics, 11*(2), 257–276.

Maudsley, G. (1999). Do we all mean the same thing by "problem-based learning"? A review of the concepts and a formulation of the ground rules. *Academic Medicine, 74*(2), 178–185.

Maudsley, R. (2001). Role models and the learning environment: Essential elements in effective medical education. *Academic Medicine, 76*(5), 432–434.

Mayo Clinic. (2009). Mayo's mission. Retrieved from http://www.mayoclinic.org/about/missionvalues.html

McDonald, F., Zeger, S., & Kolars, J. (2007). Factors associated with medical knowledge acquisition during internal medicine residency. *Journal of General Internal Medicine, 22*(7), 962–968.

McGlynn, E., Asch, S., Adams, J., Keesey, J., Hicks, J., DeCristofaro, A., et al. (2003). The quality of health care delivered to adults in the United States. *New England Journal of Medicine, 348*(26), 2635–2645.

Mechanic, R., Coleman, K., & Dobson, A. (1998). Teaching hospital costs: Implications for academic missions in a competitive market. *Journal of the American Medical Association, 280*(11), 1015–1019.

Megali, G., Sinigaglia, S., Tonet, O., & Dario, P. (2006). Modeling and evaluation of surgical performance using hidden Markov models. *IEEE Transactions on Biomedical Engineering, 53*(10), 1911–1919.

Melck, A., Weber, E., & Sidhu, R. (2007). Resident continuity of care experience: A casualty of ambulatory surgery and current patient admission practices. *American Journal of Surgery, 193*(2), 243–247.

Michaelsen, L., Knight, A., & Fink, L. (2004). *Team-based learning: A transformative use of small groups in college teaching.* Sterling, VA: Stylus.

Miflin, B., Campbell, C., & Price, D. (2000). A conceptual framework to guide the development of self-directed, lifelong learning in problem-based medical curricula. *Medical Education, 34*(4), 299–306.

Miller, G. (1980). *Educating medical teachers.* Cambridge, MA: Harvard University Press.

Mistiaen, P., Francke, A., & Poot, E. (2007). Interventions aimed at reducing problems in adult patients discharged from hospital to home: A systematic meta-review. *BMC Health Services Research, 7*(47). Retrieved from http://www.biomedcentral.com/1472-6963/7/47

Montgomery, K. (2006). *How doctors think: Clinical judgment and the practice of medicine.* New York: Oxford University Press.

Moulaert, V., Verwijnen, M., Rikers, R., & Scherpbier, A. (2004). The effects of deliberate practice in undergraduate medical education. *Medical Education, 38*(10), 1044–1052.

Moulton, C., Dubrowski, A., MacRae, H., Graham, B., Grober, E., & Reznick, R. (2006). Teaching surgical skills: What kind of practice makes perfect? A randomized, controlled trial. *Annals of Surgery, 244*(3), 400–409.

Moulton, C., Regehr, G., Lingard, L., Merritt, C., & McRae, H. (2010). Operating from the other side of the table: Control dynamics and the surgical educator. *Journal of the American College of Surgeons, 210*(1), 79–86.

Mueller, P., Segovis, C., Litin, S., Habermann, T., & Thomas, A. (2006). Current status of medical grand rounds in departments of medicine at U.S. medical schools. *Mayo Clinic Proceedings, 81*(3), 313–321.

Muijtjens, A., Schuwirth, L., Cohen-Schotanus, J., Thoben, A., & van der Vleuten, C. (2008). Benchmarking by cross-institutional comparison of student achievement in a progress test. *Medical Education, 42*(1), 82–88.

Mylopoulos, M., & Regehr, G. (2007). Cognitive metaphors of expertise and knowledge: Prospects and limitations for medical education. *Medical Education, 41*(12), 1159–1165.

Mylopoulos, M., & Regehr, G. (2009). How student models of expertise and innovation impact the development of adaptive expertise in medicine. *Medical Education, 43*(2), 127–132.

Mylopoulos, M., & Scardamalia, M. (2008). Doctors' perspectives on their innovations in daily practice: Implications for knowledge building in health care. *Medical Education, 42*(10), 975–981.

Nasca, T., Veloski, J., Monnier, J., Cunningham, J., Valerio, S., Lewis, T., et al. (2001). Minimum instructional and program-specific administrative costs of educating residents in internal medicine. *Archives of Internal Medicine, 161*(5), 760–766.

Nelson, E., Batalden, P., Huber, T., Mohr, J., Godfrey, M., Headrick, L., et al. (2002). Microsystems in health care: Part 1. Learning from high-performing front-line clinical units. *Joint Commission Journal on Quality Improvement, 28*(9), 472–493.

Nelson, E. C., Godfrey, M. M., Batalden, P. B., et al. (2008). Clinical microsystems: Part 1. The building blocks of health systems. *Joint Commission Journal on Quality and Patient Safety, 34*(7), 367–78.

Nendaz, M., & Bordage, G. (2002). Promoting diagnostic problem representation. *Medical Education, 36*(8), 760–766.

Neufeld, V., & Barrows, H. (1974). The "McMaster philosophy": An approach to medical education. *Academic Medicine, 49*(11), 1040–1050.

Newton, B., Barber, L., Clardy, J., Cleveland, E., & O'Sullivan, P. (2008). Is there hardening of the heart during medical school? *Academic Medicine, 83*(3), 244–249.

Norcini, J. (2003). Peer assessment of competence. *Medical Education, 37*(6), 539–543.

Norcini, J., Blank, L., Duffy, F., & Fortina, G. (2003). The mini-CEX: A method for assessing clinical skills. *Annals of Internal Medicine, 138*(6), 476–481.

Norman, G. (2005). Research in clinical reasoning: Past history and current trends. *Medical Education, 39*(4), 418–427.

Norman, G. (2006). Building on experience: The development of clinical reasoning. *New England Journal of Medicine, 355*(21), 2251–2252.

Norman, G., Eva, K., Brooks, L., & Hamstra, S. (2006). Expertise in medicine and surgery. In K. Ericsson, N. Charness, P. Feltovich, & R. Hoffman (Eds.), *The Cambridge handbook of expertise and expert performance* (pp. 339–353). New York: Cambridge University Press.

Norman, G., & Schmidt, H. (1992). The psychological basis of problem-based learning: A review of the evidence. *Academic Medicine, 67*(9), 557–565.

Norman, G., & Schmidt, H. (2000). Effectiveness of problem-based learning curricula: Theory, practice and paper darts. *Medical Education, 34*(9), 721–728.

Nutter, D., Bond, J., Coller, B., D'Alessandri, R., Gewertz, B., Nora, L., et al. (2000). Measuring faculty effort and contributions in medical education. *Academic Medicine, 75*(2), 199–207.

O'Brien, B., Cooke, M., & Irby, D. (2007). Perceptions and attributions of third-year student struggles in clerkships: Do students and clerkship directors agree? *Academic Medicine, 82*(10), 970–978.

Ogur, B., & Hirsh, D. (2009). Learning through longitudinal patient care-narratives from the Harvard Medical School-Cambridge Integrated Clerkship. *Academic Medicine, 84*(7), 844–850.

Ogur, B., Hirsh, D., Krupat, E., & Bor, D. (2007). The Harvard Medical School-Cambridge Integrated Clerkship: An innovative model of clinical education. *Academic Medicine, 82*(4), 397–404.

Paget, M. (2004). *The unity of mistakes: A phenomenological interpretation of medical work.* Philadelphia: Temple University Press.

Palincsar, A. (1998). Social constructivist perspectives on teaching and learning. *Annual Review of Psychology, 49*(1), 345–375.

Papa, F., & Harasym, P. (1999). Medical curriculum reform in North America, 1765 to the present: A cognitive science perspective. *Academic Medicine, 74*(2), 154–164.

Papadakis, M., Arnold, G., Blank, L., Holmboe, E., & Lipner, R. (2008). Performance during internal medicine residency training and subsequent disciplinary action by state licensing boards. *Annals of Internal Medicine, 148*(11), 869–876.

Papadakis, M., Hodgson, C., Teherani, A., & Kohatsu, N. (2004). Unprofessional behavior in medical school is associated with subsequent disciplinary action by a state medical board. *Academic Medicine, 79*(3), 244–249.

Papadakis, M., & Loeser, H. (2006). Using critical incident reports and longitudinal observations to assess professionalism. In D. Stern (Ed.), *Measuring medical professionalism* (pp. 159–174). New York: Oxford University Press.

Papadakis, M., Loeser, H., & Healy, K. (2001). Early detection and evaluation of professionalism deficiencies in medical students: One school's approach. Academic Medicine, 76(11), 1100–1106.

Papadakis, M., Osborn, E., Cooke, M., & Healy, K. (1999). A strategy for the detection and evaluation of unprofessional behavior in medical students. *Academic Medicine, 74(9),* 980–990.

Papadakis, M., Teherani, A., Banach, M., Knettler, T., Rattner, S., Stern, D., et al. (2005). Disciplinary action by medical boards and prior behavior in medical school. *New England Journal of Medicine, 353(25),* 2673–2682.

Pauwels, J., & Oliveira, A. (2006). Three-year trends in the costs of residency training in family medicine. *Family Medicine, 38(6),* 408–415.

Petrusa, E. (2002). Clinical performance assessments. In G. Norman, D. Newble, & C. van der Vleuten (Eds.), *International handbook of research in medical education* (pp. 673–709). Dordrecht, Netherlands: Kluwer.

Philibert, I. (2008). Accreditation Council for Graduate Medical Education and Institute for Healthcare Improvement, 90-Day Project. Involving residents in quality improvement: Contrasting "top-down" and "bottom-up" approaches. Retrieved from http://www.acgme.org/acWebsite/ci/90DayProjectReportDFA_PA_09_15_08.pdf

Poncelet, A., & O'Brien, B. (2008). Preparing medical students for clerkships: A descriptive analysis of transition courses. *Academic Medicine, 83(5),* 444–451.

Pradhan, A., Sparano, D., & Ananth, C. (2005). The influence of an audience response system on knowledge retention: An application to resident education. *American Journal of Obstetrics and Gynecology, 193(5),* 1827–1830.

Prawat, R. (1993). The value of ideas: Problems versus possibilities in learning. *Educational Researcher, 22(6),* 5–16.

Prince, J., Vallabhaneni, R., Zenati, M., Hughes, S., Harbrecht, B., Lee, K., et al. (2007). Increased interactive format for morbidity and mortality conference improves educational value and enhances confidence. *Journal of Surgical Education, 64(5),* 266–272.

Ramsey, P., Coombs, J., Hunt, D., Marshall, S., & Wenrich, M. (2001). From concept to culture: The WWAMI program at the University of Washington School of Medicine. *Academic Medicine, 76(8),* 765–775.

Ratanawongsa, N., Teherani, A., & Hauer, K. (2005). Third-year medical students' experiences with dying patients during the internal medicine clerkship: A qualitative study of the informal curriculum. *Academic Medicine, 80(7),* 641–647.

Regehr, G. (2001). *Report to Canadian institutes of health research committee: Research in medical education fund.* Ottawa, Canada: Association of Canadian Medical Colleges.

Regehr, G., & Mylopoulos, M. (2008). Maintaining competence in the field: Learning about practice, through practice, in practice. *Journal of Continuing Education in the Health Professions, 28*(1S), S19–S23.

Reiter, H., & Eva, K. (2005). Reflecting the relative values of community, faculty, and students in the admissions tools of medical school. *Teaching and Learning in Medicine, 17*(1), 4–8.

Reiter, H., Salvatori, P., Rosenfeld, J., Trinh, K., & Eva, K. (2006). The effect of defined violations of test security on admissions outcomes using multiple mini-interviews. *Medical Education, 40*(1), 36–42.

Rich, E., Liebow, M., Srinivasan, M., Parish, D., Wolliscroft, J., Fein, O., et al. (2002). Medicare financing of graduate medical education: Intractable problems, elusive solutions. *Journal of General Internal Medicine, 17*(4), 283–292.

Ringsted, C., Skaarup, A., Henriksen, A., & Davis, D. (2006). Person-task-context: A model for designing curriculum and in-training assessment in postgraduate education. *Medical Teacher, 28*(1), 70–76.

Robins, L., Brock, D., Gallagher, T., Kartin, D., Lindhorst, T., Odegard, P., et al. (2008). Piloting team simulations to assess interprofessional skills. *Journal of Interprofessional Care, 22*(3), 325–328.

Rogoff, B., Paradise, R., Arauz, R., Correa-Chavez, M., & Angelillo, C. (2003). Firsthand learning through intent participation. *Annual Review of Psychology, 54*, 175–203.

Rosen, J., Hannaford, B., Richards, C., & Sinanan, M. (2001). Markov modeling of minimally invasive surgery based on tool/tissue interaction and force/torque signatures for evaluating surgical skills. *IEEE Transactions on Biomedical Engineering, 48*(5), 579–591.

Rosenfeld, J., Reiter, H., Trinh, K., & Eva, K. (2008). A cost efficiency comparison between the multiple mini-interview and traditional admissions interviews. *Advances in Health Sciences Education: Theory and Practice, 13*(1), 43–58.

Rosinski, E. (1988). *The society of directors of research in medical education: A brief history.* San Francisco: University of California, San Francisco.

Ruedy, J., MacDonald, N., & MacDougall, B. (2003). Ten-year experience with mission-based budgeting in the Faculty of Medicine of Dalhousie University. *Academic Medicine, 78*(1), 1121–1129.

Salomon, G. (1993). *Distributed cognitions: Psychological and educational considerations.* New York: Cambridge University Press.

Scardamalia, M., & Bereiter, C. (2006). Knowledge building: Theory, pedagogy, and technology. In K. Sawyer (Ed.), *The Cambridge handbook of the learning sciences* (pp. 97–115). New York: Cambridge University Press.

Schackow, T., Chavez, M., Loya, L., & Friedman, M. (2004). Audience response system: Effect on learning in family medicine residents. *Family Medicine, 36*(7), 496–504.

Schauer, R., & Schieve, D. (2006). Performance of medical students in a non-traditional rural clinical program, 1998–99 through 2003–04. *Academic Medicine, 81*(7), 603–607.

Schmidt, H. (2004). Alternative approaches to concept mapping and implications for medical education: Commentary on reliability, validity and future research directions. *Advances in Health Sciences Education: Theory and Practice, 9*(3), 251–256.

Schmidt, H., & Boshuizen, H. (1993). On the origins of intermediate effects of clinical case recall. *Memory & Cognition, 21*(3), 338–351.

Schneider, J., Coyle, J., Ryan, E., Bell, R., Jr., & DaRosa, D. (2007). Implementation and evaluation of a new surgical residency model. *Journal of the American College of Surgeons, 205*(3), 393–404.

Schön, D. (1987). *Educating the reflective practitioner.* San Francisco: Jossey-Bass.

Schwartz, D., Bransford, J., & Sears, D. (2005). Efficiency and innovation in transfer. In J. Mestre (Ed.), *Transfer of learning: Research and perspectives* (pp. 1–52). Greenwich, CT: Information Age.

Schwartz, D., & Martin, T. (2004). Inventing to prepare for future learning: The hidden efficiency of encouraging original student production in statistics instruction. *Cognition and Instruction, 22*(2), 129–184.

Searle, N., Hatem, C., Perkowski, L., & Wilkerson, L. (2006). Why invest in an educational fellowship program? *Academic Medicine, 81*(11), 936–940.

Searle, N., Thompson, B., Friedland, J., Lomax, J., Drutz, J., Coburn, M., et al. (2010). The prevalence and practice of Academies of Medical Educators: A survey of U.S. medical schools. *Academic Medicine, 85*(1), 48–56.

Searle, N., Thompson, B., & Perkowski, L. (2006). Making it work: The evolution of a medical educational fellowship program. *Academic Medicine, 81*(11), 984–989.

Sharif, I., & Ozuah, P. (2001). Resident pairing: A successful way to meet RRC requirements in the ambulatory setting. *Academic Medicine, 76*(5), 569–570.

Sheehan, D., Wilkinson, T., & Billett, S. (2005). Interns' participation and learning in clinical environments in a New Zealand hospital. *Academic Medicine, 80*(3), 302–308.

Sheppard, S., Macatangay, K., Colby, A., & Sullivan, W. (2008). *Educating engineers: Designing for the future of the field.* San Francisco: Jossey-Bass.

Shuell, T. (1996). Teaching and learning in a classroom context. In D. Berliner & R. Calfee (Eds.), *Handbook of educational psychology* (pp. 726–764). New York: Simon & Schuster Macmillan.

Shulman, L. (2005a). Foreword. In M. Huber & P. Hutchings (Eds.), *The advancement of learning: Building the teaching commons* (pp. v–viii). San Francisco: Jossey-Bass.

Shulman, L. (2005b). Signature pedagogies in the professions. *Daedalus, 134*(3), 52–59.

Simpson, D., Fincher, R., Hafler, J., Irby, D., Richards, B., Rosenfeld, G., et al. (2007). Advancing educators and education by defining the components and evidence associated with educational scholarship. *Medical Education, 41*(10), 1002–1009.

Simpson, D., Marcdante, K., Duthie, E., Jr., Sheehan, K., Holloway, R., & Towne, J. (2000). Valuing educational scholarship at the Medical College of Wisconsin. *Academic Medicine, 75*(9), 930–934.

Sloan, T., Kaye, C., Allen, W., Magness, B., & Wartman, S. (2005). Implementing a simpler approach to mission-based planning in a medical school. *Academic Medicine, 80*(11), 994–1004.

Smith, C., Morris, M., Francovich, C., Hill, W., & Gieselman, J. (2004). A qualitative study of resident learning in ambulatory clinic: The importance of exposure to "breakdown" in settings that support effective response. *Advances in Health Sciences Education: Theory and Practice, 9*(2), 93–105.

Smith, C., Morris, M., Hill, W., Francovich, C., & Christiano, J. (2006). Developing and validating a conceptual model of recurring problems in teaching clinic. *Advances in Health Sciences Education: Theory and Practice, 11*(3), 279–288.

Smith, K., Saavedra, R., Raeke, J., & O'Donell, A. (2007). The journey to creating a campus-wide culture of professionalism. *Academic Medicine, 82*(11), 1015–1021.

Smith, M., Wood, W., Adams, W., Wieman, C., Knight, J., Guild, N., et al. (2009). Why peer discussion improves student performance on in-class concept questions. *Science, 323*(5910), 122–124.

Sobral, D. (2002). Cross-year peer tutoring experience in a medical school: Conditions and outcomes for student tutors. *Medical Education, 36*(11), 1064–1070.

Spear, S. (2006). Fixing healthcare from the inside: Teaching residents to heal broken delivery processes as they heal sick patients. *Academic Medicine, 81*(10S), S144–S149.

Springer, L., Stanne, M., & Donovan, S. (1999). Effects of small-group learning on undergraduates in science, mathematics, engineering, and technology: A meta-analysis. *Review of Educational Research, 69*(1), 21–51.

Stanley, A., Khan, K., Hussain, W., & Tweed, M. (2006). Disorganized junior doctors fail the MRCP (UK). *Medical Teacher, 28*(1), e40–42.

Starfield, B. (1992). *Primary care: Concept, evaluation and policy.* New York: Oxford University Press.

Stefanidis, D., Scerbo, M., Sechrist, C., Mostafavi, A., & Heniford, B. (2008). Do novices display automaticity during simulator training? *American Journal of Surgery, 195*(2), 210–213.

Steinert, Y., Cruess, S., Cruess, R., & Snell, L. (2005). Faculty development for teaching and evaluating professionalism: From programme design to curriculum change. *Medical Education, 39*(2), 127–136.

Steinert, Y., Mann, K., Centeno, A., Dolmans, D., Spencer, J., Gelula, D., et al. (2006). A systematic review of faculty development initiatives designed to improve teaching effectiveness in medical education: BME Guide No. 8. *Medical Teacher, 28*(6), 497–526.

Stern, D., & Papadakis, M. (2006). The developing physician: Becoming a professional. *New England Journal of Medicine, 355*(17), 1794–1799.

Stewart, J. (2008). To call or not to call: A judgment of risk by pre-registration house officers. *Medical Education, 42*(9), 938–944.

Stiles, B., Reece, T., Hedrick, T., Garwood, R., Hughes, M., Dubose, J., et al. (2006). General surgery morning report: A competency-based conference that enhances patient care and resident education. *Current Surgery, 63*(6), 385–390.

Stites, S., Vansaghi, L., Pingleton, S., Cox, G., & Paolo, A. (2005). Aligning compensation with education: Design and implementation of the Educational Value Unit (EVU) system in an academic internal medicine department. *Academic Medicine, 80*(12), 1100–1016.

Sullivan, W. (2004). *Work and integrity: The crisis and promise of professionalism in America* (2nd Ed.). San Francisco: Jossey-Bass.

Sullivan, W., Colby, A., Wegner, J., Bond, L., & Shulman, L. (2007). *Educating lawyers: Preparation for the profession of law.* San Francisco: Jossey-Bass.

Sullivan, W., & Rosin, M. (2008). *A new agenda for higher education: Shaping a life of the mind for practice.* San Francisco: Jossey-Bass.

Sweeney, G. (1999). The challenge for basic science education in problem-based medical curricula. *Clinical and Investigative Medicine, 22*(1), 15–22.

Tamblyn, R. (1998). Use of standardized patients in the assessment of medical practice. *Canadian Medical Association Journal, 158*(2), 205–207.

Tang, T., Hernandez, E., & Adams, B. (2004). "Learning by teaching": A peer-teaching model for diversity training in medical school. *Teaching and Learning in Medicine, 16*(1), 60–63.

ten Cate, O., & Scheele, F. (2007). Competency-based postgraduate training: Can we bridge the gap between theory and clinical practice? *Academic Medicine, 82*(6), 542–547.

ten Cate, O., Snell, L., Mann, K., & Vermunt, J. (2004). Orienting teaching toward the learning process. *Academic Medicine, 79*(3), 219–228.

Tess, A., Yang, J., Smith, C., Fawcett, C., Bates, C., & Reynolds, E. (2009). Combining clinical microsystems and an experiential quality improvement curriculum to improve residency education in internal medicine. *Academic Medicine, 84*(3), 326–334.

Teunissen, P., Boor, K., Scherpbier, A., van der Vleuten, C., van Diemen-Steenvoorde, J., van Luijk, S., et al. (2007). Attending doctors' perspectives on how residents learn. *Medical Education, 41*(11), 1050–1058.

Teunissen, P., & Dornan, T. (2008). Lifelong learning at work. *BMJ, 336*(7645), 667–669.

Teunissen, P., Scheele, F., Scherpbier, A., van der Vleuten, C., Boor, K., van Luijk, S., et al. (2007). How residents learn: Qualitative evidence for the pivotal role of clinical activities. *Medical Education, 41*(8), 763–770.

Thompson, B., Schneider, V., Haidet, P., Levine, R., McMahon, K., Perkowski, L., et al. (2007). Team-based learning at ten medical schools: Two years later. *Medical Education, 41*(3), 250–257.

Timmermans, S., & Angell, A. (2001). Evidence-based medicine, clinical uncertainty, and learning to doctor. *Journal of Health and Social Behavior, 42*(4), 342–359.

Torbeck, L., & Canal, D. (2009). Remediation practices for surgery residents. *American Journal of Surgery, 197*(3), 397–402.

Torbeck, L., & Wrightson, A. (2005). A method for defining competency-based promotion criteria for family medicine residents. *Academic Medicine, 80*(9), 832–839.

Torre, D., Daley, B., Stark-Schweitzer, T., Siddartha, S., Petkova, J., & Ziebert, M. (2007). A qualitative evaluation of medical student learning with concept maps. *Medical Teacher, 29*(9), 949–955.

Tresolini, C. (1994). *Health professions education and relationship-centered care: Report of the Pew-Fetzer Task Force on advancing psychosocial education.* San Francisco: Pew Health Professions Commission.

United States Medical Licensing Examination. (2009). Overview. *2009 USMLE Bulletin.* Retrieved from http://www.usmle.org/general_information /bulletin/2009/overview.html

van der Vleuten, C. (1996). The assessment of professional competence: Developments, research and practical implications. *Advances in Health Sciences Education, 1*(1), 41–67.

van der Vleuten, C., & Schuwirth, L. (2005). Assessing professional competence: From methods to programmes. *Medical Education, 39*(3), 309–313.

Vernon, D., & Blake, R. (1993). Does problem-based learning work? A meta-analysis of evaluative research. *Academic Medicine, 68*(7), 550–563.

Viggiano, T., Pawlina, W., Lindor, K., Olsen, K., & Cortese, D. (2007). Putting the needs of the patient first: Mayo Clinic's core value, institutional culture, and professionalism covenant. *Academic Medicine, 82*(11), 1089–1093.

Viggiano, T., Shub, C., & Giere, R. (2000). The Mayo Clinic's clinician-educator award: A program to encourage educational innovation and scholarship. *Academic Medicine, 75*(9), 940–943.

Vinson, D., & Paden, C. (1994). The effect of teaching medical students on private practitioners' workloads. *Academic Medicine, 69*(3), 237–238.

Vinson, D., Paden, C., & Devera-Sales, A. (1996). Impact of medical student teaching on family physicians' use of time. *Journal of Family Practice, 42*(3), 243–249.

Vroom, V., & Yetton, P. (1973). *Leadership and decision making.* Pittsburgh: University of Pittsburgh Press.

Wamsley., M., Julian, K., & Wipf, J. (2004). A literature review of "resident-as-teacher" curricula: Do teaching courses make a difference? *Journal of General Internal Medicine, 19*(5p2), 574–581.

Wartman, S. (2004). Revisiting the idea of a national center for health professions education research. *Academic Medicine, 79*(10), 910–917.

Watson, R. (2003). Rediscovering the medical school. *Academic Medicine, 78*(7), 659–665.

Watson, R., & Romrell, L. (1999). Mission-based budgeting: Removing a graveyard. *Academic Medicine, 74*(6), 6276–6340.

Wayne, D., Butter, J., Siddall, V., Fudala, M., Wade, L., Feinglass, J., et al. (2006). Mastery learning of advanced cardiac life support skills by internal medicine residents using simulation technology and deliberate practice. *Journal of General Internal Medicine, 21*(3), 251–256.

Wear, D., & Castellani, B. (2000). The development of professionalism: Curriculum matters. *Academic Medicine, 75*(6), 602–611.

Wear, D., & Zarconi, J. (2008). Can compassion be taught? Let's ask our students. *Journal of General Internal Medicine, 23*(7), 948–953.

Weinberg, E., O'Sullivan, P., Boll, A., & Nelson, T. (1994). The cost of third-year clerkships at large nonuniversity teaching hospitals. *Journal of the American Medical Association, 272*(9), 669–673.

Wenger, E. (1998). *Communities of practice: Learning, meaning, and identity.* New York: Cambridge University Press.

West, D., Park, J., Pomeroy, J., & Sandoval, J. (2002). Concept mapping assessment in medical education: A comparison of two scoring systems. *Medical Education, 36*(9), 820–826.

Wilen, W. (1991). *Questioning skills for teachers. What research says to the teacher* (3rd Ed.). West Haven, CT: National Education Association.

Wilkerson, L., & Irby, D. (1998). Strategies for improving teaching practices: A comprehensive approach to faculty development. *Academic Medicine, 73*(4), 387–396.

Williams, R., Klamen, D., & McGaghie, W. (2003). Cognitive, social and environmental sources of bias in clinical performance ratings. *Teaching and Learning in Medicine, 15*(4), 270–292.

Wilson, M., & Scalise, K. (2006). Assessment to improve learning in higher education: The BEAR Assessment System. *Higher Education, 52*, 635–663.

Woloschuk, W., Harasym, P., Mandin, H., & Jones, A. (2000). Use of scheme-based problem solving: An evaluation of the implementation and utilization of schemes in a clinical presentation curriculum. *Medical Education, 34*(6), 437–442.

Wolpaw, T., Wolpaw, D., & Papp, K. (2003). SNAPPS: A learner-centered model for outpatient education. *Academic Medicine, 78*(9), 893–898.

Wright, K., Rowitz, L., Merkle, A., Reid, W., Robinson, G., Herzog, B., et al. (2000). Competency development in public health leadership. *American Journal of Public Health, 90*(8), 1202–1207.

Yao, D., & Wright, S. (2005). National survey of internal medicine residency program directors regarding problem residents. *Journal of the American Medical Association, 284*(9), 1099–1104.

Zeidel, M., Kroboth, F., McDermot, S., Mehali, M., Clayton, C., Rich, E., et al. (2005). Estimating the cost to departments of medicine of training residents and fellows: A collaborative analysis. *American Journal of Medicine, 118*(5), 557–564.

Zemlo, T., Garrison, H., Partridge, N., & Ley, T. (2000). The physician-scientist: Career issues and challenges at the year 2000. *FASEB Journal, 14*(2), 221–230.

NAME INDEX

A

Aagaard, E., 95
Ackerman, A., 239
Adams, B., 126
Albanese, M., 81
Alexander, P., 50
Alford, C., 93
Alguire, P., 125
Allen, W., 183
Allison, J., 130
Ananth, C., 128
Anderson, G., 180, 181
Anderson, J., 46
Anderson, R., 150, 252
Angelillo, C., 57
Angell, A., 135, 155
Arauz, R., 57
Arky, R., 31
Arnold, G., 32
Arnold, L., 102, 108, 139, 146, 227
Arora, V., 153
Ayanian, J., 130

B

Babbott, S., 143
Backstein, D., 131
Baker, D., 223
Baker, G., 129, 132, 240
Barach, P., 223
Barber, L., 99, 183
Bardram, L., 43
Barnes, L., 128
Barnett, S., 225
Baroody, A., 225
Barrows, H., 80
Bartfield, J., 214

Batalden, P., 146, 156, 197, 245
Bates, D., 123
Batjer, H., 130
Battles, J., 223
Beard, J., 244
Beasley, B., 143
Bell, D., 94
Bell, R., Jr., 85
Bell, S., 93
Benner, P., 4, 43, 61
Benson, B., 126–127
Bereiter, C., 43, 50, 51, 52–53, 136, 152, 157, 198, 224
Berenson, R., 182
Berry, P., 129, 133
Bhandari, M., 155
Billett, S., 46, 57, 115, 223
Blake, R., 81
Blank, L., 32, 107
Bleakley, A., 62
Bligh, J., 62
Blotzer, J., 143
Bodenheimer, T., 182
Boero, J., 177
Boex, J., 158, 177, 178
Boll, A., 176
Bolman, L., 196, 197, 200
Bond, L., 4
Booher, C., 177
Boor, K., 135
Bor, D., 85
Bordage, G., 43, 79
Boshuizen, H., 42–43, 63, 84
Bosk, C., 123
Boud, D., 126
Boyer, E., 32, 207
Bragard, I., 140

285

Brancati, F., 129
Branch, W., Jr., 31, 99, 149
Bransford, J., 23, 49, 152
Brennan, R., 20
Brennan, T., 59
Brooks, L., 43
Brooks, M., 146, 214
Brown, A., 23
Brown, M., 84
Brownell, A., 249
Busari, J., 129
Buyx, A., 109

C

Cahill, L., 4
Calia, F., 183
Callahan, M., 122
Campbell, C., 215
Canal, D., 151
Carraccio, C., 107, 126–127, 146,
226, 244
Castellani, B., 41, 99, 100, 108
Cave, M., 125
Chan, T., 125
Chavez, M., 128
Chesla, C., 61
Chipman, J., 123
Chou, C., 110
Christakis, D., 110, 157
Christakis, N., 110
Christiano, J., 120
Christiansen, R., 177
Chumley-Jones, H., 93, 94
Clandinin, D., 125
Clardy, J., 99
Clark, J., 153
Cleveland, E., 99
Coates, W., 88
Cocking, R., 23
Cohen, R., 126
Cohen-Schotanus, J., 105
Colby, A., 4
Coleman, A., 20, 249
Coleman, K., 181

Collin, V., 249
Collins, J., 193, 194, 196
Colliver, J., 82
Colthart, I., 148
Colwell, N. P., 11, 12
Cook, D., 93
Cooke, M., 32, 84
Coombs, J., 87
Correa-Chavez, M., 57
Cortese, D., 141
Coulson, R., 44, 225
Coverdill, J., 118
Cox, G., 183
Cox, K., 102
Cox, M., 85
Coyle, J., 85
Crooks, K., 88
Croskerry, P., 46, 48, 124, 223
Cruess, R., 100, 102, 204
Cruess, S., 100, 102, 204
Cunnington, J., 53, 54
Custers, E., 29, 152

D

Dacey, R., 130, 244
Dario, P., 43
DaRosa, D., 85
Dat, L., 4
Davidoff, F., 156, 197
Davis, D., 23, 115, 172
Davis, M., 203
de Virgilio, C., 125, 144
Deal, T., 196, 197, 200
Derstine, P., 126–127
Desai, V., 137
Detmer, D., 253
Detsky, A., 129
Devera-Sales, A., 178
Dewey, C., 208
Dienstag, J., 19
diFrancesco, L., 157, 214
Diller, K., 224
Dobbie, A., 93
Dobson, A., 181

SUBJECT INDEX

A

About this book, 4–5, 7–8

Academic communities, 206–210

Academic health centers, 164

Academic medical centers, 164

Academic Medicine, 209

Accountability and transparency, 19

Accreditation Council for Continuing Medical Education (ACCME), 2, 250

Accreditation Council for Graduate Medical Education (ACGME), 2, 17, 22, 104, 108, 117, 121, 122, 142, 146, 148, 166–167, 168, 187, 248, 250, 252, 254

Acting: professional formation pedagogies developing, 99–103; self-reflection and habits of, 41

Adaptive expertise, 50

Admissions: Flexner's recommendations for, 13; requirements to medical school, 19–20; revising processes of, 248–250

Advances in Health Science Education, 209

Advocate and community leader, 58–59

Agencies: aligning, accrediting, certifying, and licensing, 250–251; coordinated by ACGME, 166–167

American Board of Medical Specialties (ABMS), 18, 167, 169, 250

American College of Surgeons, 59

American Educational Research Association, 209

American Hospital Association (AHA), 167

American Medical Association (AMA), 2, 5, 11–12, 14, 166–167, 168, 248, 254

Apprenticeships, 119, 124

Assessments: benchmarks of development, 109–110; clinical performance, 106–107; curriculum's effect on, 89; emphasizing situated and distributed learning, 71; integrated approaches to, 67–68; judging ability of residents, 134; learning environment, 110; licensure and certification exams, 14, 169–172; Medical College Admission Test, 20; methods in UME, 104, 105; professional formation, 108–110, 146–148; residency, 143–149, 150–151; supporting participatory learning, 69; systems of UME, 103–104

Association of Academic Health Centers (AAHC), 164

Association of American Medical Colleges (AAMC), 2, 4, 5, 15, 16, 17, 19–20, 28, 108, 164, 166–167, 173, 174, 175, 176, 177, 178, 190, 209, 248, 249, 254

Association of Directors of Medical Student Education in Psychiatry, 209

Atlantic Philanthropies, 4

Audience response system (ARS), 128

B

Basic science concepts, 135, 151–153
Board certification, 171, 250–251
Board eligible, 171
Brief structured clinical observation (BSCO), 107
Business of medical education, 18–19

C

Carnegie Foundation for the Advancement of Teaching, 2, 4, 11–12, 206–207
Case presentations and discussions: in graduate medical education, 127–129; in undergraduate medical education, 89–92
Case Western Reserve University, 16, 78
Change. *See* Organizational change
Clerkship curriculum, 82–87; disciplinary block rotations in, 84–85; evaluating student's clinical performance, 107; Flexner's influence on, 82; fourth-year advanced, 87–89; gaining patient care experience with, 82–84; longitudinal integrated clerkships, 85–86; mixed model clerkships, 86–87; pedagogy and assessment affected by, 89; professional formation pedagogies in, 102–103
Clerkship Directors in Pediatrics, 209
Clinical rotations: about, 118–119
Clinical skills: assessing, 106–107; gaining in patient care, 82–87; simulating, 130–132; teaching, 94–96; transferring into practice, 132–135; underemphasis on outpatient needs, 153–154. *See also* Clerkship curriculum
Committee on the Health Professions Education Summit, 17, 166, 206, 250

Committee on Quality of Health Care in America, 17
Committee on the Roles of Academic Health Centers in the 21st Century, 164, 251
Commonwealth Fund, 164
Communication, Curriculum, and Culture Study Group, 110
Community of practice: defined, 56; participating in, 56–58; teaching commons as, 252
Competence, 103–104, 108
Conceptual understanding, 92–94, 127–129
Consortium of Longitudinal Integrated Clerkships (CLIC), 85–86
Continuing medical education (CME) programs, 22–23
Continuity clinics, 119–120
Costs: containing medical, 165–166; graduate medical education, 180–181; reforms for GME, 254–255; student education, 22, 28, 176–178
Council on Medical Education (AMA), 11, 14
Council of Medical Specialty Societies (CMSS), 167, 169
Curriculum: clerkship, 82–87; effect of United States Medical Licensing Examination on, 171; emphasizing situated and distributed learning, 69–71; encouraging participatory learning, 69; fourth-year advanced clerkship, 87–89; future for UME, 110–112; innovative change to, 191, 196; journal club, 125; medical disciplines model for UME, 77–78; meetings and conferences, 121–124; organ systems and integrated medical sciences model of, 78–79; pedagogy and assessment affected by, 89; preclerkship, 76–82;